AACN Guide to Acute Care Procedures in the Home

DATE DUE

Gloria J. McNeal, RN, MSN, CS, PhD is a past recipient of the American Association of Critical-Care Nurses (AACN) InnoVision Project Grant Award for her creative design of a community-based mobile health care program, which was developed to improve pediatric immunization rates in urban settings. Her service to AACN has included both elected and appointed positions at the national and local chapter levels. Nationally, she has served as an appointed member of the AACN Board Advisory Team. At the chapter level, she has held elected positions as a member of the AACN Southeastern Pennsylvania Chapter Board of Directors, and as Co-Chair of the Research Committee. For over twenty years she has worked in adult critical care units, and for six of those years she held certification as a CCRN. Currently, she holds national certification as a clinical specialist (CS) in medical-surgical nursing practice. In her present position, she coordinates the acute care nurse practitioner track and supervises students in the community health practicum in the College of Nursing, at Rutgers, the State University of New Jersey. In addition, she works part-time as a field nurse for two large, urban homecare companies.

Dr. McNeal's unique mobile approach to healthcare delivery, utilizing advanced practice nurses at the head of the healthcare team, was featured on the cover of the April 1997 issue of *Critical Care Nurse*. In recognition of her work she was named recipient of the American Academy of Nursing's coveted Media Award, and the University of Pennsylvania School of Nursing's Outstanding Alumni Award. In 1993, she was invited to, and continues, membership in the Society of Critical Care Medicine.

She is the author of over 50 published abstracts, articles, book chapters, and texts. Her seminal works on community-based critical care nursing practice, published in 1979 in *AJN* and *Nursing Clinics of North America*, described the technological innovation and analyses of 24-hour ambulatory ECG monitoring. Her other published works have appeared in *Image*, *Critical Care Nurse*, *Perspectives on Community*, and *Heart and Lung*. Most recently, she served as guest editor of *Critical Care Nursing Clinics of North America*, and as an author of book chapters on burns, perioperative nursing, and community-based nursing practice.

Dr. McNeal completed her undergraduate degree in nursing at Villanova University. From the University of Pennsylvania, she attained both a master's degree in nursing and a Ph.D. in education. Her doctoral dissertation was awarded meritorious distinction for excellence in written and oral presentation. During the Vietnam War era, she served as a military officer in the U.S. Navy Nurse Corps, where she was assigned to critical care units throughout her five-year tenure.

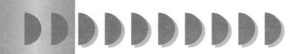

AACN Guide to Acute Care Procedures in the Home

Gloria J. McNeal, RN, MSN, CS, PhD
Assistant Professor, College of Nursing
Rutgers, the State University of New Jersey

20 CONTRIBUTORS

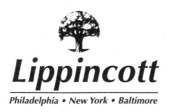

Lippincott
Philadelphia • New York • Baltimore

AACN guide to acute care
procedures in the home

Acquisitions Editor: Susan M. Glover, RN, MSN
Editorial Assistant: Hilarie Surrena
Senior Project Manager: Helen Ewan
Production Service: Pine Tree Composition
Design Coordinator: Doug Smock

ISBN: 0-7817-1816-3

9 8 7 6 5 4 3 2 1

Care has been taken to confirm the accuracy of the information presented and to describe generally accepted practices. However, the authors, editors, and publishers are not responsible for errors or omissions or for any consequences from application of the information in this book and make no warranty, express or implied, with respect to the contents of the publication.

The authors, editors and publisher have exerted every effort to ensure that drug selection and dosage set forth in this text are in accordance with current recommendations and practice at the time of publication. However, in view of ongoing research, changes in government regulations, and the constant flow of information relating to drug therapy and drug reactions, the reader is urged to check the package insert for each drug for any change in indications and dosage and for added warnings and precautions. This is particularly important when the recommended agent is new or infrequently employed drug.

Some drugs and medical devices presented in this publication have Food and Drug Administration (FDA) clearance for limited use in restricted research settings. It is the responsibility of the health care provider to ascertain the FDA status of each drug or device planned for use in their clinical practice.

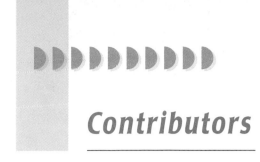

Contributors

Catherine J. Friel, RN, BSN
Role of the Nurse
Staff Development Clinical Program Management
Mercy Home Health Services
Springfield, Pennsylvania

Barbara Cornell, RN, MHA
Pediatric Homecare Unit
Clinical Manager Pediatric/PICU Diagnostic Unit
Cooper Medical Center, Children's Regional
    Hospital
Camden, New Jersey

Sandra Hartranft, BSN, RN, CDE
Home Glucose Monitoring
Director, Diabetes Disease State Management
    Program
SNI Home Care
Fort Washington, Pennsylvania

Mary Gallagher, RN, CCE, CPHQ
*Management of Preterm Labor and Non-Stress
Testing
Antepartal Assessment, Management of
Hyperemesis Gravidarum, Home Urine Monitoring,
Gestational Diabetes, and Pregnancy-Induced
Hypertension*
Clinical Manager Perinatal Services
SNI Home Care
Fort Washington, Pennsylvania

Lynn Gallagher Ford, RN, MSN
Newborn Homecare Procedures
General Manager Pediatrics Maternal Child
    Health
SNI Home Care
Fort Washington, Pennsylvania

Sharon A. Cross, RN, BSN
Colostomy Care and Gastric Tube Management
Clinical Manager
SNI Home Care
Fort Washington, Pennsylvania

Lorraine S. Dildine, RN, MSN
Developmental Assessment and Apnea Monitoring
Clinical Manager
SNI Home Care
Fort Washington, Pennsylvania

Kelly Ann Connor, RNC
*Nasogastric Tube Insertion, Failure to Thrive, Home
Phototherapy.*
Nurse Manager Pediatrics
SNI Home Care
Fort Washington, Pennsylvania

Priscilla Murphy, BSN, RNC, CPCE
*Educational Modules on Asthma Management
Smoking Cessation, Diabetes Management*
Educational Consultant
Hokessin, Delaware

Lori Jordan, RN
TPN, Chemotherapy, Chemotherapy Spill Protocol
Director of Nursing
Coram Healthcare Corporation
Denver, Colorado

Andra Adams, MA, RD, CNSD
*Nutrition Support Considerations for Hyperemesis,
Gestational Diabetes and Diabetes Mellitus,
Enteral Feeding Guides*
Pediatric and Obstetrical Dietitian
Coram Healthcare Corporation
Denver, Colorado

June Sanson, RN, BSN

*Nasogastric Tube Insertion/Removal;
Capillary Blood Sampling, Blood Component
Therapy, Phlebotomy, Blood Component Charts*

Nurse Clinician
Coram Healthcare Corporation
Denver, Colorado

Joanne Simone, BSN, MBA

*Care of the Adult with an Organ Transplant,
Tracheostomy Care and Mananagement*

Clinical Coordinator Pediatrics
Coram Healthcare Corporation
Denver, Colorado

Judy Purnell, RN, BSN

*Loop Diuretic Injection Therapy, Anticoagulant
Infusion Therapy, Inotropic Infusion Therapy*

Clinical Coordinator Cardiology Program
Coram Healthcare Corporation
Denver, Colorado

Karen Jean Feury, RN, MS,CCRN

*Loop Diuretic Injection Therapy, Inotropic Infusion
Therapy*

Injury Prevention Coordinator
Morristown Memorial Hospital
Morristown, New Jersey

Jamianne Harry, RN, BSN

Infusion Access Devices

Nurse Preceptor
Coram Healthcare Corporation
Denver, Colorado

Rebecca Roessler, RN

Medronic PumpRefill, Synchromed Pump Refill

Field Clinician
Coram Healthcare Corporation
Denver, Colorado

Pamela Berta, RN, CRNI

Insulin Administration, Home Glucose Monitoring

Field Clinician
Coram Healthcare Corporation
Denver, Colorado

Gloria J. McNeal, RN, MSN, CS, PhD

*Overview, Assessment, Adult and Geriatric
Homecare Units*

Assistant Professor, College of Nursing
Rutgers, The State University of New Jersey
Newark, New Jersey

Madeline Gervase, RN, MSN, CCRN, FNP,
PhD(c)

*Overview, Assessment, Adult and Geriatric
Homecare Units*

Clinical Instructor, College of Nursing
Rutgers, The State University of New Jersey
Newark, New Jersey

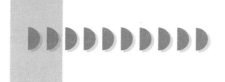

Preface

Cost containment and rapidly advancing technological development are two of the most significant factors driving the recent changes in healthcare delivery options. Procedures once performed only within the walls of the traditional intensive care unit are increasingly being implemented in the home setting. As clients return to the home environment more acutely and chronically, critically ill, a major paradigm shift has occurred dramatically impacting how and where complex nursing care is delivered. As care of the technologically dependent client moves to the home setting, different strategies must be put in place to ensure the delivery of safe, competent care. Blood transfusion, parenteral nutrition, ventilator management, peritoneal dialysis, and chemotherapy administration are but a few of the complex nursing procedures now implemented in the home setting, under the supervision of the highly trained homecare nurse.

AACN Guide to Acute Care Procedures in the Home is a clinical support text designed to serve practicing homecare nurses, faculty, and senior-level student nurses delivering care to the technologically dependent client in the home setting. The text is *not* intended to be used as the initial instruction for acute and critical care procedures. Given the complexity of nursing procedures performed in the high-technology homecare environment, nurses working in such settings must be thoroughly familiar with regulatory policies established by federal governmental agencies, state nurse practice acts, accrediting bodies, homecare companies, certification boards, and third-party payors. Prior to implementing any of the procedures contained in this text, the nurse must ensure that all actions taken comply with the rules, regulations, and guidelines of all appropriate entities. Typically, matters pertaining to regulatory issues and advanced clinical practice are covered during the homecare agency's orientation sessions for nurses, students, and faculty, and are periodically updated at ongoing inservice education programs. For some procedures, the nurse will need to hold national certification and/or be able to demonstrate competence through skills performance testing. Of necessity, the procedures presented in the text follow general guidelines. The client mix, environmental setting, and agency policy and procedures will determine the specific strategies the nurse is to use in applying the nursing process to the delivery of care in the community.

Every effort has been made to ensure the accuracy and currency of all procedures contained in the text. However, given the rapid evolution of technologic change, the reader is instructed to review manufacturer recommendations, drug and package inserts, agency policy and procedures, and to keep abreast of specialty, governmental and certification board guidelines and revisions.

Format

AACN Guide to Acute Care Procedures in the Home is divided into seven units, and each unit is subdivided into parts. Unit One provides a broad overview of the homecare setting, covering the following topics: scope of practice, role of the nurse, regulatory considerations, multidisciplinary homecare team, documentation, time management, infection control, and use of telecommunication technologies. Unit Two provides guidelines for obtaining the health history by offering an overview of body systems across the lifespan, factors to consider when assessing growth and development, tools used to assess mental health, and approaches to performing a cultural and environmental assessment. Units Three through Seven provide guidelines for implementing procedures arranged by body systems for each of the following client populations: perinatal, newborn, pediatric, adult, and geriatric. Tables, charts, and illustrations are included throughout to support the content. The units end with pertinent appendices and references. The text ends with a glossary of explanatory terms the reader may reference to clarify terminology used.

Each specific procedure in Units Two through Seven follows a structured format to provide consistency in presentation. The structured format is arranged as follows:

Description: provides brief background information relevant to the procedure described

Purpose: briefly describes the general rationale supporting use for the procedure

Equipment: lists the supplies, which serve as representative samples, needed to perform the procedure

Outcomes: identifies the client/caregiver goals for the procedure

Assessment Data: indicates the relevant client information needed by the nurse prior to implementing the procedure

Related Nursing Diagnoses: selects from a NANDA-approved list relevant nursing diagnoses specific for the procedure described

Special Considerations: addresses a variety of situational concerns and variables which might need to be taken into account when implementing the procedure

Transcultural Considerations: offers a very brief suggestion of cultural factors to consider with each procedure, a more in-depth discussion of the cultural assessment is provided in Unit Two

Interventions: uses a tabular format divided into two columns: action and rationale. The sequential steps listed in each procedure are designed to serve as general guidelines and are not intended to supersede clinical judgment or policy/procedure established by regulatory entities. It should be recognized that each intervention guideline may need to be tailored to individualize client care

Documentation: lists those clinical findings which should be included in the nursing note specific to each procedure

Interdisciplinary Collaboration: identifies members of the interdisciplinary team who will need to be consulted with regard to implementing of the procedure

Summary

The implementation of procedural skills is but one aspect of nursing care delivery. It is the belief of the editor and contributing authors that the performance of nursing skills occurs within the confines of a holistic approach to care, where nursing, health, society, and client form the metaparadigm of nursing practice. The domains of each of these four dimensions overlap in the homecare environment and must be taken into consideration when establishing the plan of care. Unlike the hospital setting, the resources of the interdisciplinary team are accessed from a community-based collaborative perspective. At the center of the interdisciplinary team is the client and caregiver. All client care is developed around mutually arrived at goals and interventional strategies. A delicate blending of the expertise of each member of the team is required in the homecare setting and is, substantively, the fundamental element that ensures a seamless care-delivery model.

Gloria J. McNeal, RN, MSN, CS, PhD
Editor

Acknowledgments

An undertaking as comprehensive as the writing of a text of this scope could not have been successfully achieved without the assistance and support of many. I would like to first thank Dr. Grif Alspach, editor of *Critical Care Nurse*, for suggesting that I even consider embarking on such a project, and for facilitating the early development of the content of the manuscript, from proposal writing to formatting. Additionally, I would like to thank Ellen French, publications director at AACN and the AACN staff, who reviewed the early outlines and supported the manuscript's further development. I am truly indebted to the leadership at AACN for never losing sight of the goal of this project.

To Sue Glover, editor, at Lippincott Williams and Wilkins and to Susan Keneally, consulting editor, I wish to extend my sincere appreciation for their assistance in taking the manuscript from its earlier versions to the finished product, complete with text design, reviewer selection, and artistic illustration.

To each of the contributing authors, I cannot express the depth of my appreciation for their commitment, attention to detail, and dedication to seeing the project through to completion, despite the seemingly neverending revisions, modifications, and painful deletions.

To the reviewers, I extend my appreciation for their thought-provoking comments, timely updates, suggestions for change, and clinical expertise in helping to critically analyze content and presentation.

Most importantly, I must thank the administrative leadership at the four participating homecare agencies, who facilitated the contribution of the clinical field homecare nurses under their employ and/or who permitted the sharing and reproduction of their agency documents: Martha J. Minniti, CEO and president, the SNI Companies; Louise Milanese, CEO and president, IAMA, Inc; Carol Quinn, CEO and president, Mercy Home Health Services; and Lori Jordan, director of nursing, and Ellen Craighead, account manager, for Coram Healthcare. Without the support and cooperation of these incredible women, the clinical expertise of the contributing authors would not have been evidenced.

Lastly, I must praise my mother, Virginia Malone, and my sister, Ida McNeal, two technologically dependent patients, who through their courage remind me daily of the challenges one must face when cardiac output and tidal volume can only be maintained with mechanical assistance and with conscious concerted effort. I must also acknowledge the memory of my two baby cousins, Kelly LeVar and Korey Lemar Graham, who died at barely one year of age both in need of daily NG tube placement and frequent feedings. They were little cherubs who introduced me to the challenges that families must face with high-tech homecare. To my little cousin, now almost a teenager, Knicole Danielle Johnston, I recognize the courage of her and her mother in dealing with central line placement and daily intravenous antibiotic therapy at such a young age. And to my husband, Lyle Severson, RN, I sincerely appreciate his willingness to share his expertise as a homecare field nurse working at the bedside to make a difference.

Gloria J. McNeal, RN, MSN, CS, PhD
Editor

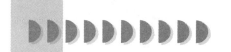

Contents

▶ UNIT 6

Adult Homecare

◗ UNIT 7

Geriatric Homecare

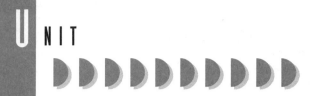

UNIT

Overview of High-Tech Homecare

1

continued

1

▷▷▷▷▷▷▷▷▷▷

Scope of Practice

Standards of Care

The practice guidelines defining the role of the high-tech homecare nurse are derived from the standards of care governing the clinical performance of the traditional homecare nursing health professional. The conventional homecare nurse is a licensed RN who functions either as a generalist prepared at the undergraduate level, or as a specialist prepared at the master's level. Both levels of health professionals practice in the client's home, site of residence, or other community-based site. Working together with the client, caregiver, and family, the ultimate aim of the professional plan of treatment is to assist the client to become self-sufficient and able to implement the prescribed medical regimen.

The role of the generalist is to teach, manage resources, supervise ancillary personnel, monitor client response to treatment modalities, collaborate with appropriate health professionals, and perform direct client care. The role of the specialist is to identify and design research projects, serve as a consultant for the generalist, educate staff, monitor and evaluate trends, develop policy and procedures, and facilitate coordination among an interdisciplinary team of health professionals.

In addition to carrying out the differentiated responsibilities of the two roles, the clinical practice of both levels of homecare nursing health professionals must also be consistent with the standard of care determined by national and regional regulatory and accrediting agencies. To become knowledgeable in the various standards of care, the high-tech homecare nurse should consult the guidelines of any of several professional organizations which publish standards for homecare practice, among which are:

► Occupational Safety and Health Administration (OSHA)
► American Nurses Association (ANA)
► Health Care Financing Administration (HCFA)
► State Boards of Nursing (SBN)
► American Society for Parenteral and Enteral Nutrition (ASPEN)
► Center for Disease Control and Prevention (CDC)
► Intravenous Nursing Society (INS)
► Oncology Nursing Society (ONS)
► Joint Commission on Accreditation of Healthcare Organizations (JCAHO)
► Community Health Accreditation Program (CHAP)
► The Association of Women's Health, Obstetric and Neonatal Nurses (AWHONN)

As in traditional acute care practice, the high-tech homecare nurse may develop expertise in any of several areas of subspecialization: high-risk perinatal/neonatal nursing, technologically dependent children/adults, infusion therapy, and the like. Nurses with nationally recognized certifications in intravenous therapy, pediatrics, perinatology, oncology, critical care, and so on are recognized as decided assets to the homecare industry [10–12, 18–19, 22, 27–29, 42, 45–48, 51, 52].

Transitioning From the Acute Care Setting to High-Tech Homecare

As the current acute care nurse prepares to practice in the high-tech homecare setting, newer role performance skills need to be developed. The homecare setting requires that the nurse perform a comprehensive health assessment, document according to guidelines established by various national regulatory and governmental agencies, manage time effectively, and work collaboratively with an interdisciplinary team of healthcare professionals. The newer concepts of care delivery place the high-tech homecare nurse at the head of a healthcare team composed of a wide variety of community-based healthcare professionals, paraprofessionals, and family members. In making the home visit, the high-tech homecare nurse carries a well-equipped nurses' bag and an array of telecommunication devices to maintain a constant link with healthcare resources: palm-held computer, dictaphone, cellular telephone, pocket pager, and portable ECG machine. Evolving telemedicine technologies are continuing to extend the traditional boundaries of the ICU to virtual critical care environments, where remote access and advanced telecommunication capability connect the most distant community-based settings with state-of-art equipment and functionality [27, 28].

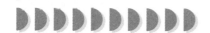

2 Role of the Homecare Nurse

The role of the high-tech homecare nurse is multidimensional and professionally challenging. For the technologically dependent and critically ill client in the home, the high-tech homecare nurse must be able to assume an advanced practice role functioning as clinician, case manager, client advocate, educator, coordinator of agency and community resources, and/or researcher. A key component in each of these nursing roles is the ability to be flexible and innovative when attempting to meet the needs of the client in a variety of home settings.

Clinician

As clinician, the skilled high-tech homecare nurse is the intermittent provider of direct care. By definition, skilled nursing care is complex, requires the knowledge and technical competence of a registered nurse and is indicated when the condition of the client dictates the need for services which cannot be provided by nonskilled nursing personnel. Skilled nursing care includes physical, mental, psychosocial, and spiritual assessment of the technologically dependent and critically ill client. An integral component of the assessment process includes appropriately reporting findings and modifying the treatment plan in collaboration with the attending physician, as the need dictates. In addition to assessment, the high-tech homecare nurse must also be able to implement a wide range of services: management of high-risk pregnancies, monitoring of cardiac dysrhythmias, administration of complex infusion therapies, and execution of home ventilator programs of care. Complex wound and ostomy care, indwelling catheter insertion and rehabilitative nursing add to the array of services now routinely offered in the homecare setting. The high-tech homecare nurse is also responsible for the supervision of ancillary personnel, whose function is to assist the client and caregiver in the performance of routine activities of daily living (ADLs).

Educator

Closely associated with the clinician nursing role is that of the role as educator. Nurses in the homecare setting must teach clients and/or caregivers how to implement complex therapies. Educating clients, families, and caregivers on self-care in the home environment is essential for several reasons. First, in most cases only intermittent nursing care will be authorized by third-party reimbursers in the community-based setting. Therefore, clients and caregivers must learn to function independently between nursing visits. Complex infusion therapies, for example, will need to be managed and maintained over a 24-hour period, even when the nurse is not in the home. Second, as the orientation of healthcare turns more toward disease management, health promotion activities will be integral components of client teaching. Attendance at smoking cessation educational programs, for example, may enable the end-stage COPD client to change aspects of his lifestyle which help to control carbon dioxide retention and improve the quality of life. As educator, the high-tech homecare nurse helps clarify for both the client and caregiver factors and lifestyle choices which may worsen or ameliorate health problems. In addition to serving as educator for clients, the high-tech homecare nurse also serves as role model and mentor for nursing students, new staff orientees, and other healthcare providers.

Case Manager

The case management role is one in which the high-tech homecare nurse is responsible for the establishment of the plan of care and coordination of community resources, following a thorough assessment of client and caregiver needs. In the case management role, the high-tech homecare nurse must have a working knowledge of the existence of community resources, and must be able to negotiate and advocate for client needs. Essential for this role is the nurse's ability to prioritize identified client problems and to work with the client and family in developing acceptable solutions for a multitude of home healthcare issues. The nurse serves as both a liaison and facilitator in identifying and accessing the most appropriate and cost-effective resources available to achieve expected client outcomes.

Coordinator

As the coordinator of agency and community resources the nurse actively collaborates with other healthcare team members in implementing the nursing process. As the coordinator of care, the high-tech homecare nurse determines client need, identifies available resources, and makes referrals with appropriate follow-up. Effectively utilizing the discharge planning process, which begins at the start of care and continues to termination of healthcare services, is an integral component of this role. Operative homecare discharge planning serves to link the client and caregiver with community resources, and ensures the safe provision of care and functioning in the home even after homecare services have ended.

Advocate

As client advocate, the high-tech homecare nurse explains the client's needs to the family, caregivers, and other health providers, and serves as an intermediary in obtaining authorization from third-party reimbursement agencies for visits and purchasing of equipment and supplies. The nurse strives to resolve care issues, and, when homecare is no longer indicated or reimbursable, assists the client and caregivers to assert their needs independently.

Researcher

The role of the nurse-researcher is vital to the expansion of homecare knowledge. It is a role which may not always be apparent in high-tech homecare nursing practice. As a member of the research team, the high-tech homecare nurse may be asked to participate in research initiatives needed to validate an agency's programs, which focus on disease management, such as congestive heart failure, sickle cell anemia, or asthma programs. The nurse may be called upon to collect and analyze data needed to increase knowledge and make changes in clinical practice supported by research findings. Research findings are heavily relied upon to document the cost-effectiveness of interventional strategies and the achievement of client outcomes. Studies have already proven the value of caring for the ventilator dependent child at home, and have demonstrated the reduction in healthcare costs associated with the client diagnosed with COPD and ALS. In order to continue to improve the quality of homecare provided and to measure the impact of nursing interventions on client outcomes, the nurse-researcher role in high-tech homecare practice must continue to be supported [2, 6, 18, 19, 22, 42, 45–48, 51, 52].

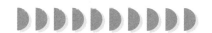

3 Regulatory Considerations

Health Care Financing Administration (HCFA)

In order to perform daily operations, homecare agencies must comply with federal and state mandated guidelines. HCFA is the department of the government responsible for implementing the Medicare and Medicaid programs. Regularly scheduled onsite review of agency functions and client care are performed by site visitors to ensure that standards are met, and that the federal funds assigned to these programs are properly disseminated. Homecare agencies must complete annual cost reports which are closely evaluated for compliance. To ensure conformity with federal guidelines, HCFA contracts with insurance companies that serve as intermediaries for certified homecare agencies. Medicare claims are submitted by the homecare agency to the intermediary which, in turn, reimburses the agency for the service provided. At any given time the medical record may be requested to document the need for reimbursement. Failure to comply can lead to stiff penalties and threat of agency closure [22, 46, 48].

Voluntary Accrediting Agencies

In addition to following the mandated guidelines for Medicare and Medicaid programs, homecare agencies may also elect to be evaluated by either of two voluntary accrediting bodies: Joint Commission on Accreditation of Healthcare Organizations (JCAHO) and the Community Health Accreditation Program (CHAP). Since 1983, JCAHO has been accrediting homecare agencies, and it outlines its standards of practice in the JCAHO Accreditation Manual for Home Care. CHAP, a subsidiary of the National League for Nursing, Inc, was granted deemed status in 1992, thus allowing all homecare agencies accredited by CHAP to be certified for Medicare reimbursement. Both CHAP and JCAHO make regular site visits to evaluate performance and award certification based on the agency's ability to demonstrate consistently high standards of care. In addition to clinical performance, the homecare agency site-visit review process will also include a review of documentation, patient satisfaction reports, quality/performance improvement activity, infection control, and evidence of adherence to national guidelines. Depending on the outcome, the homecare agency may be awarded full accreditation, provisional status, or revocation of previous certification [10–12, 22, 45, 46, 48, 52].

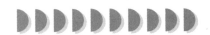

4 The Interdisciplinary Home Healthcare Team

The traditional homecare nurse is an established member of a well-defined team of community-based interdisciplinary health professionals: third-party payors, physicians, social workers, physical therapists, enterostomal therapists or wound, ostomy continence nurse, pharmacists, nutritionists, laboratory technologists, homecare aides, and others. The developing role of the high-tech homecare nurse brings an expanded scope of practice for this emerging clinical subspecialty area. The position requires that the nurse be proficient in both the provision of direct client care and knowledgeable in the vast array of reimbursement mechanisms specific to a wide variety of third-party payors. As a key member of the homecare team, the high-tech homecare nurse collaborates with other healthcare disciplines as the need arises and appropriately documents all care to facilitate the reimbursement process [28].

Third-Party Payors

A host of agencies are responsible for the direct reimbursement of client healthcare services: Medicare, Medicaid, private insurance companies, no-fault insurance, workmen's compensation, self-pay, HMO's and charity care. A vital function of the high-tech homecare nurse is to ensure that services provided will be covered by the client's third-party payor. As the client's case manager, the nurse will interface directly with the client's insurer to obtain the necessary authorization for treatment prior to rendering service [28].

Third-party payors typically reimburse the cost of care for skilled nursing services (SN), physical therapy (PT), occupational therapy (OT), speech-language pathology and audiology (S-LP), social work services (SW), home health aides (HHA), durable medical equipment (DME), and medical supplies. The skilled services of nursing, PT, OT, and S-LP are reimbursable when the services rendered are complex and in need of the expertise of the highly trained and educated healthcare professional. The services of the HHA are reimbursable when the client is unable to independently perform activities of daily living (ADLs): bathing and grooming, preparing meals, transfer activities, and the like. If one other skilled professional service is present in the home, the medical social worker will be covered to perform: counseling, financial evaluation, psychosocial assessment, and acquisition of community resources. The high-tech homecare nurse determines the need for all members of the intra- and interdisciplinary teams and documents their visit patterns and skilled activities on the HCFA form 485 [28].

The Intradisciplinary Homecare Team

Often the homecare agency will have, as either consultants or employees, other members of the discipline of nursing to assist the high-tech homecare nurse in the provision of services. Enterostomal therapists (ETs), or wound, ostomy, continence (WOC) nurses, nurse practitioners (NPs), and clinical nurse specialists (CNSs) may be accessed by the high-tech homecare nurse to assist in developing and implementing the Plan of Treatment (POT). Additionally, to help the client perform ADLs, the home health aide (HHA) under the supervision of the professional nurse may be assigned to assist the client and caregiver in the delivery of basic care [28].

The Interdisciplinary Homecare Team

Depending on the complexity of care required at the initiation of homecare services, the high-tech homecare nurse may need to collaborate with other health professionals in the provision of services: the pharmacist, the laboratory technician, the physician, the social worker, the physical therapist, the speech language pathologist and audiologist, the respiratory therapist, the nutritionist, and others. Ongoing and throughout the period of certification, the nurse may need to obtain changes in orders and to update the physician with regard to laboratory results and general client progress. Lastly, in the event of life-threatening situations, the high-tech homecare nurse will need to interface directly with the community's emergency medical system to access the services of paramedics and EMTs. Typically, standing orders and protocols will be followed in determining the need for urgent care, and client advance directives will specify the end-of-life treatment modalities to be followed [10–12, 22, 28, 45, 46, 52].

5 ▷▷▷▷▷▷▷▷▷
Documentation

Standardized Data Collection Forms

The technologically dependent or critically ill client receiving homecare services must be under the direct care of a primary care physician (PCP), who writes the orders for treatment. The nurse collaborates with both the physician and the client in developing the treatment plan. The nurse determines, prior to admission to homecare service, that the client has met the guidelines for homecare status established by both regulatory and governmental agencies. The client must be able to comply with all ordered treatment modalities. At the time of admission and through to discharge from homecare service, the high-tech homecare nurse continually assesses suitability of the home setting and the client's compliance with agency and payor policy and procedures [28].

The Health Care Financing Administration (HCFA) government agency created the following series of forms to be used as standardized data collection forms for the delivery of care in the homecare setting. The HCFA-485, Home Health Certification Plan of Care, is the form used to meet all regulatory and national survey requirements in the establishment of the plan of treatment (POT), and documents the start of the certified authorization for care. The HCFA-487, Addendum to the Plan of Treatment/Medical Update, is used to provide additional data to support information appearing on the HCFA-485. The HCFA-488, Intermediary Medical Information Request, contains supplemental data that may be requested by regulatory agencies when the information provided on the HCFA-485, and/or 487 is insufficient [28].

OASIS

HCFA now mandates that all Medicare-certified homecare agencies uniformly collect client data and use the information to improve clinical outcomes. HCFA has developed a standardized data set containing approximately 80 items. The methodological approach to measuring these outcome data is known as the Outcome and Assessment Information Set (OASIS). Homecare agencies are currently incorporating OASIS data sets into assessment forms, clinical pathways, care plans, documentation, and the Home Health Certification and Plan of Care (the 485). At the start of care, OASIS data are collected in the areas of demographics and health history, living arrangements, supportive assistance, sensory, integumentary, respiratory, elimination, neurological/emotional status, ADLs and IADLs, medications, equipment management and emergent care. OASIS identifiers are coded with an M0 number and grouped under each of the major headings (See Table 1-1). A follow-up and discharge version of the start of care OASIS form is used to track client progress.

The paradigm to improve clinical outcomes using OASIS is referred to as outcome-based quality improvement (OBQI). In the OBQI model an outcome is measured as a change in patient status from baseline to two or more subsequent points in time. Precisely quantified scales generate reports that show improvement or stabilization for each OASIS outcome measure. The homecare agency can use the scores to identify problematic or stable outcomes for each of its clients [1, 36, 44].

TABLE 1-1 Outcomes and Assessment Information Set (OASIS)

OASIS Identifier	OASIS Item	OASIS Identifier	OASIS Item
Clinical Record Items			
M0010	Agency Medicare Number	M0012	Agency Medicaid number
M0020	Patient ID Number	M0030	Start of care date
M0032	Resumption of Care Date	M0040	Patient name
M0050	Patient residence	M0060	Patient zip code
M0063	Medicare number	M0064	Social Security number
M0065	Medicaid number	M0066	Date of birth
M0069	Gender	M0072	Referring physician
M0080	Discipline Completing Form	M0090	Date assessment completed
M0100	Reason for Completion of Form		
Demographics and Patient History			
M0140	Race/Ethnicity	M0150	Current payor
M0160	Financial Factors	M0170	Recent inpatient facilities
M0180	Inpatient Discharge Date	M0190	Inpatient diagnoses
M0200	Change in medical treatment	M0210	Changed medical diagnoses
M0220	Conditions prior to change in medical regimen/inpatient stay	M0230/M0240	Diagnoses/severity index
M0250	Therapies at home	M0260	Overall prognosis this episode
M0270	Rehabilitative Prognosis	M0280	Life expectancy
M0290	High risk factors		
Living Arrangements			
M0300	Current residence type of home	M0310	Structural barriers
M0320	Safety Hazards	M0330	Sanitation hazards
M0340	Patient lives with		
Supportive Assistance			
M0350	Assisting persons other than home care agency staff	M0360	Primary caregiver
M0370	Frequency of assistance from primary caregiver	M0380	Type of primary caregiver assistance
Sensory Status			
M0390	Vision	M0400	Hearing and ability to understand spoken language
M0410	Speech and oral expression of language	M0420	Frequency of pain
M0430	Intractable pain		
Integumentary Status			
M0440	Skin lesion or open wound	M0445	Pressure ulcer
M0450	Number of pressure ulcers at each stage	M0460	Stage of most problematic ulcer
M0464	Status of most problematic ulcer	M0468	Stasis ulcer formation
M0470	Number of observable stasis ulcers	M0474	Unobservable stasis ulcer

(continued)

TABLE 1-1 Outcomes and Assessment Information Set (OASIS) *(Continued)*

OASIS		OASIS	
Identifier	*Item*	*Identifier*	*Item*
M0476	Status of most problematic observable stasis ulcer	M0482	Surgical wound
M0484	Number of observable surgical wounds	M0486	Unobservable surgical wounds
M0488	Status of most problematic observable surgical wound		
Respiratory Status			
M0490	Shortness of breath	M0500	Respiratory treatments
Elimination Status			
M0510	Urinary tract infection	M0520	Urinary incontinence/ catheter
M0530	When does urinary incontinence occur	M0540	Bowel incontinence frequency
M0550	Ostomy for bowel elimination		
Neuro/Emotional/Behavioral Status			
M0560	Cognitive functioning	M0570	When confused
M0580	When anxious	M0590	Depressive feelings reported or observed
M0600	Reported/observed behaviors	M0610	Behaviors reported at least weekly
M0620	Frequency of behavior problems	M0630	Psychiatric nursing services
ADL/IADLs			
M0640	Grooming	M0650	Ability to dress upper body
M0660	Ability to dress lower body	M0670	Bathing
M0680	Toileting	M0690	Transferring
M0700	Safety in ambulation/locomotion	M0710	Feeding and eating
M0720	Planning/preparing light meals	M0730	Transportation
M0740	Laundry	M0750	Housekeeping
M0760	Shopping	M0770	Ability to use telephone
Medications			
M0780	Management of oral medications	M0790	Management of inhalant-mist medications
M0800	Management of injectable medications		
Equipment Management			
M0810	Patient management of equipment	M0820	Caregiver management of equipment

Adapted from Spearling, R & Humphrey, C. (1999). *OASIS and OBQI: A guide for education and implementation.* Philadelphia: Lippincott, Williams and Wilkins. Used with permission.

THE 485

Upon admission to homecare service, the nurse completes the HCFA form 485 (Display 1-1). The form contains the signatures of both the admitting nurse and attending physician and verifies the collaborating plan of treatment. The form contains 28 sections numbered consecutively in a one-page format. It is vitally important that each section of the form be accurately completed. Any discrepancy in the completion of the form will render the document invalid and will result in a denial of the request for reimbursement. The 485 contains 28 fields that must be completed at the start of care. OASIS M0 numbers directly relate to several of the 28 fields on the 485. The following description of the information to be entered/reviewed by the nurse in each of the 485's 28 sections follows. OASIS M0 numbers appear in bold to serve as a guide to indicate their relationship with the corresponding fields of the 485:

- ▶ Section 1: Health Insurance Claim Number [**M0063**]

  In this section, the nurse inputs the client's medical insurance number, which is typically found on the client's insurance card [28].
- ▶ Section 2: Start of Care (SOC) Date [**M0030**]

  The SOC date is the date of admission to homecare service and will be the date used on all subsequent forms until the client is discharged from homecare service. This field requires the entry of six digits, e.g., 120499 for December 4, 1999. Whenever the client is discharged from homecare service and subsequently readmitted, the SOC date will change for each readmission [28].
- ▶ Section 3: Certification Period

  The certification period covers 2 months of service, if required, beginning with the Start of Care (SOC) Date. If beyond the 2-month period, the client continues to require care, a request for recertification must be filed. The dates are entered as six-digit numbers, e.g., from 120499 to 020400 [28].
- ▶ Section 4: Medical Record No [**M0020**]

  The homecare agency may assign a medical record number to facilitate record keeping and filing of client information within the agency. The record number differs from the health insurance claim number and is entered in this field [28].
- ▶ Section 5: Provider Number

  A unique number to be used in the processing of claims for reimbursement is assigned to each homecare agency by the regulating insurer. The number contains two digits, a hyphen, and four digits (00-9000), and is entered in this field [28].
- ▶ Section 6: Client's Name and Address [**M0040, M0050, M0060**]

  The client's last name first, full address and telephone number are entered in this field. The information must coincide with the client's health insurance card [28].
- ▶ Section 7: Provider's Name, Address, and Telephone Number

  The name of the homecare agency, its address and business telephone number are entered in this block [28].
- ▶ Section 8: Date of Birth [**M0066**]

  The client's birthdate is entered as a six-digit number, e.g., 022453, for February 24, 1953 [28].
- ▶ Section 9: Sex [**M0069**]

  A check mark is placed in the box which correctly identifies the client's gender [28].
- ▶ Section 10: Medications: Dose/Frequency/Route (N)ew (C)hanged [**M0200, M0500, M0780, M0790, M0800**]

  All ordered medications are placed in this block with the correct dose, frequency and route of administration. Oxygen therapies are also placed here. The nurse is to indicate if the order is new within the last 30 days or changed within the last 60 days. The list of medications must include all drugs used for the treatment of the medical diagnoses appearing in Sections 11 and 13 [28].

Department of Health and Human Services
Health Care Financing Administration

Fo.m Approved
OMB No. 0938-0357

HOME HEALTH CERTIFICATION AND PLAN OF CARE

1. Patient's HI Claim No.	2. Start of Care Date	3. Certification Period		4. Medical Record No.	5. Provider No.
		From:	To:		

6. Patient's Name and Address

7. Provider's Name, Address and Telephone Number

8. Date of Birth	9. Sex ☐ M ☐ F	10. Medications: Dose/Frequency/Route (N)ew (C)hanged

11. ICD-9-CM	Principal Diagnosis	Date

12. ICD-9-CM	Surgical Procedure	Date

13. ICD-9-CM	Other Pertinent Diagnoses	Date

14. DME and Supplies	15. Safety Measures:

16. Nutritional Req.	17. Allergies:

18.A. Functional Limitations

1	☐ Amputation	5	☐ Paralysis	9	☐ Legally Blind
2	☐ Bowel/Bladder (Incontinence)	6	☐ Endurance	A	☐ Dyspnea With Minimal Exertion
3	☐ Contracture	7	☐ Ambulation	B	☐ Other (Specify)
4	☐ Hearing	8	☐ Speech		

18.B. Activities Permitted

1	☐ Complete Bedrest	6	☐ Partial Weight Bearing	A	☐ Wheelchair
2	☐ Bedrest BRP	7	☐ Independent At Home	B	☐ Walker
3	☐ Up As Tolerated	8	☐ Crutches	C	☐ No Restrictions
4	☐ Transfer Bed/Chair	9	☐ Cane	D	☐ Other (Specify)
5	☐ Exercises Prescribed				

19. Mental Status:

| 1 | ☐ Oriented | 3 | ☐ Forgetful | 5 | ☐ Disoriented | 7 | ☐ Agitated |
| 2 | ☐ Comatose | 4 | ☐ Depressed | 6 | ☐ Lethargic | 8 | ☐ Other |

20. Prognosis:

| 1 | ☐ Poor | 2 | ☐ Guarded | 3 | ☐ Fair | 4 | ☐ Good | 5 | ☐ Excellent |

21. Orders for Discipline and Treatments (Specify Amount/Frequency/Duration)

22. Goals/Rehabilitation Potential/Discharge Plans

23. Nurse's Signature and Date of Verbal SOC Where Applicable:	25. Date HHA Received Signed POT

24. Physician's Name and Address	26. I certify/recertify that this patient is confined to his/her home and needs intermittent skilled nursing care, physical therapy and/or speech therapy or continues to need occupational therapy. The patient is under my care, and I have authorized the services on this plan of care and will periodically review the plan.

27. Attending Physician's Signature and Date Signed	28. Anyone who misrepresents, falsifies, or conceals essential information required for payment of Federal funds may be subject to fine, imprisonment, or civil penalty under applicable Federal laws.

Form HCFA-485 (C-3) (02-94) (Print Aligned)

PROVIDER

DISPLAY 1-1 ▶ Home Health Certification and Plan of Care (HCFA-485)

▶ Section 11: ICD-9-CM Code, Principal Diagnosis, and Date [M0230]

The medical diagnosis listed here must be the principal diagnosis which supports admission to homecare service. The International Classification of Diseases, 9th edition, Clinical Modification (ICD-9-CM) code source book is the reference used to assign diagnostic code numbers [28].

▶ Section 12: ICD-9-CM Code, Surgical Procedure, and Date

In this section, the nurse must indicate all recent surgical interventions specific to the principal diagnosis and must enter the dates for all corresponding interventions and correct ICD-9-CM code numbers [28].

▶ Section 13: ICD-9-CM Code, Other Pertinent Diagnoses, and Dates [M0240, M0210, M0220]

In this section, the nurse lists all current diagnoses, in order of priority, supporting the need for homecare service [28].

▶ Section 14: Durable Medical Equipment (DME) and Supplies [M0250, M0500, M0520, M0810, M0820]

The nurse lists in this section all billable equipment and supplies currently in use for the client's care [28].

▶ Section 15: Safety Measures [M0310, M0320, M0330, M0390, M0400, M0410, M0560, M0700]

All safety measures identified by the nurse or physician needed to keep the client safe in the homecare environment are listed in this section [28].

▶ Section 16: Nutritional Requirements [M0710, M0720]

All dietary orders are listed in this section and include any special diets, fluid restrictions or requirements, enteral feedings, and supplements [28].

▶ Section 17: Allergies

Include in this section all allergens: food, drugs, insect bites, pollen, dust, etc. If none are known enter NKA (no known allergies) [28].

▶ Section 18A: Functional Limitations [M0390, M0400, M0410, M0490, M0520, M0540, M0700]

In this field are listed eight functional limitations: amputation, bowel/bladder incontinence, contracture, hearing, paralysis, endurance, ambulation, speech, legally blind, dyspnea with minimal exertion, and other. Check all limitations that apply to the client [28].

▶ Section 18B: Activities Permitted [M0640-0700]

The nurse will confer with the primary care physician prior to indicating any of the following activities: complete bedrest, bedrest BRP, up as tolerated, transfer bed/chair, exercises prescribed, partial weight bearing, independent at home, crutches, cane, wheelchair, walker, no restrictions, other (specify) [28].

▶ Section 19: Mental Status [M0560-0590]

The nurse will evaluate the client's mental status and check the appropriate box: oriented, comatose, forgetful, depressed, disoriented, lethargic, agitated, other [28].

▶ Section 20: Prognosis [M0260]

Enter the client's expected response to the plan of treatment: poor, guarded, fair, good, excellent [28].

▶ Section 21: Orders for Discipline and Treatments (Specify Amount/frequency/duration) [M0220, M0250, M0410, M0440-0488, M0500, M0550, M0780-0820]

The duration and frequency of the homecare visits are determined by the nurse in collaboration with the physician at the time of admission to service. The visit pattern is based on the nature of the illness and the level of skilled care required. For the critically ill client, the initial visit pattern will need to be daily, then tapered as the client responds to therapy. A large component of the visit will be devoted to educating the client and caregiver in the correct administration of ordered therapies and evaluation of client response. Time considerations must be made for the client and caregivers learning capacity, cultural or language barriers to communication, and willingness to participate in the treatment plan. Orders must reflect the medical diagnoses, the clinical assessment and goals for treatment. (See Display 1-2) [28].

▶ Section 22: Goals/Rehabilitation Potential/Discharge Plans [M0270, M0640-0820]

The high-tech homecare nurse in collaboration with the physician and client will determine the goals for care. All goal statements must be related to the diagnoses, client specific, and measurable. The nurse will describe the achievable goals for the client, determine the client's ability to meet those goals, and provide an estimated date of goal achievement. Examples of appropriately defined goals follow:

Within one week, client/caregiver will perform dressing changes as ordered.

Within one day, client/caregiver will safely administer nebulizer therapy with bronchodilator as ordered.

Within two weeks, client/caregiver will correctly prepare and administer TPN therapy as ordered.

Also, within this locator, specification should be made of the client's rehabilitation potential [28].

DISPLAY 1-2 *Documenting the Visit Pattern on HCFA Form 485*

A specific client care situation may serve to clarify the appropriate documentation which must be entered Section 21: Orders for Discipline and Treatment:

In caring for the client status post CVA, complicated by a history of COPD and acute respiratory infection in need of intravenous antibiotic therapy might read as follows:

Skilled Nursing (SN)

SN7 wk1, 3wk2, 2–4wk6 (Skilled nursing needed 7 times per week for 1 week, then 3 times per week for 2 weeks, then 2 to 4 times per week for 6 weeks); for :

Skilled observation and assessment of the cardiovascular, respiratory and integumentary systems, and client response to medications and all ordered therapies

Teaching and training of intravenous medication administration, signs and symptoms of infection, fluid volume overload, and oxygen therapy

Performance of the following skilled procedures: intermittent intravenous medication administration via peripheral site, daily oral medication administration, and safe management of oxygen therapy

Management and evaluation of the plan of care

Home Health Aide (HHA)

HHA3wk4×2hrs, & 2wk5×2hrs (Home Health Aide needed 3 times per week for 2-hour visits for 4 weeks, then twice per week for 2-hour visits times 5 weeks) for:

Assistance with personal care, meal preparation and home exercises ordered by physical therapist

Physical Therapy (PT)

PT1-3wk9 (Physical Therapy needed 1 to 3 times per week for 9 weeks) for:

Instruction in endurance training

Medical Social Worker (MSW)

SW1wk1 (Social Worker needed for a one-time assessment within first week) for:

Assessment of the family's financial status and evaluation of need to contact other community resource systems [28]

▶ Section 23: Nurse's Signature and Date of Verbal Start of Care (SOC)
   The nurse signs and dates this entry upon obtaining the medical orders, and upon receiving approval for authorization of the visit patterns from a representative of the client's insurance provider [28].
▶ Section 24: Physician's Name and Address
   Enter the name, address, and telephone number of the physician who is responsible for the client's care, writes and verifies all orders, and certifies the visits and services [28].
▶ Section 25: Date Home Health Agency (HHA) Received the Signed Plan of Treatment (POT)
   The physician reviews the form 485, dates and signs in the appropriate field and returns the form to the home health agency. Upon receipt of the form from the physician's office, the agency inserts the date in this locator [28].
▶ Section 26: Physician Certification
   The nurse will circle the appropriate notation to indicate whether the plan of treatment is for the initial certification period or for the recertification period beyond the first 60–62 days [28].
▶ Section 27: Attending Physician's Signature and Date Signed [M0072]
   The physician signs and dates the form in this field to certify all care to be received by the client [28].
▶ Section 28: Penalty Statement
   This field contains notification of all penalties associated with the knowing misrepresentation, falsification, or concealment of information related to payment of federal funds for healthcare delivery [28].

The HCFA Form 485 is completed as part of the admission process. The form provides a record of the estimated plan of treatment (POT) over the initial 60–62 day certification period. Each POT is client specific and documents the need for third-party payor reimbursement for the services provided. Should additional space be required the nurse will complete a form 487, the addendum to the POT [28].

Should the client require continuous care beyond the initial SOC period, the recertification process will need to be initiated. To recertify, the same HCFA 485 will be completed with updates and modifications to the original plan as needed. The physician orders treatments for the next 60–62 day period which must then be submitted to the client's insurer for authorization for payment. The SOC date will remain the same, however the certification period will extend through the next continuous 60–62 day period. Should there continue to be a need for further clarification, the HCFA-488 form may also be requested. The individual homecare agency will establish guidelines for the completion of the summary note, which documents the client's medical progress [28].

Consent Form

On admission to homecare service, the client will be asked to sign a consent form, which permits the start of care, verifies accuracy of insurance information, authorizes release of medical records, assigns direct payment of third-party reimbursement to the homecare agency, and establishes financial liability for unpaid services.

Advance Directives

The client will be informed of the need to make end-of-life decisions, and encouraged to prepare an advance directive/living will and to assign a durable power of attorney. A copy of the appropriate forms should be maintained on file with the homecare agency. Living wills become operational only after a copy has been filed with the client's attending physician. Typically, the client will be asked to sign a form indicating that an explanation regarding advance directives/living wills has been given and that information regarding state and federal regulations has been provided (see the Advance Directive Declaration).

Comprehensive Health Assessment

At the time of admission to service, a complete history and physical examination will be made. The high-tech homecare nurse will assess the family dynamics and the bio-psychosocial, spiritual, cultural, and environmental dimensions. All body systems will be evaluated and need for interdisciplinary collaboration documented. Unit 2 provides guidelines for an in-depth assessment of all systems.

Medication List

A medication profile will be compiled by the nurse listing drug name, classification, dosage, route, frequency, and allergies. The medication form documents the name and contact telephone numbers of the attending physician and pharmacist. A copy of the medication list will be maintained in the home and reviewed for accuracy and completeness at each visit (see the Medication Profile, Appendix 1-1).

Nursing Note

Depending on the format in use, the documentation of the nursing assessment may be written as a narrative note, SOAP note, checklist, or computerized medical record. Regardless of format, all notes will contain goals, interventions, evaluation of treatment response, complex equipment settings, discharge plans, and summary of interdisciplinary collaboration. Client teaching will be an integral component of the note, documenting the client's and caregiver's abilities to implement the medical regimen. Comprehensive body system assessments are documented at each visit, and plans for emergency preparedness are constantly reevaluated (see Appendix 1-3).

Telephone Orders

Periodically, depending on need, the high-tech homecare nurse may determine that a change in the plan of care is required. Any deviation from the orders written on the initial 485 must be accompanied by a written medical order. At the time of the change, the nurse will telephone the client's attending physician to obtain the necessary verbal order. Verification of the verbal order will be documented on a telephone order form. The form contains the client's name, address, insurance numbers; the physician's name address and telephone number; date and time of the order; and the nurse's signature. A copy of the order is maintained in the medical record. The original is mailed to the physician for signature, and then returned to the homecare agency for placement in the client's file.

Coordination Log

Consultation with other member's of the healthcare team, family or caregivers, school nurse, and so on will be documented on the coordination or communication log. The purpose of the entry is to maintain an ongoing record of discussions held regarding the client's treatment or goals for care. The form is used to document need for unscheduled visits, missed visits, or untoward events [10–12, 18, 19, 22, 27, 28, 45–48, 52].

6 ▷▷▷▷▷▷▷▷▷ Time Management

Depending on the complexity of the case, the homecare industry standard requires that five to six client visits be made daily, and that the nurse complete 25 to 30 visits per week. Generally, 90 to 120 minutes are allocated for admissions, and 45 to 60 minutes for all revisits. However, in addition, several other factors need to be taken into consideration in planning the daily visitation schedule. First, plan for clients needing BID wound care or glucometer assessments, for example, they will need to be seen early in the day and then again in the late afternoon or early evening. Second, any emergent situations which may arise during the day will need a priority visit. Blocked drainage tubes, acutely developed clinical symptoms, infiltrated intravenous lines, and the like require immediate attention. Third, the homecare visit may need to be timed around the client's visit to his or her primary care physician; the caregiver's availability; the homecare aide's mandated, scheduled nurse-supervised visit, which occurs bimonthly; or, the physical therapist's need to visit jointly with the client's primary nurse. Fourth, geographical distance will increase the length of time needed to reach a client. Part of the daily visit schedule will depend on the physical distance between client home locations, and the feasibility of traveling over many miles to reach each home. A well-planned daily visit schedule considers priority of care needs, ability to postpone visits to a later date for the stabilized client, travel distance, interdisciplinary team conferencing, telephone calls to clients and healthcare team members, and completion of paperwork (see Display 1-3) [28].

Preparing for the Initial Home Visit

The client will be referred from the acute care setting to the homecare agency typically by the hospital discharge planner, case manager, or homecare coordinator. The homecare agency will complete a referral form and provide the nurse assigned to the case with a copy. The form usually contains the client's name, address and telephone number; name, address and telephone number of the significant other; medical diagnoses; treatment protocols; list of medications; special equipment needs; dietary regimen; mobility aids; and, name, address and telephone number of the primary care physician.

Prior to the visit, the nurse will make an introductory telephone call to the client to establish the visit time. The purpose of the call is to verify the client's location, determine the need to bring any additional supplies, and to familiarize the client with the names of the agency and nurse (s) assigned to the case. Upon arrival at the home, the nurse will begin the elaborate admission process. The following forms comprise the typical admission packet:

Consent (see Appendix 2-1)
Patient Homecare Bill of Rights (see Appendix 2-3)
Verification of Insurance
Environmental Assessment (see Table 2-1)
Physical Assessment (see Appendix 1-3B)
Plan of Treatment (see Display 1-1)
Medication List (see Appendix 1-1)
Satisfaction Survey

DISPLAY 1-3 *Sample Daily Log*

The Visitation Sequence

The following is a chronicled, anecdotal log of a typical day in the clinical field. The log details the complex critical decision making strategies that must be implemented by the nurse, the level of nursing skills required, time management considerations, and the coordination of urgent care services.

0800—The nurse arrives at the home of Mr. and Ms. T. Mr. T is a 58-year old Caucasian American, who has returned home 1 week following a cervical fusion for a herniated cervical disc. During the course of his hospital stay he developed a post-operative staphloccal infection. He is to begin a 6-week course of IV vancomycin therapy. The nurse obtains Mr. T's vital signs and assesses his integumentary, pulmonary, cardiovascular, and neurological systems. A peripherally inserted central catheter (PICC) line was placed by the nurse on the previous day, and twice daily IV vancomycin therapy was initiated as ordered. Mr. T is to wear a Philadelphia collar at all times, administer his own IV vancomycin therapy, and assess both the right groin donor site and the operative site incision lines for evidence of infection. Because Mr. T was out of work for several weeks prior to surgery and will be out of work for an additional 2 months, he and his wife express concerns regarding their financial status. A social work consult is ordered. Mr. T is to begin administering his IV medication today, however both he and his wife are very apprehensive. While they are both comfortable with flushing the line, they are not yet ready to manage the IV pump system. The nursing decision is made to allow them both time to ventilate their feelings, and to permit several days of observing the nurse's technique in preparing the drug for administration. Blood urea nitrogen, creatinine, and trough vancomycin levels are drawn by the nurse, and the infusion is started. A peak vancomycin level will be drawn on the return visit three hours later. The nurse teaches the couple signs and symptoms of infection and evaluates their learning by permitting them time to verbalize understanding. Duration of the visit: 45 minutes

0915—The nurse arrives at the home of Mr. and Ms. S. Mr. S is a 78-year old, middle-class Caucasian American, who is status post bilateral knee replacements for degenerative joint disease. The nurse obtains vital signs and performs a physical assessment. The physical therapist has just completed gait training, stair climbing, and range of motion exercises with Mr. S. The therapist discusses the client's progress with the nurse and a collaborative note is written. Today the skin staples are to be removed by the nurse, who will also draw blood for prothrombin Times (PT) and international normalized ratio (INR) levels to monitor coumadin therapy. The nurse reviews the medication regimen and teaches the family methods of pain control. Because the wife must continue to leave the home daily to maintain employment as a cashier in a local department store, Mr. S's sister assists in caring for Mr. S. The nurse removes the skin staples and applies steri-strips to both incision sites. The nurse reinforces the family's understanding of wound care and assessment, and observes and evaluates the wife's return demonstration. Visit duration: 60 minutes

1030—The nurse arrives at the home of Mr. and Ms. W. Mr. W is a 60-year old African American suffering with congestive heart failure, obesity, and sleep apnea. The W's are an indigent family living in a low-income neighborhood ravaged by unemployment, illicit drug use, and burglaries. Mr. W uses an oxygen concentrator to maintain nasal oxygen at 4L/min while awake, and sleeps with nasal continuous positive airway pressure (CPAP) to stimulate ventilation. The nurse obtains vital signs and performs a physical assessment. The nurse provides dietary instruction to assist Ms. W with weekly menu planning to maintain a 2-gram sodium, low-fat diet. Over the past month, Mr. W has lost 30 pounds, is much less edematous, and has no S3 gallop or adventitious lung sounds. Mr. and Ms. W share concerns that they have regarding an unemployed adult son who lives with them, and the fact that they must assume total responsibility for their grandson. The nurse permits them time to ventilate their concerns. The nurse assists them to establish realistic limit-setting behaviors, to help the son assume some of the responsibilities of caring for his child. The W's also express pride for their daughter, who

(continued)

DISPLAY 1-3 *Sample Daily Log* (Continued)

has just bought a new home and works for the postal service. Mr. W is stable. Visit duration: 45 minutes

1130—The nurse returns to the home of Mr. & Ms. T to obtain vancomycin peak levels, and to instruct Ms. T in the daily technique to change the damp Philadelphia collar after the morning shower and apply a spare. Mr. T is to lie in a flat position and during the collar change he is not to move, cough, or speak until the second collar is securely in place. While a bit apprehensive, Ms. T is able to use excellent technique in making the change. Mr. T remains stable. Visit duration: 20 minutes.

1200—The nurse arrives at the home of Ms. P a newly diagnosed insulin-dependent diabetic, status post a recent cerebral vascular accident with right-sided weakness. Ms. P is a divorced 50-year old, middle-class African American, who lives alone in a private two-story home. The physician has placed her on decreasing doses of prednisone to control cerebral edema. Because she is unable to care for herself at this time, her sister visits daily to administer medications and provide activities of daily living (ADLs). Vital signs are obtained and blood pressure is found to be 200/100 mmHg with an apical pulse rate of 110/minute. Ms. P's sister reports a morning glucometer reading of 390 mg/dl. A neurological assessment reveals diminished deep tendon reflexes on the right, pupils equal and reactive to light, blurred vision, intact mental status, a right-sided facial droop, and no complaints of headache. After reviewing with Ms. P's sister the morning medications, the nurse calls Ms. P's physician to discuss the hypertensive findings, and elevated blood glucose. The physician orders a repeat dose of her morning lasix, an increase in her evening insulin dose, and a stat dose of regular insulin. The nurse writes the verbal order on the medical order sheet, and observes Ms. P's sister's ability to accurately administer the ordered dose of subcutaneous insulin. The nurse reinforces the new medication orders with the sister, and reviews the signs and symptoms of hyperglycemia and hypoglycemia. The client voids approximately 500 cc of clear yellow urine. A half hour later the blood pressure is down to 180/90 mmHg, the pulse is 100/minute, and the blood glucose is 200 mg/dl. Ms. P's sister is given clear instructions regarding findings that would indicate the need to contact the nurse prior to the next visit scheduled for the following day. Visit duration: 60 minutes

1300—On the way to the next visit, the nurse receives a stat page from the home care office. Mr. S's wife has called to say the Mr. S's left knee incision line as opened and is draining a large amount of fluid. From the car, the nurse returns the call to Ms. S, and informs her that she is in the area and will arrive shortly.

1315—The nurse returns to the home of Mr. S and finds a 1-inch opening at the proximal end of the left knee incision site. The wound is draining a copious amount of serous fluid. Vital signs remain stable. The client is assisted to a position of comfort and a pressure dressing is applied to the site. The physician is called and informed of the client's status. The physician instructs the nurse to have the client transported to the emergency room where he will meet the client upon arrival. The operating room is placed on standby alert. Because the situation is urgent, but not life-threatening, the decision is made to call a local ambulance service to transport the client to the hospital, which is approximately 45 minutes away. Vital signs are obtained every 15 minutes until the ambulance arrives at 1400.

1420—The nurse arrives at the home of Mr. B, an elderly middle-class Caucasian gentleman, who is status post pacemaker insertion for sick sinus syndrome. He lives in a private two-story home and is the sole caregiver for his wife, who has a mild case of dementia. Concerned neighbors stop by periodically to provide any needed assistance with food shopping and the like. Today, the sutures are to be removed and a 12-lead electrocardiogram (ECG) obtained. The nurse finds that Mr. B's vital signs are stable and the wound edges are well approximated. The sutures are removed, and wound care and follow-up assessment instructions are given to Mr. B by the nurse. The ECG reveals paced rhythm with

(continued)

DISPLAY 1-3 *Sample Daily Log* (Continued)

good capture. The ECG report is simultaneously transmitted to the physician's office while the nurse is still in the home. The nurse applies a Holter monitor to review 24-hour electrocardiographic data, reviews the pacemaker surveillance system, and instructs Mr. B on potential sources of electrical interference to be avoided. Visit duration: 40 minutes

1530—The nurse arrives at the homecare office to update plans of care, review medical orders, dictate nursing notes for transcription, arrange for pickup of blood specimens, plan the next day's visits, and confer with the evening nurse, who will administer Mr. T's 8 P.M. dose of vancomycin. Pharmacy is called to review intravenous orders and to arrange for home delivery of: saline flush kits, bags of vancomycin, and heparin lock solution. The nurse telephones Mr. S's physician for an update of his status. Mr. S was sent to the operating room for wound closure. He is to return home on post-operative day three.

1700—End of the day

McNeal, GJ. (1996). High-tech homecare: An expanding critical care frontier. *Critical Care Nurse* Vol 16, No 5, pp. 52–57. Used with permission.

Advance Directives (see Appendix 1-2)
Nursing Note and Care Plan (see Appendices 1-3 and 1-4)
Teaching Plan
Doctor's Order Sheet
Communication Log
Discharge Summary

Depending on need the following forms may also be required:

Wound Care Assessment
Blood Transfusion Form
Nutritional Assessment

After completing the admission process, the nurse will collaborate with the pharmacist to ensure accuracy of physician orders for complex infusion therapies, and with the enterostomal therapist or Wound, Ostomy Continence Nurse for all complex wound care treatment. Other members of the interdisciplinary team will be consulted as the need arises.

The Re-Visit

All subsequent visits following admission will adhere to a strict schedule of times documented on the initial Plan of Treatment (POT). Any changes to the time schedule must be accompanied by a physician order and authorized by the third-party insurer. Follow-up visits are made to assess client progress, to teach and evaluate client's and/or caregiver's abilities to perform complex treatment tasks, to review any changes in orders, to obtain laboratory specimens, and to update other members of the interdisciplinary team with regard to the client's status. Emergency unscheduled visits will be made as the need arises to attend to occluded infusion lines or drainage tubes, deteriorating changes in the client's status, malfunctioning equipment, and the like. For all life-threatening situations, the client and caregiver will be instructed to access the community's emergency medical system.

Discharge from Homecare Service

When all goals and outcomes for care have been met, the client will be discharged from homecare service. At the time of discharge the client will be medically stable. If ongoing therapy is required, the client or caregiver must demonstrate the ability to assume care. The nurse will need to carefully document all teaching and will need to evaluate the client's or caregiver's ability to implement the medical regimen. The nurse will complete the discharge summary, documenting all of the following: the achievement of all goals, the client's knowledge of the disease process, the client's compliance with medication administration and adherence to the dietary regimen, and the client's understanding of all untoward symptoms, which must be reported to the physician [10–12, 18, 19, 42, 45–48, 52].

7 Infection Control

Federal Guidelines

The Center for Disease Control and Prevention (CDC) publishes guidelines, for use by health professionals, which contain procedural protocol for infection control. The CDC recommends that *Standard Precautions* be used for all clients, and that *Transmission-based Precautions* be used for all clients diagnosed with conditions that can be transmitted by air, droplet, or contact routes. The nurse should adhere to the following CDC guidelines to maintain infection control in the home setting:

STANDARD PRECAUTIONS
Wash hands prior to initiating direct client contact and after touching body fluids, using an antimicrobial or waterless antiseptic agent
Wear nonsterile gloves when touching body fluids, changing gloves as necessary between tasks on the same client
Wear personal protective equipment (goggles, masks, gowns, shields) for all activities where splashing or spraying of body fluids will occur
Ensure that all equipment coming in contact with contaminated body fluids is properly discarded or disinfected
Use appropriate environmental controls to ensure that proper protocol is followed by all personnel
Handle contaminated linen in a manner which prevents the transmission of microorganisms
Use correct techniques to prevent injury from contaminated sharps, needles, and scapels [10–12, 45–48]

Source of Contamination

THE CLIENT
The homecare client may be admitted to service for treatment of an infection occurring throughout all body systems or contained within one area of the body. The plan of care may include administering intravenous antibiotic therapy, topically applying anti-infectious agents, and teaching infection control strategies. Often the stress of disease renders the client immune compromised and at risk for the development of infection. The nurse must be alert to the signs and symptoms of undiagnosed infection, and must take appropriate precautions to prevent its spread. Any evidence of redness, pain, fever, purulent exudate, or swelling must be reported to the primary care provider, and appropriate monitoring of febrile states, culture and sensitivity reports, complete blood counts, and x-ray findings must be immediately implemented. Clients on long-term antibiotic therapy must be closely monitored for the development of super infection. Tuberculosis, hepatitis, and HIV/AIDS are three of the most troubling infectious diseases currently causing concern because of their increasing incidence [10–12, 45–48].

THE NURSE

The homecare nurse, traveling from home to home, may be at risk for transmitting disease from one setting to another. It is imperative that homecare personnel follow strict infection control procedure when carrying supplies into the home, when transporting biohazardous waste, and when disposing of contaminated supplies in the home. Because of the risk of transmission, most homecare agencies have strict guidelines for the provision of alternate assignments for the sick employee. Nurses harboring viral infections, herpetic lesions, or contaminated wounds on exposed body surfaces endanger the safety of all clients, especially those with immunocompromised disease states [10–12, 45–48].

Infection Control Strategies

HANDWASHING

Handwashing is the single most effective intervention in the prevention of spread of infection by contact transmission. In the display of appropriate handwashing technique, nurses serve as role models for clients and their caregivers. All jewelry should be removed from hands and hands should be vigorously scrubbed with bacteriocidal cleanser for three minutes, from fingers to wrists while held under running water. Keep fingers in an upright position during the procedure to permit draining of water from the cleanest area of the fingertips. Complete the procedure by drying hands with a paper towel, and using the towel to turn off the faucets.

In those home settings where running water and soap may not be available, the nurse should carry a waterless bacteriocidal cleanser to maintain good handwashing technique. Because of the drying tendency of waterless cleansers, the nurse should apply lotion frequently to the skin surfaces of the hands to prevent excessive drying and potential breaks in the skin, which will serve as portals of entry for contaminants [10–12, 45–48].

BAG TECHNIQUE

The nurse's bag is used to carry necessary supplies and small items. To reduce the possibility of transmission of infectious agents, the nurse must attend to proper bag technique. The bag must contain interior compartments for storage of clean and sterile supplies and external compartments for reusable equipment that does not typically come in contact with body fluids [stethoscope, digital thermometer, sphygmomanometer, antiseptic soap, and the like] (see Display 1-4) [10–12, 45–48].

 Procedural Protocol for Removing and Replacing Bag Equipment and Supplies

- ▶ Upon entering the home a protective barrier is removed from the external compartment of the bag, and placed on a hard surface.
- ▶ The nurse's bag is placed on the protective barrier, never on the floor.
- ▶ Wash hands.
- ▶ Remove only those items to be used during the visit, then close the interior compartments.
- ▶ At the completion of the visit, clean all reusable equipment and wash hands before replacing items and closing the bag.
- ▶ Contaminated items are never carried inside the bag.

PERSONAL PROTECTIVE EQUIPMENT

As part of the equipment included in the nurses' bag, gowns, gloves, masks, and eyewear are required standard supplies. These items should be disposable and used only once before discarding. They must be readily available at all times in the event that the nurse must follow transmission-based precautions. Because of the increase in outbreaks of tuberculosis, CDC guidelines now mandate that healthcare professionals who may be potentially exposed to TB must be fitted with a high efficiency particulate air (HEPA) respirator (Figure 1-1). Homecare agency policy will define the type of respirator required [10–12, 45–48].

NEEDLESTICK PRECAUTION

Needlestick injuries predispose the nurse to exposure to bloodborne pathogens. Most such injuries occur from attempts to recap the needle after use when starting intravenous lines, performing venipuncture, and after administering an injection. Guidelines prohibit the recapping of needles and instruct the nurse to immediately dispose of sharps in puncture-proof disposable containers, which must be carried at all times. When the sharps container becomes more than two-thirds full it should be appropriately replaced according to agency protocol. Nurses should report all needlestick injuries immediately to the appropriate supervisor for follow-up care. Many agencies use needleless systems to reduce the threat of needlestick injury [10–12, 45–48].

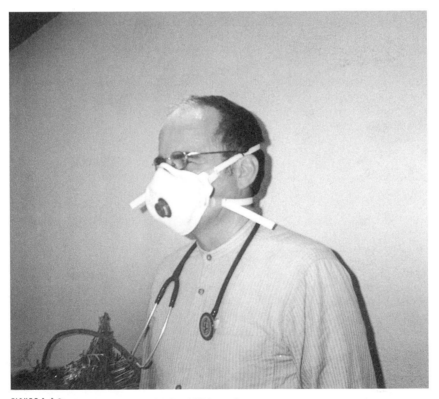

FIGURE 1-1 ▶ Homecare nurse wearing HEPA mask.

Client Education

Nurses must reinforce with clients and caregivers the importance of strictly following infection control procedures. Clients and their caregivers must be instructed in appropriate handwashing techniques, and in standard and transmission-based precautions. It is important for clients and caregivers to understand that personal items, such as toothbrushes, combs and brushes, razors and the like, should never be shared. The client's dishes and utensils should be washed separately in hot soapy water. Toys of pediatric clients should be cleaned regularly and kept separate from those of other siblings. All surfaces in the bathroom, kitchen, and sick room should be washed frequently. Trash cans, supplies, and durable medical equipment used by the client should be frequently disinfected [10–12, 45–48].

Clothing and linen contaminated with body waste should be washed immediately and handled with gloves. All such materials should be contained in plastic bags until they can be washed. The wash cycle should last at least 30 minutes, and a cup of bleach should be added to the detergent used. Clothing and linens should be dried in a hot dryer or hung in direct sunlight to dry.

Appropriate disposal of all contaminated trash must follow the rules of the community department of sanitation. All such trash should be placed in plastic bags and disinfected with a 10% bleach solution. Sharps containers should be returned to the agency for proper disposal. Lastly, the need for maintenance of personal hygiene for the client and caregiver must be reinforced. Daily bathing, oral hygiene, frequent handwashing, and avoidance of colds and other infectious diseases are requisite strategies in reducing spread of infection [10–12, 18, 19, 45–48].

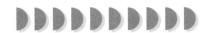

Telecommunication Technologies

With the advent of telecommunication technologies, the high-tech homecare setting has become a virtual electronic environment. Telemedicine capability and functionality have spearheaded the delivery of complex healthcare services to meet the needs of the critically ill client at home. Electronic networks, using Windows®-based programs and Internet access, have revolutionized the manner by which intricate clinical procedures can be implemented in the home setting. Video conferencing technology now uses cable linkages and wireless remote systems to transmit video and digital imaging from the home to the agency. The computerized medical record, via the laptop, is now on the road and in use to download or export data from the home to the agency. In addition to computerization, the miniaturization of ventilators, dialysis systems, cardiac monitors, infusion pumps, and so on has significantly expanded the range of healthcare services once available only within the walls of the traditional intensive care unit. It goes without saying that computer literacy is a requisite skill for today's high-tech homecare nurse.

The Computerized Medical Record

As accrediting bodies, payors, and government agencies demand more and more clinical evidence to support interventional strategies, documenting findings and outcomes has gained paramount importance. To assist the high-tech homecare nurse to document all critical data, the computerized medical record is rapidly becoming the manner by which the nurse charts clinical findings in the homecare setting. The laptop or palmtop (hand-held) computer is carried in the nurses' bag. Upon entering the home, the nurse may choose to connect the computer directly into the client's telephone line for instant documentation or retrieval of information, or the nurse may choose to store the data findings on the hard drive or disk, for transmission to the homecare agency at a later time. As systems become more user friendly, the computerized medical record will soon be an integral component of documentation nationwide.

Home Telemedicine Systems

Teleconferencing systems are currently being configured to enable the homecare health professional to directly interface with the client from remote access sites. The Personal Telephone System (PTS1) and the Home Assisted Nursing Care (HANC) Device are two systems which use a video television screen, camera, and telephone line to connect the client directly to the homecare agency for constant surveillance and real-time communication. With additional add-on technology these units can be equipped to monitor heart sounds and lung sounds (telestethoscope); obtain pulse oximeter readings; transmit 12-lead ECG recordings; obtain blood pressure, pulse and temperature readings; and, administer continuous and intermittent infusions (tele-infusion). From remote sites, infusion rates can be changed, pumps can be reprogrammed, and wounds and intravenous sites can be directly viewed. Most importantly, all electronic information can be saved and stored for later retrieval.

Transtelephonic Monitoring

HUAM—In caring for the client with preterm labor, the high-tech homecare nurse monitors the client using a home uterine activity monitoring (HUAM) unit. The nurse instructs the client in the correct application of the unit and linkage of the client's telephone lines with the homecare agency's network for daily monitoring. Such units have demonstrated their usefulness in assisting the nurse to closely observe for evidence of preterm uterine contractions.

Pacemaker Surveillance—Clients with implanted cardiac pacemakers are able to periodically evaluate pacemaker function and monitor the presence of erratic cardiac activity. Systems, which typically use the client's telephone line, can transmit an ECG recording indicating pacemaker function to the agency or physician office. The high-tech homecare nurse is responsible for instructing the client in the correct application of the pacemaker surveillance system.

Dysrhythmia Detection—Transtelephonic monitoring of cardiac activity was implemented in the 1960s with the advent of ambulatory monitoring devices, which captured data over a 24-hour period. More current technology utilizes a miniature three-lead ECG machine with modem that is capable of storing and transmitting cardiac information over a 4-week period. The client is taught how to apply the device and how to connect the device to a telephone line at home or work, to transmit information to the agency or physician office. In the event of an abnormal rhythm, the client is instructed in the self-administration of emergency medications while the nurse activates the emergency medical system from the agency or the command center.

Transtelephonic Defibrillation—Still in the experimental stages of development are devices which can halt erratic cardiac activity over telephone lines. For clients with automatic implanted cardioverter defibrillator (AICD) devices, a tone can be transmitted over the receiver of the telephone placed on the client's chest to signal the detonation of a defibrillating electrical charge. The caregiver can dial into the monitoring agency and by placing the telephone over the client's chest, the cardiac pattern is transmitted and, if indicated, the critical care clinician can initiate the charge.

It is clear that telecommunication technologies have significantly contributed to the current evolution of high-tech homecare nursing practice. Increasing advances in information science will continue to facilitate the transition of the ICU to the homecare environment [3–5, 7–9, 13, 14, 16, 17, 20, 21, 23–26, 30, 31, 33–35, 37–41, 49, 50, 53].

REFERENCES

1. Adams, CE, Wilson, M., Haney, M., et al. Using outcomes-base quality improvement model and OASIS to improve HMO patient's outcomes. *Home Healthcare Nurse* 16: 395, 1998
2. Ark, PD & Nies, M. Knowledge and skills of the home healthcare nurse. *Home Healthcare Nurse* 14: 292, 1996
3. Baff, M. Enhancing homecare's off-site operations through Internet technology. *Health Care Innovation* 7: 18, May–June 1997
4. Barrell, JM. Telemedicine: you can't do that at home. *Infusion* 4: 29, 1997
5. Benson, JA, Michelman, JE, Radjenovic, D. Using information technology strategically in home care. *Home Healthcare Nurse* 14: 977, 1996
6. Bohny, GJ. A time for self-care: Role of the home healthcare nurse. *Home Healthcare Nurse* 15: 281, 1997
7. Braunstein, ML. Electronic patient records for homecare nursing. *Computers in Nursing* 12: 232, 1994

8. Bruderman, I & Abboud, S. Telespirometry: Novel system for home monitoring of asthmatic patients. *Telemedicine Journal* 3: 127, Summer 1997

9. Carrol, P. Using pulse oximetry in the home. *Home Healthcare Nurse* 15: 88, 1997

10. Clark, MJ. *Nursing in the community,* 2nd edition. Stanford, CT: Appleton & Lange, 1996

11. Clemen-Stone, S, Eigati, DG, & McGuire, SL. *Comprehensive community health nursing: Family aggregate and community practice,* 4th edition. St. Louis, MO: Mosby Inc., 1995

12. Green, K. *Home care survival guide.* Philadelphia, PA: Lippincott, 1998

13. Dalzell GW, McKeown PP, Roberts JM, & Adgey AA: A cellular transtelephonic defibrillator for management of cardiac arrest outside of the home. *American Journal of Cardiology* 68: 909, 1991

14. Flaherty RJ. Electronic bulletin board systems extend advantages of telemedicine. *Computers in Nursing* 13: 8, 1995

15. Freudenheim, M. An exam for home health care. *The New York Times* D 1-2, September 15, 1995

16. Gee, PM. The Internet Part II: A home care nursing clinical resource. *Home Healthcare Nurse* 15: 175, March 1997

17. Hoss, S. Back to the future. *Home Care* 17: 145, 1995

18. Jaffe, MS & Skidmore-Roth, L. *Home health nursing: Assessment and care planning,* 3rd edition. St. Louis, MO: Mosby, 1997

19. Johnson, JY, Smith-Temple, J, & Carr, P. *Nurses' guide to home procedures.* Philadelphia, PA: Lippincott, 1998

20. Kingsley, PA, Backinger, CL, & Brady, MW: Medical-device users instructions. *Home Healthcare Nurse* 13: 31, 1995

21. Kinsella, A: Home 'tele-infusion': Emerging trends in today's telecare industry. *Infusion* 4: 16, 1997

22. Marrelli, TM. *Handbook of home health standards and documentation guidelines for reimbursement,* 3rd edition. St Louis, MO: Mosby, 1998

23. McConnell, EA. The future of technology in critical care. *Critical Care Nurse Supplement* 3–16, June 1996

24. McManamen L & Hendrickx L. Telemedicine: tuning in critical care's future? *Critical Care Nurse* 16: 102, 1996

25. McNeal, GJ. Twenty-four hour ambulatory monitoring: A new electrocardiographic tool. *Nursing Clinics of North America* 13: 3, 437–448, 1978.

26. McNeal, GJ. Tracing arrhythmias. *American Journal of Nursing* 79: 1, 98–100, 1979

27. McNeal, GJ: High-tech home care: an expanding critical care frontier. *Critical Care Nurse* 16: 51, 1996

28. McNeal, GJ. Care of the critically-ill client at home. *Critical Care Nursing Clinics of North America* 10(3): 267, 1998

29. McNeal, GJ. Diversity issues in the homecare setting. *Critical Care Nursing Clinics of North America* 10(3), 1998

30. McNeal, GJ. Telecommunication Technologies in high-tech homecare. *Critical Care Nursing Clinics of North America* 10(3):279, 1998

31. Mersch, J & Cook, K. Technology whose time has come: The Stanford Transtelephonic arrhythmia network. *Stanford Nurse* 18: 4, 1996

32. Moulton, PJ, Wray-Langevine, J, & Boyer, C. Implementing clinical pathways: One agency's experience. *Home Healthcare Nurse* 15: 343, 1997

33. O'Neal, P & McFarlin, P. Home care goes high tech. *Stanford Nurse* 18: 8, 1996

34. Pait EP & Pallesen, BJ. Fundamental considerations in home chemotherapy administration. *Infusion* 2: 24, 1996

35. Pitts, M: Finding a niche. *Home Care* 17: 151–154, November, 1995

36. Polzien, G, Kendall, BJ, & Hindelang, M. The challenge of implementing OASIS. *Home Healthcare Nurse* 16: 805, 1998

37. Rice, R. Home mechanical ventilator management. *Home Healthcare Nurse* 13: 73, 1995

38. Romano, CA. Imaging: an innovative technology. *Computers in Nursing* 11: 222, 1993

39. Saladow, J. Welcome to the Twenty-first century. *Infusion* 2: 10, 1996

40. Saltzman, KM & Lammers KA: Telemedicine: where health care services meet technology. *Infusion* 4: 23, 1997

41. Schlachta, LM & Pursley-Crotteau, S. Leveraging technology: telemedicine in disease management and implications for infusion services. *Infusion* 4: 36, 1997

42. Schwartz, R & Grier P. Caring comes home. *Advanced Practice Nurse.* Fall/Winter: 38, 1994

43. Shaffer, C & Houser, K. The big boom theory. *Infusion* 2: 21, 1996

44. Sperling, R. Frequently asked questions about OASIS: Answers from a rural agency participant. *Home Healthcare Nurse* 15: 340, 1997

45. Spradley, BS & Allender, JA. *Community health nursing: Concepts and practice.* Philadelphia, PA: Lippincott, 1996

46. Stackhouse, JC. *Into the community: Nursing in ambulatory and home care.* Philadelphia, PA: Lippincott, 1998
47. Stanhope, M & Knollmueller, RN. *Handbook of community and home health nursing: Tools for assessment, intervention and education,* 2nd edition. St Louis MO: Mosby, 1996
48. Stanhope, M & Lancaster, J. *Community health nursing: Promoting health of aggregates, families, and individuals,* 4th edition. St. Louis, MO: Mosby Yearbook Inc., 1996
49. Susman, E. Telemedicine permits overnight dialysis at home. Health care workers watch for problems from office. *Telemedicine Virtual Reality* 2: 13, February 1997
50. Warner, I. Introduction to telehealth care. *Home Healthcare Nurse* 14: 790, 1996
51. Yuan, JR. Using standards and guidelines in your daily practices. *Home Healthcare Nurse* 16: 753, 1998
52. Zang, SM & Bailey, NC. *Home care manual: Making the transition.* Philadelphia, PA: Lippincott, 1997
53. Zerwekh, JV: High-tech home care for nurses: Questioning technologies. *Home Healthcare Nurse* 13: 9, 1995

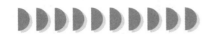

Appendices

MEDICATION PROFILE

Patient _____

Height _____ Weight _____ D.O.B. _____

Allergies _____

DX _____

Pharmacy _____

Address _____

Phone _____

Physician_____ Phone _____

Dates Reviewed / Initials ____ / ____   ____ / ____   ____ / ____   ____ / ____   ____ / ____   ____ / ____

NEW / CHANGED	START DATE	DESCRIPTION	DOSE	ROUTE	FREQUENCY	CLASS	D/C DATE

DRUG CLASSIFICATION

A   **A**

SE

CI

FI

ANALGESIC   G

A   Neural impulses are decreased in the hypothalamus, limbic system, thalmus and the central nervous system through action of neurotransmitters.
SE   N/V, anorexia, dry mouth, constipation, urinary retention, changes in libido, antidiuretic effect, flushing, tachycardia, hypertension, dizziness, sedation, headache, rash, respiratory depression.
C/I   Epilepsy, asthma, hepatic disease, respiratory depression, G.I. disorders, pregnancy. Use cautiously with alcohol, MAO inhibitors, other narcotics, tricyclic antidepressants, CNS depressants and anticoagulants.

A   **B**

SE

C/I

FI

ANTACID   H

A   Magnesium chloride is produced as a reaction of magnesium with stomach acid. Pepsin is inhibited as a result of calcium raising the gastric pH. Increased gastric pH results from aluminum reducing acid concentration and pepsin activity
SE   Constipation, N/V/D, fecal impactions, iron deficiency, anemia, malaise, anorexia, muscle weakness, negative Ca+ balance, mental depression, hypercalcemia, hypercalciuria, hypomagnesia, hypermagnesia, hypophosphatemia.
C/I   Sensitivity, sodium restriction, hypercalcemia and hypercalciuria, GI hemorrhage or obstruction, colostomy, or ileostomy, dehydration, ventricular fibrillation, cardiac disease. Cautious use in renal impairment, gastric outlet obstruction, elderly, decreased bowel activity, history of CHF.

A   **C**

SE

C/I

FI

ANTIANGINAL   I

A   Coronary vessels are relaxed and dilated through action on cardiac smooth muscle.
SE   N/V, rash purpuric eruptions, erythema, abdominal pain, tachycardia, hypotension, headache, dizziness, weakness.
C/I   Hypersensitivity, pregnancy, children.

ADRENERGIC   D

A   Increased myocardial force, rate and contraction, vasodilation, vasoconstriction, bronchial dilation, decreased insulin output, nasal decongestion, results from Alpha and Beta stimulation.
SE   N/V, anorexia, cramps, insomnia, tremors, anxiety, dizziness, pallor, flushing, sweating, poly & dysuria, sphincter spasm, tachycardia, palpitations, chest pain, C.V. collapse.
C/I   Glaucoma, arrhythmias, severe hypertension. Enhanced by other adrenergics, antihistamines, MAO inhibitors, tricyclic antidepressants.

ANTIARRHYTHMIC   J

A   The decreased electrical impulses in the myocardium and conduction in the atrium results in a slowing and strengthening of the contraction of the heart muscle.
SE   Anorexia, N/V/D, abdominal pain, hepatomegaly, bitter taste, fever, chills, weakness, depression, rash, hypotension, ventricular asystole, ventricular fibrillation.
C/I   Aortic stenosis, AV block, CHF. Enhanced by antihypertensive and neuro-muscular blockers.

ADRENOCORTICAL STEROID   E

A   Inflammation is inhibited secondary to the adrenal gland stimulation of secretion of adrenocortical hormones.
SE   Pancreatitis, esophagitis, N/V, headache, convulsion, intracranial pressure, hypertension, CHF, skin rash, poor wound healing, petechiae, cataracts, glaucoma, weakness, compression fractures, muscle atrophy, menstrual irregularities, hirsutism, latent diabetes mellitus.
C/I   CHF, T.B., glomerulonephritis. Enhanced by CNS depressants, oral contraceptives, and salicylates.

ANTIARTHRITICS / ANTIGOUT   K

A   An antiinflammatory effect results from decreased synthesis of prostaglandin.
SE   N/V, abdominal pain, flatulence, rash, purpura, alopecia, CHF, hypertension, pericarditis, tachycardia, chest pain, arrhythmias, edema, hematuria, headache, drowsiness, agitation, tinnitus, blurred vision, renal detachment, deafness, anemia and hemotologic changes.
C/I   Hypersensitivity, GI disease, renal disease, hepatic disease, pregnancy, lactation, children under 14, asthma, peptic ulcer.

ANABOLIC STEROID / ANDROGEN / ESTROGEN / PROGESTIN   F

A   Exact mechanism of androgens and progestins is not known. Estrogen counters the androgenic influence by competing for receptor sites and binding to intracellular receptors which stimulate DNA and RNA to synthesize proteins, others are synthetic derivatives of testosterone. These suppress the gonadotropic function of pituitary and may exert a direct effect on testicles.
SE   Deepening of the voice, acne, facial hair growth, clitoral enlargement, amenorrhea, glossitis, anorexia, N/V, jaundice, maculopapular erythema, edema, alopecia, nervousness, insomnia, leg cramps, risk of thrombosis including nonfatal M.I. in men when used forprostatic cancer, C.V.A.
C/I   Hypersensitivity, carcinoma of the male breast, premenopausal women, active thrombophlebitis or thromboembolic disorders. May increase the effects of oral anticoagulants. Glucose tolerance may decrease. Blood pressure elevations may occur.

ANTIBIOTIC / ANTIBACTERIAL   L

A   Growth of microorganism is inhibited as a result of inhibition of folic acid production or, mucoprotein or cell wall synthesis.
SE   N/V/D, anorexia, abdominal pain, proteinuria, oliguria, increased BUN, dysuria, veginitis, hematuria, anuria, anemia, hematologic changes, urticaria, dermatitis, photosensitivity, headache, dizziness, fleuropathy, psychosis, depression, confusion.
C/I   Hypersensitivity, blood dyscrasias, psychosis. Enhanced by other antibiotics, oral anticoagulants, salicylates, Phenylbutazone, Tolbutamide, Chlorpropamide. Use cautiously in asthma, renal and hepatic disease, myasthenia gravis, convulsive disorders. Action of oral contraceptives may be decreased.
Due to variety of agents and potentially different A, SE and C/I, please refer to specific drug reference for additional information.

Initials	Signature/Title	Date	Initials	Signature/Title	Date

A   Actions
SE   Side Effects / Adverse Reactions
C/I   Contrainidications / Interactions
FI   Food Interaction

*NOTE: Classifications are not inclusive of all actions, side effects, contraindications and interactions.

WARNING: This form is registered with the U.S. Copyright Office. No part of this form may be copied or reproduced in any form or by any means without the express prior written consent of Healthcare Concepts, Inc.

FORM 1340

APPENDIX 1-1A ▶ Medication Profile (*Source: Reprinted by permission of Healthcare Concepts*)

ANTICHOLINERGIC M

A Intestinal motility and relaxation of specific muscles from the inhibition of acetylcholine at parasympathetic neuroeffector sites.

SE N/V/D, heartburn, constipation, urinary hesitancy, retention, dysuria, impotence, tachy & bradycardia, palpitations, nervousness, headache, drowsiness, rash, blurred vision, photophobia, mydriasis.

C/I Myasthenia gravis, hepatic and renal disease, glaucoma. Enhanced by antihistamines, alphaprodine, bucizine, meperidine, orphenadrine, tranquilizers, tricyclic antidepressants, nitrates, procainamide, quinidine and MAO inhibitors, increases intraocular pressure with corticosteroids, haloperidol, increases adverse reactions of digitalis, cholinergics, levodopa and neostigmine.

ANTICOAGULANT N

A Decreases the conversion of prothrombin to thrombin, or decreases the prothrombin time or decreases the production of Vitamin K.

SE N/V/D, hemorrhage, leukopenia, thrombocytopenia, GI bleed, rash, alopecia, urticaria, hematuria, heavy menstrual flow, decreased renal flow, asthma, rhinitis, lacrimation.

C/I Bleeding disorders, hepatic or renal disease, psychosis, pregnancy, lactation, TB. Use cautiously in allergies, elderly, CHF, diabetes, alcoholism, pregnancy and postpartum salicylates.

FI Vitamin K-rich foods may decrease effects of oral anticoagulants. (e.g., leafy green vegetables, broccoli)

ANTICONVULSANT O

A Convulsive activity is decreased through action on the motor cortex.

SE N/V/D, nystagmus, slurred speech, confusion, dizziness, insomnia, nervousness, fatigue, urticaria, rash, dermatitis, hematologic changes.

C/I Hepatic and renal disease, heart block, blood dyscrasias. Barbiturates enhance, anticoagulants, Isoniazid and Chloramphenicol inhibit. Tricyclic antidepressants may increase seizure activity.

ANTIDEPRESSANT P

A The action of catecholamines is potentiated as a result of the blocking of the re-uptake of serotonin and brain amines in the CNS.

SE Orthostatic hypotension, hypertension, arrhythmias, tachycardia, headache, confusion, anxiety, extrapyramidal symptoms, dry mouth, N/V/D, constipation, anorexia, urinary retention, breast enlargement, change in libido, hematologic changes, rash, photosensitivity, edema.

C/I Myocardial infarction, hepatic or renal disease, glaucoma. Death may result when used with MAO inhibitors. Used with CNS depressants, oversedation may occur. Used with thyroid meds, arrhythmias may occur. Phenothiazines inhibit metabolism of this drug.

FI Tyramine-rich foods may cause increased blood pressure / hypertensive crisis / hemorrhagic stroke within 4 weeks of MAO inhibitors.

* Examples of Tyramine rich foods: Aged, overripe, fermented foods and drinks (cheese, caviar, wine, beer, anchovies, pepperoni, salami,bananas, chocolate, caffeine, avocados, fava beans)

ANTIDIABETIC Q

A Glucose is transported across the cell membrane or the pancreas is stimulated to synthesize and release insulin.

SE Hepatic toxicity, jaundice, allergic reactions, rash, weakness, headache anemia, hematologic changes.

C/I Hypersensitivity, acidosis, hepatic or renal disease. Thiazides may increase diabetic state. Action enhanced when taken with MAO inhibitors, salicylates, dicumoral, butazone. Action decreased with alcohol.

FI Sulfonylureas, disulfuram-like reaction with alcohol.

ANTIHISTAMINE R

A Acts in competition with histamine and the receptor sites.

SE N/V/D, epigastric pain, anorexia, constipation, urinary frequency or retention, menstrual irregularities, sedation, dizziness, nervousness, insomnia, euphoria, headache, urticaria, rash, blurred vision, tinnitus, confusion.

C/I Asthma, glaucoma, prostatic hypertrophy, coma. May be enhanced by CNS depressants, other antihistamines and alcohol. Use cautiously with convulsive disorders.

ANTIHYPERTENSIVE S

A Various actions which may include depletion of dopamine, decrease of renin and angiotension, relaxation of vascular smooth muscle or the decrease of norepinephrine.

SE N/V/D, constipation, liver disorders, paralytic ileus, peptic ulcer, sedation, headache, weakness, extrapyramidal symptoms, orthostatic hypotension, bradycardia, myocarditis, CHF, tachycardia, angina, nasal congestion, eczema, glaucoma, anemia, hematologic changes, rash, impotence.

C/I Heart block, children, pregnancy, lactation, hypersensitivity, electroshock therapy, depression, myocardial infraction, blood dyscrasias. Use cautiously in renal or cardiac disease, seizure disorders, CVA.

ANTIINFLAMMATORY / NON-STEROIDAL T

A Decreases prostaglandin synthesis by inhibiting an enzyme needed for biosynthesis. Ketorolac, inhibits synthesis of prostaglandins and may be considered a peripherally acting analgesic.

SE GI disturbances including pain, bleeding, gastritis, peptic ulcer, N/V, fatigue, dizziness, fluid retention, abdominal pain, tinnitus, visual disturbances, decreased appetite, depression, blurred vision, impaired renal / hepatic function, insomnia, blood dycrasias.

C/I Hypersensitivity to ASA and other non-steroidal drugs which produce acute asthma attacks, urticaria, or rhinitis with use of these products.

ANTINEOPLASTIC U

A Cell replication is decreased or blocked by a variety of methods including inhibition of cell division, blocking of folinic acid participation in cell division, inhibition of DNA and RNA synthesis and purine metabolism, etc.

SE N/V/D, myelosuppression, anorexia, leukopenia, thrombocytopenia, bleeding dyscrasias, alopecia, colitis, hepatic dysfunction, fibrosis, dermatitis, rash, pigmentation, thromobophlebitis, anaphylaxis, peripheral neuropathy, depression, malaise, stomatitis, renal failure, cardiac myopathies, fever.

C/I Hepatic or renal disease, hypersensitivity, bone marrow depression, bacterial infections, leukopenia, pregnancy, thrombocytopenia, caution with radiation.

FI Procarbazine (Matulane) with tyramine-rich foods may cause flushing and increased blood pressure.

* Due to a variety of agents and potentially different A, SE and C/I, refer to specific drug reference for additional information.

ANTIPARKINSON V

A Increase in dopamine resulting in decreased Parkinson's effects.

SE N/V, anorexia, abdominal pain, urinary incontinence, dark urine, adventitious movements, headache, hand tremors, numbness, weakness, confusion, anxiety, insomnia, delusions, hallucinations, euphoria, palpitations, orthostatic hypotension.

C/I Glaucoma, melanoma, psychosis, lactation. Vit. B6 may lower effectiveness. Sympathomimetics may potentiate. Use cautiously with tricyclic antidepressants.

FI Selegiline (Eldepryl®): with tyramine-rich foods may cause increased blood pressure.

ANTIPYRETIC W

A Action on the hypothalmus or vasodilation results in decrease of temperature.

SE N/V/D, GI bleed, heartburn, anorexia, rash, increased prothrombin time, leukopenia, neutropenia, tinnitus, dizziness, confusion, headache, convulsions, flushing, thirst.

C/I Hypersensitivity, GI bleed, bleeding disorders, Vit. K deficiency, children under 3, pregnancy, lactation. Use cautiously in gout, allergies, cardiac or renal disease, pulmonary disease.

ANTIULCER X

A Inhibits / suppresses basal gastric secretions by inhibiting histamine (H_2 blocker), by inhibiting the H^+/K^+ ATPase enzyme system or by various other methods protects the gastric mucosa.

SE Diarrhea, headache, nausea, vomiting, constipation, dizziness, flatulence, abdominal pain, neutropenia, somnolence, reversible impotence, gynecomastia, rash.

C/I Pregnancy, lactation. Decrease dose in renal or hepatic failure. May interact with diazepam, phenytoin, warfarin, antacids, tricyclic antidepressants, calcium channel blockers and others too numerous to list. Refer to specific drug.

BRONCHODILATOR Y

A Stimulates the central nervous system at the cortex or bronchial dilation results from stimulation of beta receptors.

SE N/V, anorexia, GI bleed, epigastric pain, restlessness, anxiety, headache, hypertension, palpitations, tachycardia, arrhythmias, circulatory failure, tachypnea, poly & dysuria, diuresis.

C/I Renal or hepatic disease, myocardial infraction. Do **NOT** use with other sympathomimetics or MAO inhibitors. Potentiated by tricyclic antidepressants, antihistamines and levothyroxine. Antihypertensive action may be reduced.

CARDIAC GLYCOSIDE Z

A The refractory period and the force of the cardiac contraction is increased.

SE N/V/D, anorexia, cramps, headache, drowsiness, apathy, confusion, muscular weakness, arrhythmias, visual disturbances.

C/I Ventricular tachycardia and fibrillation. Use cautiously with antihistamines, anticonvulsants, barbiturates, hypoglycemic agents and phenylbutazone. Thiazides and furosemide can cause hypokalemia. Levels of digitoxin may be increased by propantheline bromide, spironolactone, and quinidine.

CHOLINERGIC AA

A A slowing of the heart, increased intestinal and urinary tone and movement, sweating, decreased blood pressure or salivation result indirectly from increased levels of acetylcholine at the cholinergic receptor sites or directly at the cholinergic receptor sites.

SE Stinging, burning, blurred vision, headache, nervousness, dizziness, rash. If taken internally, N/V/D, urinary frequency & urgency.

C/I Eye abrasions, asthma, diabetes, eye inflammation, cardiac disease. Succinylocholine may increase effects. anticholinergics may decrease effects.

DIURETIC BB

A Decreased water reabsorption in the kidneys resulting in diuresis.

SE Dysuria, hematuria, frequency, hypokalemia, hyponatremia, vomiting, diarrhea, hepatic failure, anorexia, flushing, paresthesia, confusion, lethargy, convulsions, headache, nervousness, rash, tinnitus, hearing loss, orthostatic hypotension.

C/I Anuria, hepatic or severe kidney disease, COPD, pregnancy, infants, lactation, electrolyte imbalances. May be enhanced by cholestryamine, diazoxide, lithium and steroids.

FI K^+ sparing agents: with Vitamin K-rich foods (leafy green vegetables, broccoli) or salt substitutes may result in hyperkalemia.

LAXATIVE / STOOL SOFTENER CC

A Various mechanisms which could include irritating the intestinal mucosa, adding fatty substances to the stool, lubricating the intestines or retention of water.

SE Cramps, electrolyte imbalances, rash, N/V.

C/I Intestinal obstruction, lower abdominal pain, fecal impaction. Use cautiously in third trimester of pregnancy, N/V, renal disease. May increase effect of drugs in intestinal tract.

MUSCLE RELAXANT DD

A Muscle relaxation 2° to CNS depression or decrease in number of impulse transmissions.

SE Headache, dizziness, lethargy, uncoordination, N/V, hypotension, thrombophlebitis, bradycardia, blurred vision, diplopia, sedation.

C/I Myasthenia gravis, cardiac disease, infants, hyperthyroidism. Enhanced by alcohol, CNS depressants or psychotropics.

NUTRITIONAL ADDITIVE / IV FLUID / ELECTROLYTE EE

A Provides the body with essential fats, carbohydrates, protein, vitamins, minerals, electrolytes, water and additives which assist in digestion, metabolism and synthesis, maintenance of desirable body composition, and which promote growth.

SE N/V/D, anorexia, allergic reaction, urticaria, jaundice, dehydration, metabolic acidosis, hepatomegaly, spleenomegaly, restlessness, lethargy, infection, intestinal perforation, EKG changes, decreased B/P, arrhythmias, palpitations, confusion, tingling of extremeties, paralysis, weakness, sensation of body swelling, peripheral vascular thrombosis, pulmonary edema, CHF, inflammation at the injection site, hypercalcemia, hyperkalemia.

C/I Hypersensitivity, inborn errors of metabolism, encephalopathy, allergies, prematurity, use of oral iron. Use cautiously in renal or cardiac disease, dehydration, severe burns, hyperkalemia, gout, anemia, peptic ulcer, enteritis, colitis, pregnancy, pulmonary disease, osteoporosis, pernicious anemia, Zollinger-Ellison syndrome. Spironolactone, Triaterene, salt substitutes, Penicillin G, Potassium, Lithium, diuretics, Antabuse, salicylates, cardiac glycosides.

SEDATIVE / HYPNOTIC FF

A The central nervous system is depressed by disturbance of transmission of impulses in the cerebral cortex of the thalmus.

SE N/V/D, anorexia, epigastric pain, headache, dizziness, drowsiness, excitement, confusion, hypotension, circulatory collapse, respiratory depression, apnea, urticaria, rash, edema, hematologic changes.

C/I Contraindicated in patients with history of manifest or latent porphyria, mental depression, drug abuse, hepatic damage, aspirin sensitivity, CNS depressants, alcohol use.

THYROID AGENT GG

A Restores thyroid hormone which is necessary in regulating metabolic activity and in mental and physical growth and development.

SE Palpitations, arrhythmias, angina, headache, tremors, insomnia, nervousness, menstrual irregularities, anorexia, weight loss.

C/I Nephrosis, hyperthyroidism, thyrotoxicosis. May increase effects of anticoagulants. May decrease effects of insulin or hypoglycemic agents.

FI Levothyroxine: with enternal nutrition may cause hypothyroidism.

TRANQUILIZER / ANTIPSYCHOTIC HH

A A calming effect is produced through depression at the subcortical level or through production of dopamine resulting in depression of the cerebral cortex.

SE Laryngospasm, dyspnea, postural hypotension, hypertension, cardiac arrest, anemia, extrapyramidal symptoms, seizures, drowsiness, headaches, confusion, agitation, insomnia, dizziness, catatonia, psychosis, depression, N/V/D, anorexia, constipation, blurred vision, photosensitivity, impotence, urinary retention.

C/I Renal, hepatic or cardiac disease, coma, blood dyscrasias, glaucoma, psychosis, pregnancy. CNS depressants or alcohol may cause oversedation. Potentiated by phenothiazines, MAO inhibitors, antidepressants and CNS depressants. Trihexphenidyl and lithium may decrease the effect.

FI Antacids and food decrease absorption rate.

VASODILATOR II

A Cardiac blood flow is increased as a result of beta cell stimulation causing dilation of the arteries in skeletal muscle.

SE N/V, abdominal distension, hypotension, tachycardia, dizziness, rash.

C/I Postpartum, tachycardia, pregnancy, lactation. Use cautiously in cardiac disease and myocardial infractions.

APPENDIX 1-1B ▸ Medication Profile

ADVANCE DIRECTIVE
DECLARATION

I_____, being of sound mind, willfully and voluntarily make this declaration to be followed if I become incompetent. This declaration reflects my firm and settled commitment to refuse life-sustaining treatment under the circumstances indicated below.

I direct my attending physician to withhold or withdraw life-sustaining treatment that serves only to prolong the process of dying if I should be in a terminal condition or in a state of permanent unconsciousness.

I direct that treatment be limited to measures to keep me comfortable and to relieve pain, including any pain that might occur by withholding or withdrawing life-sustaining treatment.

In addition, if I am in the condition described above, I feel especially strongly about the following forms of treatment:

I DO	I DO NOT	
☐	☐	want cardiac resuscitation.
☐	☐	want mechanical respiration.
☐	☐	want tube feeding.
☐	☐	want other artificial or invasive form of nutrition (food).
☐	☐	want other artificial or invasive form of hydration (water).
☐	☐	want blood or blood products.
☐	☐	want any form of surgery.
☐	☐	want any invasive diagnostic tests.
☐	☐	want kidney dialysis.
☐	☐	want antibiotics.
☐	☐	other:

I realize that if I do not specifically indicate my preference regarding any of the forms of treatment listed above, I may receive that form of treatment.

Other instructions:

I DO	I DO NOT	
☐	☐	want to donate my organs upon death.
☐	☐	want to designate a surrogate to make medical treatment decisions for me if I should be incompetent and in a terminal condition or in a state of permanent unconsciousness. *Surrogate (name & address):* *Substitute surrogate (name & address):*

I made this declaration on the _____day of _____ (month, year).

Your signature: _____ Address: _____

The above named individual or a person on behalf of and at the direction of the individual knowingly and voluntarily signed this writing by signature or mark in my presence.

Witness's signature: _____ Witness's signature: _____

Address: _____ Address: _____

APPENDIX 1-2 ▶ Advance Directive Declaration. (*Source:* Reproduced as a public service announcement by the Foundation for Critical Care.)

Visiting Nurse
Association
of Essex Valley

Bringing Quality Health Care To Your Home Since 1902
33 Evergreen Place · East Orange, NJ 07018 · 201-673-0158

Patient Name _____

ID # _____

Start of Care _____

CARDIAC/VASCULAR I CareMap
(CHF, Disorders in Cardiac Output)

ASSESS/OBSERVE EACH VISIT:

Complete cardiovascular assessment with vital signs, wieght, lung sounds. Assess for fatigue, dyspnea, chest pain, cough, orthopnea, anorexia, mobility, emotional status, and orientation.

NURSING DIAGNOSES:

☐ 1. Fluid volume excess related to decreased cardiac output.

☐ 2. Activity intolerance related to decreased cardiac output.

☐ 3. Ineffective management of therapeutic regimen related to lack of knowledge of disease process, home management, activity/rest schedule, and pain.

☐ 4. High risk for impairment of skin integrity related to edema.

☐ 5. Ineffective individual/family coping related to responses to diagnosis and prognosis.

Collaborative Problems:

☐ 1. PC: Decreased Cardiac Output*

☐ 2. PC: Dysrhythmia

☐ 3. PC: Pulmonary Edema

☐ 4. PC: Deep Vein Thrombosis

    * PC = Potential Complication

LONG-TERM GOALS:

1. Patient/caregiver will demonstrate understanding of disease process and self-care managment.

2. Patient will have improved cardiac output.

3. Patient will minimize fluid retention.

4. Patient will have intact skin surface (or absence of S/S of infection from skin breakdown.)

5. Patient's vital signs, weight and cardiovascular status are normal for patient range for 3 weeks without major treatment plan changes.

GOAL	PROJECTED DATE	DATE MET	SIGNATURE
1			
2			
3			
4			
5			

RECOMMENDED FREQUENCY: 3-4 wk x 2.2 wk x 3, 1 wk x 4
(16 visits total)

NOTE: It is anticipated that most patients may stablize quickly and learn quickly, and meet all outcomes and long-term goals by the end of Visit 12. Some patient's, however, will require additional visits. Visits 13-16 will be used to complete instruction not yet accomplished because of variances, to do additional teaching for concurrent diagnoses, to assess and evaluate cardiovascular status, and to monitor response to treatment.

Home Health CareMaps™ are designed to address the patient's acute episode of illness. Visit intensity and frequency may also be influenced by the patient's unique set of circumstances, including but not limited to the home environment, resources, presence of life-supporting therapies, and the presence of other chronic illnesses or limiting handicaps.

FORM NO. 901 5/94   PRINTED BY STANDARD REGISTER U.S.A.

APPENDIX 1-3A ▶ Cardiac/Vascular I CareMap. (*Source:* Moulton, PJ, Wray-Langevine, J, & Boyer, C. Implementing clinical pathways: One agency's experience. *Home Healthcare Nurse* 15:343, 1997)

Visiting Nurse Association of Essex Valley

CLINICAL PROGRESS NOTE

CARE MAP: CARDIAC/VASC I

T _____	RP _____	EDEMA	
BP _____	R _____	R	L
_____	LS (R) _____	I __	I __
_____	(L) _____	A __	A __
AP _____	WT _____	C __	C __

PATIENT NAME:	ID #:	VISIT DATE:	VISIT #: 1

SUBJECTIVE FINDINGS:

CIRCLE OR FILL IN BELOW AS APPROPRIATE

CNS: L.O.C.: alert   lethargic   other _____
Orientation: Person   Place   Time
Mood/Beh: Irritable   Restless   or Nervous?
Headache/Dizzy?   Location _____
Frequency _____

SKIN: Color: wnl   abnl   Turgor: wnl   taut   tenting
Cyanosis?   N   Y: lips   mucous membranes

CV: Pain?   N   Y: Chest?   N   Y
other location? _____
with exertion?   N   Y
freq. _____ duration _____
relieved by: rest?   N   Y
medications?   N   Y _____
Palpitations?   N   Y: _____
Other: _____

CP: S.O.B. at rest?   N   Y: After act.?   N   Y: desc. _____
Orthopnea?   N   Y _____ # of pillows: _____   PND?   N   Y ____
Endurance: Good   Fair   Poor
Cough?   N   Y: Productive?   N   Y: Sputum?   N   Y: desc. _____
Oxygen used?   N   Y: Rate _____ L/min., Freq/Dur _____
Equip: _____

GI: Food & Fluid intake: _____
BMs: freq. _____ wnl   ABN   Other:

GU: Nocturia?   N   Y: freq. _____
Output appropriate to intake and any medications?   N   Y
Other: _____

PV: Pedal pulses: L.   wnl   faint   absent   R: wnl   faint   absent
T°: L: Foot   warm   cool   Coloring: L: wnl   abn: _____
R: Foot   warm   cool   Coloring: R: wnl   abn: _____

MOBILITY: BB   WC   Amb. stdy/unstdy with assist of _____ persons &/or _____ device(s): _____

Medications: Changed?   N   Y   Pt. Knowledgeable?   N   Y   Compliant?   N   Y   Exhibiting side effects?   N   Y

CARE ELEMENTS

		DONE	NOT DONE	COMMENTS
DISEASE PROCESS	Provide brief definition and causes of cardiac disease.			
MEDICATION	Establish basic medication schedule in writing and leave in home (name of medication, times.)			
NUTRITION/ HYDRATION	Assess prior knowledge regarding dietary and fluid restrictions.			
ACTIVITY	Avoid exertion; instruct frequent rest periods.			
SAFETY	Assess for environmental hazards, including O₂; provide emergency phone numbers.			
TREATMENTS	Weigh patient (on patient's own scale, if available.)			
TESTS	Ask MD for orders for electrolytes, digoxin level, others as indicated by medications/diagnosis.			
PSYCHOSOCIAL				
INTERDISCIPLINARY SERVICES/COMMUNITY REFERRALS	HHA, if unable to do ADLs; MSW for social factors interfering with care.			

PATIENT OUTCOMES

	MET	NOT MET	EXPLAIN VARIANCE
States definition of CHF.			
Verbalizes understanding of simple medication schedule.			
States/how when to call for help.			
Identifies need to avoid exertion and to rest frequently.			
Adequate cardiac output as evidenced by *pulse pressure >30 mm Hg; lungs clear; warm dry skin. (If not met, nurse will notify MD.)			

CHECK HERE FOR COMAP ☐

SIGNATURE

*Pulse pressure is the difference between the systolic and diastolic blood pressure.

PRINTED BY STANDARD REGISTER U.S.A

FORM NO. 901 5/94

APPENDIX 1-3B ▶ Cardiacac/Vascular I CareMap

Visiting Nurse Association
of Essex Valley

CLINICAL PROGRESS NOTE
Continuation Sheet

PATIENT NAME:	ID #:	VISIT DATE:	VISIT #:

FINDINGS

Check Box(es): ☐ Subjective ☐ Objective ☐ Care Elements ☐ Outcome (includes additional professional evaluation of findings)

HHA SUPERVISION

Y/N	ORIENT HHA	Y/N	HHA UNDERSTANDS ASSIGNMENT/ ASSIGNMENT FOLLOWED	Y/N	FREQUENCY OF VISITS OK	Y/N	PT CARE NEEDS BEING MET
Y/N	SUP HHA	Y/N	PROPER PROCEDURES FOLLOWED IN GIVING CARE	Y/N	LENGTH OF VISITS OK	Y/N	PT/FAMILY SATISFIED WITH HHA CARE
Y/N	HHA PRESENT						

COORDINATION/CASE CONFERENCE

Check Box(es): ☐ PT ☐ OT ☐ ST ☐ MSW ☐ HHA ☐ MD ☐ Diet ☐ Other

Change of visit frequency needed? N Y   New frequency: _____
Change in plan of treatment? N Y   I/O sent? N Y

PLAN FOR THE NEXT VISIT

DISCHARGE PLAN

Discussed with: (Check all that apply) ☐ Patient ☐ Family ☐ MD ☐ Community-Based Services ☐ Other

NEXT M.D. APPOINTMENT:

SIGNATURE	DATE

Patient Name _____

ID # _____

Start of Care _____

Cardiac/Vascular CoMap

NURSING DIAGNOSES

☐ 1. Fluid volume excess related to compromised regulatory mechanism.

☐ 2 Activity intolerance related to decreased cardiac output.

☐ 3. High risk for ineffective management of therapeutic regimen related to lack of knowledge of disease process, home management, medication regimen, and activity/rest schedule.

LONG-TERM GOALS

Patient/caregiver will demonstrate understanding of disease process and self care management and follow through with therapeutic regimen.

PATIENT OUTCOMES

Patient/caregiver will: DATE MET

1. State 3 signs and symptoms of cardiac decompnsation.   _____

2. Follow through with medication regimen.   _____

3. State actions and major side effects of cardiac medications.   _____

4. Demonstrate follow through with therapeutic diet.   _____

5. Demonstrate compensated fluid volume balancc.   _____

* Signs and symptoms may include: edema, dyspnea, orthopnea, cough, weakness, fatigue, chest pain, PND, cyanosis, activity tolerance. Specific signs and symptoms must be documented in the narrative.

DATE	CARE ELEMENTS	SIGNATURE

Reformatted CoMap.

□ama°		PAGE 1 OF 4	CLINICAL NOTE INITIAL ASSESSMENT

+ = Problem   − = Adequate   NA = Not Applicable

History of Present Illness (Onset of events, symptoms, complications, other significant factors related to primary problem(s) for which patient was referred)

Past Medical History (significant chronic acute medical/surgical, psychiatric — dates of onset)

Patient's Understanding of Diagnosis − Treatment − emotional response to current health

General Appearance

Temp: _____   Pulse: _____   Resp: _____   BP: L _____ R _____   Ht: _____   Wt: _____
        Oral Ax Rectal   AP / RAD

Usual Daily Food Intake (include supplements)   At Nutritional Risk? ☐ Yes   ☐ No

Number of Meals   Usual Daily
Per Day   Fluid Intake   Snacks

	SYSTEMS	CODE	DESCRIPTIVE DATA — COMMENTS
SKIN	Color		
	Temp.		
	Turgor		
	Rash		
	Scars		
	Pressure Areas		
	Open Areas		
	Nails		
SENSES	Vision		
	Hearing		
	Smell		
	Taste		
RESPIRATORY	Cough		
	SOB		
	Chest Configuration		
	Use of Accessory Muscles		
	Breath Sounds		
	Tracheostomy		
CARDIOVASCULAR	Oxygen		
	Chest Pain		
	Fatigue		
	Orthopnea		
	Paroxysmal Nocturnal Dyspnea		
	Jugular Vein Distention		
	Edema		
	Dizziness		
	Heart Sounds		
	Rhythm		
	Pacemaker		
LOWER EXREMS.	Pedal Pulses		
	Temperature		
	Color		
	Sensation		

Patient Name _____   Date _____   Record # _____

APPENDIX 1-4A ▶ Clinical Note Initial Assessment (*Source:* Used with permission IAMA, Inc., Philadelphia, PA)

□ama		PAGE 2 OF 4	INITIAL ASSESSMENT

	SYSTEMS		CODE	DESCRIPTIVE DATA — COMMENTS
GI/ELIM	Dentition/Chewing			
	Oral Mucosa			
	Swallowing			
	Appetite / Eating Patterns			
	Food Intolerance / Preference			
	Enteral Feedings			
	Abd. Distention			
	Nausea/Vomiting			
	Bowel Patterns			
	Ostomy (Type)			
MUSCULAR-SKELETAL	Joints (pain, swelling, deformities)	Upper		
		Lower		
	Muscle Strength	Upper		
		Lower		
	ROM	Upper		
		Lower		
	Contractures			
	Spine			
NEURO.	Headaches			
	Tremors			
	Speech			
	Vertigo			
	Seizures			
	Numbness			
	Tingling			
	Ataxia			
	Rigidity			
G.U.	Bladder Function (incontinence, retention, urgency, frequency)			
	Urine (odor, color, usual output)			
	Foley Catheter (size, date last changed)			
	Suprapubic Catheter (size, date last changed)			
	Other			
REPRODUCTION	Male/Female Genitalia	Discharge		
		Pain		
		Bleeding		
	Pap Test — GYN Exam			
	Breasts — Mammogram date			
	Prostate Exam date			
HIGH TECH.	Peripheral IV			
	Central Venous Catheter			
	Portacath			
	Biliary Tube			
	Other			
MENTAL STATUS	Oriented			
	Affect			
	Ability to communicate and understand			
PAIN	Pain (describe): 0 1 2 3 4 5			
	— Type			
	— Location			
	— Onset			
	— Duration			
	— Relieved by			
OTHER HEALTH FACTORS	Use of: Alcohol			
	Drugs			
	Tobacco			
	Sleep Patterns			
	Caffeine			

Patient Name _____   Date _____   Record # _____

APPENDIX 1-4B ▶ Clinical Note Initial Assessment

□ama   PAGE 3 OF 4   CLINICAL NOTE
                                                                  INITIAL ASSESSMENT

Mark Areas with lesions

Dermal lesions/scars _____

Other _____

INTEGUMENTARY

Problems: ❏ YES ❏ NO

History of: ❏ YES ❏ NO

Turgor: ❏ YES ❏ NO ❏ Good

Rash: ❏ YES ❏ NO

Bruises: ❏ YES ❏ NO

Pruritis: ❏ YES ❏ NO

Scars: ❏ YES ❏ NO

Incision: ❏ YES ❏ NO ❏ Location: _____

Wound: Site: _____

         Odor: _____ Size: ._____

         Drainage/Color: _____

         Amount: SM.___ MOD.___ LG.___

Description / Comments:

Pertinent Lab Test Results (as available):

Preventive and Periodic Health Screenings:

Communication Skills: Short-term memory   ❏ Good   ❏ Fair   ❏ Poor

   What languages do you speak?

   Do you have difficulty understanding what is said by others?   ❏ YES   ❏ NO

   Do you have difficulty reading?   ❏ YES   ❏ NO

   Do you have any problems with attention or memory?   ❏ YES   ❏ NO

   Do any cultural or religious practices limit your ability to learn?   ❏ YES   ❏ NO

   Explain any "YES" responses:

		Can't Do	ASSISTANCE				DME
			Min.	Mod.	Max.	Ind.	
A.D.I.	Ambulation						
	Stairs						
	Dressing						
	Feeding / Food Prep						
	Household Activity						
	Transfer Ability						
	Personal Care						
	Toileting						
	Ability to operate/ maintain equipment						

Patient Name _____   Date _____   Record # _____

APPENDIX 1-4C ▶ Clinical Note Initial Assessment

□ama° PAGE 4 OF 4

CLINICAL NOTE
INITIAL ASSESSMENT

Directions to Locate Home and/or Gain Entry

Emergency Contact — Name | Relationship

Home Phone | Work Phone

ALLERGIES: — Medications:

— Food:

— Environmental:

Date of Last Chest X-ray and/or PPD Test and Results:

FAMILY DYNAMICS:

Primary Caregiver:

| name | relationship | age | education level |

Ability to care for patient: ❑ YES ❑ NO

Willingness to care for patient: ❑ YES ❑ NO

Availability to care for patient: ❑ YES ❑ NO

Other Household Members/Support:

Other Organization involved:

Does patient wish to have family involved with care? ❑ YES ❑ NO

Explain:

Strengths/Weaknesses in Support System:

Pets: Access to Transportation? ❑ Public ❑ Private

SOCIAL–ENVIRONMENTAL–CULTURAL FACTORS

HOUSING: Private House ❑ Apartment ❑ Boarding Home ❑ Single Level ❑ Multi Level ❑

Phone ❑ Electric ❑ Heat ❑ Fan/A/C ❑ Smoke Detector ❑ Emergency Phone Numbers ❑ Doorlocks ❑

POTENTIAL SAFETY HAZARDS/BARRIERS: Electrical/Plumbing/Structural Hazards ❑ Rugs/Runners/Mats ❑ Space Heater ❑

Lighting ❑ Bathroom Hazards ❑ O₂ ❑ Stairs ❑ Clutter ❑ Unsafe Equipment Use ❑ Location in High Crime Area ❑

PERSONAL: Current or Previous Occupation:

Hobbies/Exercise:

Cultural Ethnic, Religious Practices

Anticipated Post-Discharge Community Resource Needs:

Finances Appear: Comfortable ❑ Adequate ❑ Poor ❑ Indigent ❑

Patient Instructed in:

	YES	NO		YES	NO	
Emergency Procedures/Copy in Home	❑	❑	Grievance/Complaint Procedure	❑	❑	
Bill of Rights	❑	❑	Patient has A/D	❑	❑	Where kept? _____
Advance Directive	❑	❑	Patient has Durable Power of Attorney	❑	❑	
Emergency Preparedness	❑	❑	Who is Healthcare Representative?	❑	❑	
			Patient Teaching Handouts	❑	❑	

Discipline Referrals: PT ❑ OT ❑ ST ❑ MSW ❑ Nutritionist ❑ HHA ❑ Psych ❑ Other ❑

Instruction / Intervention / Response to Instruction:

Progress Toward Goals / Response Toward Treatment / Patient Care Conference:

Measurable Goals / Date for Next Visit:

Interdisciplinary Communications:

Signature: _____ Date: _____ Time In: _____ Out_____

Patient Name: _____ Record #: _____

*Used with permission IAMA, Inc.

APPENDIX 1-4D ▷ Clinical Note Initial Assessment

UNIT

▶▶▶▶▶▶▶▶▶

2

Advanced Physical Examination and Health Assessment

continued

References

Appendices

    A2-1 Consent for Treatment, Release of Information, Assignment of Benefits, Notice of Client Rights

    A2-2 Client Responsibilities

    A2-3 Home Healthcare Client's Bill of Rights/Responsibilities

    A2-4 Newborn Universal Home Risk Assessment Form

    A2-5 Denver Developmental Screening Test II and Denver Articulation Screening Examination

    A2-6 Infant and Child Growth Charts

    A2-7 Home Care Needs Assessment Tool for the Child

    A2-8 Pediatric Assessment and Care Screening for Function

    A2-9 Culturological Assessment Guide

    A2-10 Mini-Mental State Examination

    A2-11 Glasgow Coma Scale

The Assessment Process

In implementing the ordered treatment modalities, the high-tech homecare nurse will need to plan for and assess the client encounter. Toward that end, the nurse will typically perform an environmental assessment, which documents the client support systems and adequacy of the home setting, and a client advanced physical examination and health assessment, which documents physical and psychosocial findings. The importance of a complete, comprehensive assessment to establish the client's baseline clinical data cannot be overemphasized. Deviation from the client's norm, progress toward recovery, and maintenance at an optimum level of wellness are factors which will be derived from and compared with the baseline clinical findings obtained during the initial visit. All subsequent visits will be evaluated against the clinical data obtained at the time of admission to service. Moreover, because the initial comprehensive assessment of the client is a rather time-consuming process, the nurse must plan to devote 1-1/2 to 2 hours to complete the admission process. More than one home visit may be required to complete all assessment forms. Consequently, time allocation for the initial homecare visit must be carefully managed, permitting flexibility in the visit schedule to allow for all necessary adjustments in time.

Environmental Assessment Overview

The goal of homecare is to assist the client to achieve self-sufficiency through the coordination of a collaborative system of care involving interdisciplinary health professionals, the family, and designated caregivers. Client outcomes, determined by standardized criteria, are oriented toward returning the client to his/her optimum level of wellness. A safe and supportive home environment is a requisite condition for the attaining of all care objectives. The home and community environments are assessed for suitability. Environments determined not to be safe for delivery of high-tech homecare will be documented and alternative settings will be sought. Safety of the home setting is determined by assessing the adequacy of the structural facility, electrical wiring, heating and cooling systems, water and sewage disposal, assistive devices, and the presence of smoke detectors and emergency call systems. A safe community is one which has adequate community resources, plans for disaster preparedness, and can dispatch emergency medical teams within adequate time limitations.

To ensure that the goals of the plan of care are met, the client must have a reliable family support system capable of rendering safe care. The high-tech homecare nurse will evaluate client relationships with family and significant others, and will evaluate the ability and willingness of caregivers to assist with and implement the plan of treatment. The high-tech homecare nurse will continually observe and document the client/caregiver's ability to perform and implement the plan of care, reinforce learning throughout the duration of homecare service, select teaching modalities that meet the educational needs of the client/family unit, and identify barriers to care and document measures taken to eliminate same.

Client Physical Examination and Health Assessment

The high-tech homecare nurse will begin the history-taking process with the client interview. The nurse will obtain and record information related to the client's biographical data, chief complaint, history of the present illness, past medical and surgical history, family history, psychosocial history, allergies, immunizations, and the review of systems. The nurse will perform a complete physical examination and record findings associated with each body system and functional area of the high-risk client.

The high-tech homecare nurse working with special client populations must also be aware of the comprehensive assessment data needed for the high-risk perinatal client, neonatal client, and geriatric client [4, 5, 7, 10, 17, 19, 31, 37–41].

PROCEDURE
The Interview and Health History

DESCRIPTION
The health history is obtained to collect subjective client information, and uses an interviewing format to allow the client the opportunity to describe symptoms and clinical findings in his own words. The history begins with the orientation phase of the interview process and is facilitated by using open-ended statements. During the implementation phase, the nurse utilizes therapeutic communication techniques to elicit client responses to questions concerning body system functioning. The interview ends with the termination phase at which time an overall summary of what has been learned by the clinician is offered for client corroboration.

PURPOSE
To gather pertinent client information to be utilized in the formation of the plan of care, and in the documentation of client progress

EQUIPMENT
Health history forms

OUTCOMES
The client/caregiver will:

▶ Relate information to be documented in the health history
▶ Verbalize feelings and concerns regarding the plan of care
▶ Participate in the mutual development of goals and expected outcomes

ASSESSMENT DATA
Document the client's native language
Determine the client's proficiency and literacy in use of the English language

Assess the client's level of education
Observe the client's use of verbal and nonverbal cues
Ascertain the availability of health-related materials in the client's native language

RELATED NURSING DIAGNOSES
Impaired communication
Knowledge deficit
Powerlessness
Sensory perceptual alteration
Social isolation
Altered thought process
Altered self-concept

SPECIAL CONSIDERATIONS
The history should be obtained in an environment which supports privacy and permits the inclusion of family and significant others. For the client with severe psychiatric disturbance, impaired cognitive function as a complication of the illness state, sensory-perceptual deficit (hearing, sight, speech), or developmental delay, the nurse will need to obtain an accurate history from a caregiver.

TRANSCULTURAL CONSIDERATIONS
The client's cultural and ethnic background must be taken into consideration when addressing questions or issues of an intimate nature. Consider use of the AT&T Language Line. See Culturological Assessment procedure for general overview of cultural considerations.

▶ **INTERVENTIONS**
Conducting the Interview

The Orientation Phase	*Establishment of trust*
1. Begin the interview by addressing the client by his/her surname.	*In many cultures use of first names is inappropriate.*
2. Use broad, open-ended statements.	*To facilitate the communication process.*
The Implementation Phase	*Exploration of areas of concern*
3. Engage in therapeutic communication techniques.	
a. Silence	*The technique of silence allows the client opportunity to collect and organize thoughts. A natural pause in verbal communication permits the client to introduce a topic of concern and conveys the nurse's sincere interest in the client.*
b. Facilitation	*Comments such as "go on" or nodding affirmatively indicate that the nurse is following the topic of conversation and is encouraging the client to continue.*

c. Reflection

The technique of reflection is used to assist the client to review a comment just made to permit introspective thought and to acknowledge understanding of the client's feelings. When the client expresses feelings and ideas, the nurse can recognize those feelings by reflecting them back to the client, e.g., "You think that . . ." or "You feel that . . ."

d. Clarification

When thoughts or ideas are ambiguous, the technique of clarification is used to help the client explain unclear statements. The nurse should seek clarification when a statement becomes misunderstood by using such phrases as, e.g., "Could you tell me more about what you mean when you say . . ."

e. Empathy

When the nurse puts into words what has been implied or said indirectly, the client can be assisted to feel that his or her thoughts are being accepted and that he or she will be encouraged to express any concerns openly.

f. Confrontation

When the client appears perplexed, angry, or depressed, this technique may be used to verbalize what is perceived. By focusing the client's attention, the nurse is able to make the client more aware and to encourage mutual understanding through discussion. "You seem upset today. Let's talk about some of your concerns."

g. Inference

This technique seeks to verbalize feelings which are being expressed only indirectly.

The technique of inference links situations, correlates events, or implies cause. For example, the client who views the healthcare environment as "cold" and impersonal is probably feeling socially isolated by comparison. By introducing the notion of isolation or alienation into the conversation, the nurse is more likely to have a more therapeutic interaction than by discussing the "cold" environment as such.

h. Explanation

This technique is used to offer factual information regarding the client's diagnoses, treatment modalities, and so on. Offering information helps to build a trusting relationship, helps the client to anticipate the probable sequence of events, and serves to demystify the healthcare milieu.

4. Avoid using of the following non-therapeutic communication techniques.
   a. Reassuring

This non-therapeutic technique indicates that there is no need for anxiety. Statements such as "everything is going to be all right" have little meaning, can be very damaging, devalue the client's feelings, trivialize the source of the anxiety, and may terminate the discussion.

b. Advising

This technique is used to tell the client how he or she should perform. It implies that the client is incapable of any self-direction, and shifts the accountability for decision-making from the client to the nurse. The client must be given the op-

c. Using authority

portunity to work out his/her own solutions. Implying that the doctor, nurse, or other authority figure knows what is best for the client promotes feelings of dependency and inferiority. The client should be assisted to participate in the decision-making process, and all goals should be mutually developed by both the client and members of the healthcare team.

d. Using avoidance language

This technique is used to ignore the existence of a problem or to explain away a matter of importance. The nurse may unknowingly use this technique to avoid discussion of a topic, which the nurse feels is nonexistent, meaningless, or frightening. Often discussions regarding death and the dying process, for example, are expressed as euphemistic sayings, sometimes used to avoid the anxiety associated with death and the grieving process.

e. Engaging in distancing

To put space between the client and the nurse, this technique may be employed to avoid helping the client to identify and explore a problem. The technique is used to put distance between a threatening thought or concept and self.

f. Using professional jargon

Similar to the technique of advising, use of professional jargon establishes a paternalistic relationship that implies that the client is unable to make decisions for himself.

g. Using leading or biased questions

Use of this technique forces the client to give the "correct" response rather than the response that is true in his situation. "You don't engage in unprotected sexual activity, do you?" tends to lead the client to respond in the negative, even if the affirmative response is true in his or her case.

h. Talking too much

Those who are uncomfortable with silence may feel the need to engage in constant meaningless conversation. Such conversations may be disconcerting for some clients, especially when the subject matter does not address the concerns of the client.

i. Interrupting

This technique may be inadvertently used by the nurse to anticipate the client's feelings by stating his or her thoughts for him or her. The client is not given the opportunity to express fully his or her concerns, and the nurse runs the risk of jumping to conclusions that the client has not been given opportunity to corroborate.

j. Using "why" questions

Using the "why" question asks the client to explain rather than describe a situation. Requesting explanations for actions may imply blame and may put the client on the defensive. The nurse should try instead to use broad, open-ended statements to elicit reasons for client behavior.

The Termination Phase

Summarization of the Visit

5. Conclude the visit.
   Summary

This technique is used to organize and sum up what has transpired. Summarization is a necessary part of the communicative process. The technique allows for both the client and the nurse to depart with the same ideas in mind and provides a sense of closure to the interviewing process.

Obtaining the Health History

1. Obtain client consent [See Appendix 2-1].

    A signed consent documents that the client has been given information regarding the parameters of care and has been given the opportunity to make informed healthcare decisions

2. Review client responsibilities and bill of rights [See Appendices 2-2 & 2-3].

    Establishes the client's rights and outlines the procedures to follow in the event of a dispute

3. Obtain and record demographic data.
    Name
    Address
    Telephone number
    Age
    Birthdate
    Sex
    Race/Ethnicity
    Occupation

    Provides baseline identifying data

4. Identify source of information.
    Client or caregiver

    Names the person serving as informant

5. Permit the client to describe in his or her own words the reason for the visit.

    Subjective data are critical components of the history-taking process and provide a personal account of the client's health status

6. Obtain the history of the current illness.
    Onset of symptoms
    Symptom characteristics
        location
        quality
        duration and frequency
        setting
        factors which improve or worsen symptoms
        influencing factors
        client's perception of meaning of symptoms

    Provides baseline data against which later clinical findings can be compared

7. Obtain past history.
    Illnesses
    Hospitalizations
    Surgeries
    Immunizations
    Health promotion activity: blood pressure screening,
        dental/vision/hearing examinations, etc
    Allergies
    Current medications
	Identifies previous health problems which may be related to current illness

8. Obtain family history. Construct a family genogram and indicate health status of client's siblings, spouse, offspring, parents, and grandparents	*Identifies hereditary factors that may affect health status*
9. Perform review of health systems.	*Provides baseline objective data of clinical findings*
a. Perform a developmental assessment	*Evaluates the client's ability to attain age appropriate growth and developmental milestones*
b. Perform a culturological assessment	*Identifies the client's health care practices, family/kinship composition, support network, spiritual beliefs, food sanctions/avoidances, socioeconomic level, and educational background*
c. Perform a Mental Status Assessment	*Documents the client's level of consciousness, emotional status, and cognitive functioning*
d. Assess the structures of the eye	*Evaluates the client's visual acuity, optic disk, retinal vessels, macula, pupillary response, extraocular movement, condition of cornea and conjunctiva, and presence of discharge or discoloration*
e. Assess the structures of the ear	*Evaluates the condition of the client's auditory canal, tympanic membrane, hearing acuity, and external ear structures*
f. Assess the cardiovascular peripheral vascular and hematologic system	*Evaluates the quality of the first and second heart sounds, and detects the presence of third or fourth heart sounds, murmurs, rubs, and splitting of the second heart* *Evaluates the quality of the peripheral pulses and capillary refill*

	Detects presence of neck vein distension, bleeding tendencies, and lymph node swelling
g. Assess the respiratory system	*Evaluates the presence of normal and adventitious breath sounds, vocal resonance, tactile fremitus, respiratory excursion, percussion tones, anterior-posterior diameter of the chest, cough, character of sputum production, use of accessory muscles of respirations, orthopnea and activity intolerance*
h. Assess the sensory and motor system	*Evaluates the client's proprioception, tactile sensation, coordination, balance, hand and leg strength, and deep tendon reflexes*
i. Assess the musculoskeletal system	*Evaluates the client's gait, joint range of motion, spinal curvature, and strength and balance*
j. Assess the head and neck	*Evaluates the client's cranial nerve function, cerebral function, lymph nodes, sinuses, thyroid gland, trachea, oral cavity, and nasal passages*
k. Assess the breast and axilla	*Detects the presence of abnormal masses and lesions*
l. Assess the integumentary system	*Provides baseline data for hair growth patterns, vascularity, color and temperature*
	Detects presence of lesions, ecchymosis, petecchiae, and edema
m. Assess the abdominal area	*Evaluates peristaltic activity, level of discomfort, and condition of ostomy sites*
	Detects presence of fluid retention, masses, or lesions
n. Assess the genitourinary system	*Evaluates the structures of the internal and external genitalia and function of urinary catheters, and client's knowledge and practice of safe sex techniques*
	Detects presence of edema, discoloration, vaginal/penile

10. Obtain a functional assessment.
    Include the following assessment areas:
    Ability to perform activities of daily living (ADLs)
    Self-esteem/self concept
    Activity/exercise
    Sleep/rest
    Nutrition/elimination
    Role function
    Coping strategies
    Spiritual practices
    Hobbies
    Recreational activities
    Drugs/alcohol/tobacco abuse
11. Record client's perception of illness.

discharge, odor, character of urine and menstrual flow
Evaluates the client's role function, self-concept, religiosity, coping strategies, level of independence, diversional activities, elimination patterns, nutritional status, and patterns of rest and exercise

Documents the client's health beliefs

DOCUMENTATION

The following information should be included in the nursing note:

Date and time of the interview
Name of person from whom the clinical information was obtained
Identify presence of any communication barriers
Indicate use of any nonverbal cues or gestures
Note use of interventional strategies to facilitate communication
Document clinical findings
Report all abnormal findings, inform physician, and document related interventions

INTERDISCIPLINARY COLLABORATION

Depending on the findings associated with all body systems the nurse will discuss with the client's physician the need to consult with the social worker; physical or occupational therapist; wound, ostomy, continence nurse; nutritionist; or other health discipline in meeting client needs [3, 10, 13, 17–20, 28, 31, 32, 36–38, 41, 43].

PROCEDURE

Environmental Assessment

DESCRIPTION:

An assessment of the client's home and community is performed by the nurse, and typically follows guidelines established by the homecare agency. The home is assessed to determine adequacy of the client's support mechanisms and the home's physical setting. The surrounding neighborhood is assessed to document issues related to safety, accessibility of community emergency medical services, and adequacy of sewage and trash disposal.

PURPOSE:

To detemine suitability and adequacy of the home and neighborhood environments in supporting the plan of care.

EQUIPMENT
Health history forms to include:

Environmental Assessment Form (see Table 2-1)
Safety Assessment Form
Family Assessment Form

OUTCOMES
The client/caregiver will:

▶ Render care in a safe and supportive environment
▶ Participate in the modification of the home environment to support safe care delivery
▶ Have sufficient support to follow the plan of treatment as ordered

ASSESSMENT DATA
Note client relationships with family member, neighbors, friends and other community resources
    (religious institutions, support groups, volunteer and governmental agencies)
Record willingness and ability of caregiver and others to implement the treatment plan
Document the status of the current environment on appropriate assessment forms
Check for barriers to access or potential risks for falls and injury
Determine who will serve as an emergency contact and the location of the client's emergency tele-
    phone numbers
Assess the client/caregiver's plan for emergency preparedness

TABLE 2-1 Environmental Assessment

TYPE OF HOME	Private, apartment, condominium, trailor, shelter. Number of rooms.
NUMBER OF FLOORS, STAIRS	Accessibility of stairs, elevators, fire escape, fire extinguisher, number of exits, fire evacuation plan
NUMBER OF OCCUPANTS IN THE HOME	Adequacy of sleeping arrangements, functional toilet and bathing facilities
AVAILABILITY OF PUBLIC UTILITIES	Running water, electricity, heat
CLEANLINESS OF HOME AND ENVIRONMENT	Interior and exterior
ENVIRONMENTAL HAZZARDS	Chipped paint, rodents, vermins, insects, poor sanitation, faulty waste disposal, pollution
HOME SAFETY	Window and door locks or bars, security gaurds, electronic surveillance, window screen locks, smoke and carbon monoxide detectors (number of detectors and where), electric outlet caps, proper lighting, clean and dry pathways, secured rugs
AVAILABILITY OF PHONE	Nearest phone, emergency numbers (MD, hospital, relatives and emergency contacts, ambulance)
MEDICATION STORAGE	Out of the reach of children properly stored or refrigerated, medical supplies in clean, organized container
PETS	Number and what kind
PLAY AREAS	Fenced play area, locked, fenced pool area
CAREGIVERS KNOWLEDGE	Safety guidelines, CPR, First aid

Author: Cornell, B. Clinical Manager of Pediatrics. Cooper Medical Center, Camden, New Jersey.

RELATED NURSING DIAGNOSES
At risk for injury
Self-care deficit
Impaired home maintenence management
Altered family process
Ineffective coping
At risk for lonliness
Anxiety
Altered parenting skills
Caregiver role strain
Potential for violence

SPECIAL CONSIDERATIONS

Community assessment—The homecare agency will provide the nurse with protocols to follow in caring for the client who resides in an unsafe neighborhood. The nurse will be instructed to observe for signs of unsafe activity in high crime areas. An escort service may be required for some neighborhoods during the day, and other neighborhoods may be designated as unsafe after dark. In all circumstances, the nurse will be instructed to use judgment in avoiding or leaving questionable situations, and to report unsafe incidents to supervisory personnel.

Disposal of biohazardous waste will follow regulations established by the community department of sanitation. The homecare agency will keep the nurse informed of those regulations and will provide updates as rules change over time.

As part of the community assessement, the nurse will need to know how to activate the emergency medical system for assistance in the event of a life-threatening change in the client's status. For fire or other emergencies, the nurse will need to know how to contact the fire or law enforcement departments for assistance.

Home assessment—As part of the home assessment, the nurse will note the structural integrity of the home's foundation. If floorboards, roofing, walls, stairways, or plumbing fixtures are in need of repair, the nurse will need to consult with the social worker. The MSW will be able to assess the client's financial status and determine the client's eligibility for special community programs that provide housing repair services, lead/asbestos removal, and so on. Similarly, should the nurse note the presence of rodent or insect infestation, the client may qualify for the exterminating services of certain government and public agencies. Again, the MSW can assist the nurse in locating these community resources. The home must be able to safely support the ordered treatment modalities. Toward that end, fire safety guidelines for the use of oxygen, electrical safety guidelines for power sources, functional telephone equipment to call for assistance, and operational plumbing facilities for laundering and adherence to universal precautions must be available and maintained at all times.

Client support systems—The client who is unable to implement the treatment plan without assistance will need to rely on the help of family and significant others. In observing the client's interactions with others the nurse will need to assess the quality of those interactions. Any evidence of substance or client abuse, or the potential for such abuse, must to documented and appropriate follow-up protocol must be initiated. The homecare agency will provide the nurse with detailed guidelines for assessing and reporting abuse findings.

TRANSCULTURAL CONSIDERATIONS

The nurse must be aware of all cultural and healthcare practices which may need to be modified to maintain a safe environment. The lighting of candles for some religious practices, the social isolation associated with some "shameful" disease states, and the degree of privacy and limited disclosure maintained by some ethnic groups will be challenging situations for the nurse. Ever mindful of the importance of the client's religious and cultural orientation, the nurse will need to assist the client to adapt those practices which may compromise the safety of the environment. Enlisting the services of religious and cultural leaders may be an effective way to help the client change his environment to meet necessary safety guidelines. Consider use of the AT&T Language Line. See Culturological Assessment procedure for general overview of cultural considerations.

▶ INTERVENTIONS

1. Develop a trusting nurse-client relationship during the initial home visit.

   Facilitates exchange of information

2. Explain the importance of adhering to safety protocol.

   Enhances client understanding and promotes compliance

3. Perform an assessment of the home documenting the physical setting and record findings in health record.

   Establishes baseline information of the home environment

   Note external entrances and exits and suggest ramps if needed for access

   Observe internal barriers to mobility and suggest removal of throw rugs, avoidance of stair climbing by moving bed furnishings and commode chair to first floor, placement of grab bars in bathroom, use of safe transfer techniques from bed to chair, etc.

   Assess cooking area and note cleanliness of kitchen, adequacy of refrigeration and food storage, operation of oven and stove, client's ability to prepare meals, etc.

   Note functionality of electrical system throughout the house, note adequacy of three-pronged plugs, presence of frayed wiring, use of extension cords, lighting, and document alternate plan in case of power outage

   Note heating, cooling, and plumbing systems for safe use of heaters, fans and availability of running water

   Observe fire safety measures and document presence of smoke detectors and plan for exiting the home in the event of a fire

   Document the presence of rodent or insect infestation and arrange for exterminating services

   Determine adequacy of telecommunication devices (telephone, intercom, emergency call system, etc.)

   Document presence of allergens (dust, dander, plants, sprays, powder, etc.)

4. Assess the client's support systems and record findings in the health record

   Documents roles, relationships, and responsibilities of support persons

   Evaluate family roles, note evidence of role conflict, role incompetence, or role strain

   Examine relationships by actively listening to and observing family interactions

   Observe communication skills

Observe for signs of physical/emotional abuse

Examine parenting role

Identify family member or significant other who will
    serve as caregiver

If client lives alone, identify neighbor or friend who will
    serve as caregiver

If no support system can be identified, refer client to
    MSW for assistance with transportation, housekeep-
    ing, food preparation, shopping, etc.

DOCUMENTATION

The following should be included in the nursing note:

Findings of safety check and environmental assessment

Modifications needed and approaches taken to ensure correction of unsafe conditions

Consultations and referrals made to other disciplines and agencies regarding adaptations

Client's/caregiver's ability to maintain a safe environment

Availability and willingness of support person(s) to follow the plan of care

Evidence of abuse, reporting mechanism, and follow-up plan

INTERDISCIPLINARY COLLABORATION

Initiate consult with the MSW to identify community resources and to determine the client's eligi-
    bility for assistance with modification of the home environment, transportation services, and
    meal preparation

Obtain orders for home health aide if needed to assist with ADLs

Initiate consult with physical therapist to assist client in performance of safe transfer techniques
    and to improve mobility

Inform the physician and homecare agency of all uncorrected safety conditions and threat of vio-
    lence for follow-up [2, 3, 13, 17, 19, 36–38]

PROCEDURE

Developmental Assessment

DESCRIPTION:

From infancy to adolescence and early adulthood, the growing child is assessed for his/her ability
to attain age-appropriate developmental milestones. Significant physical, psychosocial, and mental
achievements occur during normal growth and development. Assessing the developing infant,
child, and adolescent is an integral component of the health history and physical examination. The
assessment includes examining the relationship between the parent/caregiver and child, a relationship which forms the basis for the process of parenting. The high-tech homecare nurse observes interactions between the child and caregiver, documents all developmental findings, and notes deviations from the norm. In obtaining baseline assessments, the nurse notes and is aware that
developmental delays may be caused by the presence of bulky equipment, tubes and wires; physically compromising disease states; factors causing inadequate nutritional intake; or, disturbances in
the parent/child attachment. Using standardized tools, see Appendices 2-5 and 2-6, the nurse com-
pares the child's development with age-appropriate guidelines and charts, documents the findings,
and collaborates with other members of the interdisciplinary team in the implementation of developmental interventions.

In addition to explaining the physical and psychosocial changes associated with the development of the young child and teenager, developmental theorists also address the physical and psychosocial changes associated with the mature and elderly adult. While such theorists tend to agree that physical, psychosocial, and cognitive changes occur in each phase of adult life, there are varying views regarding the consistency and predictability of those changes toward the end of the life cycle. As the American population grows older than ever before and becomes more culturally diverse, the applicability of current developmental theories has been called to question. As research continues on the growth and development of the healthy elderly and culturally diverse groups, more accurate information should emerge. This chapter will focus on the growth and development issues related to the infant, child, and adolescent.

PURPOSE
To determine the presence of normal and abnormal developmental findings, to identify the child at risk for inability to master age-appropriate milestones, and to collaborate with other members of the interdisciplinary team in the management of developmental delays

EQUIPMENT
Health Assessment Forms (see Appendices 2-4, 2-7, & 2-8)
Weight scale
Stethoscope
Tape measure
Vision screening chart
Tuning fork
Otoscope and ophthalomoscope
Sphygmomanometer
Tongue blade
Denver Developmental Screening Test II (see Appendix 2-5)
Denver Articulation Screening Examination (see Appendix 2-5)
Infant and Child Growth Charts (see Appendix 2-6)

OUTCOMES
The client/caregiver will:

▶ Be knowledgeable in ways to facilitate attainment of developmental goals
▶ Meet age-appropriate developmental milestones as able
▶ Be referred to other members of the interdisciplinary health team, as appropriate, to assist in meeting developmental goals

ASSESSMENT DATA (see Appendices 2-4 & 2-8)
Document the client's respiratory status and presence of respiratory disorders causing impairment and physical compromise
Record use of technologic equipment (ventilators, oxygen, suction, tracheostomy)
Assess baseline vital signs and physical findings to appropriately plan for intensity and duration of developmental interventions
Document the client's neurological status and presence of any deficits (seizures, increased intracranial pressure)
Note the client's feeding and nutritional status and determine adequacy of caloric intake to meet energy demands for growth and development
Determine need for hearing or visual aids
Assess the parent/caregiver-child relationship and document evidence of inappropriate parental attachment

Observe for signs of stress and evidence of abnormal responses: autonomic (vital signs, visceral signs), motor (posturing, muscle tone and movement), and attention-interaction (ability to respond appropriately to stimuli)

RELATED NURSING DIAGNOSES
Activity intolerance
Impaired gas exchange
Altered growth and development
Altered sensory perception
Compromised family coping
Ineffective breast feeding
Altered parent-infant attachment
Altered parenting

SPECIAL CONSIDERATIONS

It is important for the nurse to note that in many cases, depending on the primary diagnosis, children who have been hospitalized for an extended period of time, and have been diagnosed with developmental delays, make substantial gains once they are in the home environment. While performing the assessment, it is important to have the child's full cooperation. Utilizing familiar items/toys in the child's environment will help establish trust. The nurse should offer suggestions to the family in ways that will stimulate the child's ability to attain developmental milestones, i.e., play games like "peek-a-boo," "where's your nose, mouth, . . ." and so on.

Many technologically dependent children require the professional services of the physical, speech, and/or occupational therapist. For the hearing impaired, a translator who is fluent in sign language will need to be consulted. The nurse will be responsible both for consulting with the physician in making needed referrals, and for coordinating the care of other members of the interdisciplinary team. In assessing the presence or absence of developmental delays, the more time that the parent/caregiver or nurse can spend with the child observing activity, the more opportunity there will be to identify those activities the child can or cannot perform.

Each family and child carries a unique set of variables that all nurses need to appreciate. How the caregiver was parented often plays an important role in how the caregiver will parent his/her own child. Assessment of the parental/caregiver-child bond requires astute skills in observing and interviewing. The following guiding questions will serve to assist the nurse in helping the family to acquire therapeutic developmental interventions:

Does the parent/caregiver:

Call the child by name
Identify the child as special or different
Maintain body contact when holding or touching the child
Express concerns or feel uncomfortable in providing care
Display affection for the child
Comfort the child when the child cries or becomes upset
Stimulate the child, as appropriate, with use of verbal communication, music, touch or direct eye contact

The nurse can positively intervene and influence the development of the bonding process. Through the offering of guidelines or suggestions, the nurse can assist in promoting the development of the parenting role.

TRANSCULTURAL CONSIDERATIONS

It will be important for the nurse to note that in many cultures the bond between the mother-child and father-child is very different. In some families, the grandparent assumes the major caregiver role, so that bonding occurs between the child and grandparent. As the nurse in the home, recognizing the family as a whole unit, and establishing lines of communication with all members of the family who are involved in the care of the child, will help to appropriately identify bonding relationships.

In developing the teaching plan, the nurse will need to carefully distinguish between culture-driven healthcare practices and a real lack of parent/caregiver understanding in implementing the treatment regimen. Consider use of the AT&T Language Line. See Culturological Assessment procedure for general overview of cultural considerations.

▶ INTERVENTIONS

Intervention	Rationale
1. Establish a trusting parent/caregiver-professional relationship.	*Facilitates the development of mutually developed goals*
2. Observe the relationship between the parent/caregiver and child.	*Allows for an assessment of the bonding process*
3. Explain the purposes of the developmental assessment and use of screening tools.	*Reduces anxiety and fosters receptivity*
4. With the assistance of the parent/caregiver, perform a developmental assessment of the child.	*Involves the parent/caregiver in the identification of developmental findings*
5. Obtain baseline vital signs and observe for signs of stress prior to implementing the developmental plan.	*Monitors child's ability to tolerate planned activities*
6. With the parent/caregiver and older child, set realistic measurable goals.	*Promotes client participation*

For the Infant/Toddler

Intervention	Rationale
1. Encourage the parent/caregiver to use tactile, visual, and verbal stimulation.	*Engages the child in social interaction*
2. If appropriate, promote nonnutritive sucking for the infant unable to swallow.	*Provides oral gratification*
3. Use extension tubing, cords, etc. with technologic equipment.	*Enhances the child's mobility*
4. Facilitate the development of the bonding process.	*Promotes a positive caregiver/child relationship*
5. Maintain a safe environment.	*Reduces threat of injury*
6. Allow the toddler to exercise control of the environment, as appropriate.	*Reduces fear and anxiety.*
7. Provide the toddler with simple explanations of equipment and procedures.	*Reduces anxiety.*
8. Use play therapy.	*Promotes understanding and acceptance of treatment modalities*

For the School-Aged Child

Intervention	Rationale
1. Involve the child's teachers, school nurse, and classmates in the plan of care.	*Ensures a collaborative approach to the child's health care needs at school*
2. Allow appropriate outlets for the expression of anger and frustration.	*Channels aggressive behavior into constructive activities*

3. Permit the child to assist with procedures.	*Promotes involvement of the child in meeting healthcare needs*
4. Help the child develop alternative methods of communication when speech impaired.	*Use of augumentative communication devices and methods enhance the child's ability to communicate nonverbally*
5. Encourage use of motorized wheelchairs and other similar equipment.	*Enhances mobility*
6. Help the child to master self-care.	*Promotes independence*
7. Train the child in performance of emergency procedures.	*Reduces time delay in administration of medication or implementation of life-saving interventions*
8. Encourage use of board games, computers, and so on when mobility must be restricted.	*Promotes diversional activity*
9. Assist the child to socialize with peer groups.	*Appropriate peer interaction shapes the child's social development*
10. Identify and contact appropriate support groups.	*Support organizations serve as community resources offering information, client advocacy, and assistance*

For the Adolescent

1. Involve the adolescent in decision-making.	*Ensures that the client goals will be mutually developed*
2. Maintain self-esteem.	*Facilitates the development of self-worth and value*
3. Accept rebellion.	*Mild rebellion is a necessary component of maturation*
4. Discuss adult issues [tobacco and drug use, sexual activity] openly and honestly.	*Encourages ongoing dialogue regarding controversial issues*
5. Identify and contact technologically-dependent support groups.	*Support organizations serve as community resources offering information, client advocacy and assistance*

DOCUMENTATION

The following information should be included in the nursing note:

▶ Date and time of the interview
▶ Name and relationship of the person assisting with the assessment
▶ Identification of the presence of any communication barriers
▶ Identification of all technologic equipment
▶ Documentation of all clinical findings

► Report of all abnormal findings, information for the physician and documentation of related interventions
► Modifications needed and approaches taken to ensure client safety
► Consultations and referrals made to other disciplines and agencies
► Client's/caregiver's ability to maintain a safe environment
► Availability and willingness of caregiver to follow the plan of care

INTERDISCIPLINARY COLLABORATION

Depending on the findings associated with each body system, the nurse will discuss with the client's physician the need to consult with the social worker; physical or occupational therapist; wound, ostomy, continence nurse; nutritionist; or other health discipline in meeting the client's needs

Identify and contact community resources needed for social support, transportation, meal preparation, schooling, etc.

Obtain orders for home health aide to assist with activities of daily living, if needed [2, 3, 7, 10, 15, 18, 20, 25, 33, 37, 42]

PROCEDURE
The Culturological Assessment

DESCRIPTION

Assessing the client's cultural beliefs and health practices affords the nurse the opportunity to develop culturally sensitive plans of care. Knowledge of the client's religious practices, kinship network, dietary sanctions and restrictions, educational background, language use, and racial and ethnic group membership will assist the nurse in developing mutually derived goals for the plan of care which take into consideration the client's cultural background. Appendix 2-9 provides guidelines for the nurse to follow in making a cultural assessment.

PURPOSE

To develop a culturally competent plan of care

EQUIPMENT

Culturological Assessment Guide (see Appendix 2-9)
Health Assessment Forms

OUTCOMES

The client/caregiver will:

► Relate folk-care practices and beliefs
► Participate in the planning/implementation phases of care
► State that decisions regarding health regimen were supported
► Express satisfaction with treatment modalities

ASSESSMENT DATA

Identify racial and ethnic group membership
Determine communicative competence
List health beliefs and folk practices
Document religious and spiritual needs
Note dietary restrictions/sanctions
Identify family structure and social networks

Ascertain level of education
Determine socioeconomic status
Identify client's Explanatory Model of Illness Causation

RELATED NURSING DIAGNOSES
Powerlessness
Anxiety
Altered family process
Ineffective coping
Fear
Grieving
Spiritual distress

SPECIAL CONSIDERATIONS
Language barriers may require the use of a translator. The nurse may access the AT&T Language Line at 800-752-6096. To utilize this service the homecare agency must have an access code. The Language Line offers a variety of interpreters who are available to provide translation over the telephone. Sensitive issues such as religious practice and concerns regarding death and dying are difficult subjects to approach. There is no "right" way to address such matters. It may be easier for the nurse to begin with open-ended questions that permit the client to respond in his/her own manner of expression. Once trust has been established the nurse will be able to proceed with more sensitive questioning as the client's level of comfort permits. The nurse will need to keep in mind that in some cultures the nature of the questioning may be too intrusive and will need to be deferred.

A large component of the nursing visit involves use of the teaching-learning process. To ensure that all prescribed treatment plans are carried out between nursing visits, the nurse will need to devote a significant amount of time to ensuring that the client/caregiver fully understands the protocol and can carry out procedures. Adherence to the principles of teaching will facilitate the learning process (See Table 2-2).

TABLE 2-2 Principles for Maximizing the Teaching Learning Process

Teaching Principles	Learning Principles
Adapt teaching to the clients' level of readiness	The learning process makes use of the clients' experience and is geared to their level of understanding
Determine the clients' perceptions about subject matter before and during teaching	Clients are given opportunity to provide frequent feedback on their understanding of the material taught
Create an environment conducive to learning	The environment for learning is physically comfortable, offers an atmosphere of mutual helpfulness, trust, respect, and acceptance and allows for free expression of ideas
Involve clients throughout the learning process	Clients actively participate. They assess their needs, establish, goals, and evaluate learning progress
Make subject matter relevant to clients' interests and use	Clients feel motivated to learn
Ensure client satisfaction during the teaching process	Clients sense progress toward their goals
Provide opportunities for clients to apply material taught	Clients integrate the learning through application

Source: Spradley B, Allendin, J. *Community Health Nursing.* Phila. PA: Lippincott-Raven.

▶ INTERVENTIONS

1. Complete the culturological assessment guide. (see Appendix 2-9)

   Provides a structured approach to eliciting sensitive information

2. Support use of alternative methods of therapy.

   Nursing interventions and expected outcomes should generally provide for a continuation of healthcare practices.

3. Support client/family in the ability to make informed decisions.

   The nurse should encourage the use of family as support

4. When possible, delay treatment until culturological needs are met.

   The treatment plan should match the client/family expectations of care

5. Allow client/family to ventilate feelings

   Recognize that some cultures have definitions of health and illness, as well as practices that attempt to promote health and cure illness, that may differ significantly from western medical practices

6. Permit client/family to participate in the planning and implementation of healthcare.

   Fosters receptivity and facilitates modification of the treatment plan, as needed, to ensure that approaches to care are consistent with the client's health beliefs and care practices

7. Allow the client/family to demonstrate ability to implement all procedures.

   Documents client/family learning

DOCUMENTATION
The following should be noted in the nursing note:

The client/caregiver's:
  cultural beliefs and folk healthcare practices
  ability to read, write, or communicate using the English language
  food sanctions/restrictions
  family support system
  religious practices
  ability to perform all prescribed therapies
teaching aids used

INTERDISCIPLINARY COLLABORATION
Consider need to include religious representatives, and translators in the plan of care
Consult with the nutritionist in the planning of therapeutic diets that include cultural foods
Consult with the social worker to determine client's eligibility for economic support and to assist in identifying cultural support groups [1, 3, 8, 9, 11, 12, 14, 21–23, 25–28, 30, 34, 35, 37–40]

Mental Status Assessment

DESCRIPTION
The mental status assessment evaluates the client's orientation, memory, use of language, cognitive functioning, and level of consciousness Throughout the nurse-client interaction, the client's mood, emotional status, ability to establish goals and implement care activities, and monitor body response to therapy all will be constantly evaluated. A major focus of the examination is the identification of the client's strengths and ability to interact with others in implementing the treatment plan.

PURPOSE
To assess the client's emotional, motor, and cognitive functioning

EQUIPMENT
Health Assessment Forms
MiniMental Exam (see Appendix 2-10)
Glasgow Coma Scale (see Appendix 2-11)
Pen and pencil
Blank sheet of paper

OUTCOMES
The client will:

► Respond appropriately to all questions, as able
► Demonstrate ability to recall recent and past events, as able
► Interpret abstract concepts, as able
► Carry out motor function as able

ASSESSMENT DATA
Note client's general appearance
Identify level of consciousness
Determine mood and affect
Elicit client's perceptions and thought processes
Measure cognitive functions

RELATED NURSING DIAGNOSES
Altered thought process
Ineffective coping
Anxiety
Impaired communication
Fear
Knowledge deficit
Hopelessness
Powerlessness
Role performance
Self-concept disturbance
Social isolation

SPECIAL CONSIDERATIONS

Determine if client has taken any medications or substances which may alter mood or consciousness

Ascertain that client is relatively free of pain or other distractions

Infants and toddlers will be unable to complete the MiniMental Examination

The visually or hearing impaired client will need to use assistive aids

The physically compromised client may be unable to respond appropriately, especially if the underlying disease pathology causes confusion or disorientation

TRANSCULTURAL CONSIDERATIONS

Language and cultural barriers may limit the nurse's ability to obtain an accurate assessment. Consider use of the AT&T Language Line. See Culturological Assessment procedure for general overview of cultural considerations.

▶ INTERVENTIONS

1. Assess the client's level of consciousness (LOC).

   The terms used to describe LOC define states of consciousness that exist along a continuum, ranging from fully alert to comatose. Reduced LOCs are associated with impaired cerebral function

2. Use the Glasgow Coma Scale (GCS) to objectively measure LOCs.

   Mental status is an inferred assessment that is subject to individual interpretation. The GCS is a quantitative assessment that defines the LOC by assigning a numerical value to client responses.

3. Use the MiniMental State Examination to assess client.

   The MiniMental State Exam is a standard assessment tool used to detect the presence of organic disease and to screen for dementia and delirium

4. Have the client interpret the meaning of a proverb e.g. "people who live in glass houses should not throw stones."

   The client with impaired mentation will provide a literal translation or simply repeat the sentence

DOCUMENTATION

The following information should be noted in the nursing note:

The client's:
   level of consciousness
   score on the Glasgow Coma Scale
   Score on the MiniMental State Examination

INTERDISCIPLINARY COLLABORATION

Inform physician of abnormal findings. Discuss with the physician the possible need to obtain referrals for a psychiatric clinical nurse specialist; social worker; occupational, or physical therapist; psychiatrist; speech-language pathologist and audiologist; or neurologist [3, 10, 12, 17, 18, 32, 37, 43].

PROCEDURE
Head and Neck Assessment

DESCRIPTION

The head and neck provide the protective bony structure for the brain and the special senses: vision, smell, hearing, and taste. The examination includes an assessment of the hair and scalp, ears, eyes, nose, mouth, and the structures in the neck.

PURPOSE

To evaluate the structures of the head, face, and neck and the function of the special senses

EQUIPMENT
Opthalmoscope
Otoscope
Tuning fork
Snellen Eye Chart
Health Assessment Forms

OUTCOMES
The client/caregiver will:

▶ Report any signs of upper respiratory tract infection
▶ Demonstrate correct use of assistive devices (eye glasses, hearing aids, dentures, etc)
▶ Identify presence of skin lesions/irritation, growths or lice,
▶ Indicate changes in sight or hearing

ASSESSMENT DATA
Document the presence of any upper respiratory tract infections, or sensory-perceptual impairment
Check for node and thyroid enlargement
Determine need for hearing or visual aids
Note status of dentition
Observe condition of hair and scalp

RELATED NURSING DIAGNOSES
Impaired skin integrity
Impaired gas exchange
At risk for infection
Altered sensory perception
Ineffective airway clearance
Ineffective breathing patterns
Self-care deficit

SPECIAL CONSIDERATIONS
Detailed assessments will need to be made on the initial visit and for all acutely ill clients
In life-threatening situations body assessment areas will need to prioritized

TRANSCULTURAL CONSIDERATIONS
An interpreter will be needed for clients unable to speak or understand English
Darker skin pigmentation may obscure clinical findings in persons of color
Consider use of the AT&T Language Line
See Culturological Assessment procedure for general overview of cultural considerations.

▶ **INTERVENTIONS**

1. Wash hands.	*Prevents transmission of microbes*
2. Explain procedure.	*Allays anxiety*

Head

1. Inspect and palpate the head and scalp.	*Detects presence of irregular shape, masses, lesions, or lice*
2. Have client touch chin to chest and each shoulder, touch ear to corresponding shoulder, and tilt head back, forward and from side to side.	*Evaluates range of motion of cervical spine*

Eyes

1. Check visual acuity using Snellen Chart.	*Determines presence of visual disturbances*
2. Inspect eyes, eyelids, eyebrows, lacrimal ducts, conjunctiva, and sclera or cataracts.	*Determines presence of visual disturbances or identifies presence of infection.*
3. Test for pupillary reaction to light.	*Detects possible central nervous system injury*
4. Test for extra ocular movements.	*Determines presence of nystagmus*
5. Test for accommodation	*Detects the ability of the eye to adjust for distance through modification of the lens*
6. Locate optic discs: note vessels, cup margins, retinal surface, vitreous humor (see Figure 2-1).	*Detects evidence of increased intracranial pressure, hypertensive or diabetic changes, macular abnormality*

Ears

1. Inspect and palpate the ear and surrounding area.	*Determines presence of impaired hearing, ear infection*
2. Inspect tympanic membrane.	*Determines presence of bulging or ruptured tympanic membrane*
3. Test for hearing acuity (see Display 2-1).	

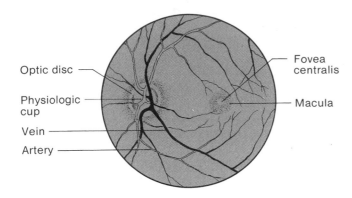

Optic disc

Physiologic cup

Vein

Artery

Fovea centralis

Macula

FIGURE 2-1 ▶ The fundus

DISPLAY 2-1 *Types of Hearing Losses*

Sensorineural Hearing Loss (Perceptive Deafness)

Associated Conditions

Conditions that disrupt *neural* hearing pathways: the cochlea, cranial nerve VIII, or the auditory portions of the cerebral cortex (bilateral lesions).

Causative Factors
- Congenital defects
- Maternal rubella
- Erythroblastosis fetalis
- Traumatic injury involving the inner ear or cranial nerve VIII
- Vascular disorders involving the inner ear
- Ototoxic drugs
- Bacterial and viral infections (meningitis, encephalitis, mumps, etc.)
- Meniere's disease
- Severe febrile illness
- Posterior fossa tumors
- Multiple sclerosis
- Presbycusis
- Prolonged or repeated exposure to loud sounds

Signs and Symptoms
- Delayed language and speech development (infants)
- Hearing loss that may be more severe in noisy environments
- May be associated with speaking loudly

Hearing Tests
- Whisper test and watch-tick test may indicate hearing loss
- Weber test usually shows sound lateralization to the good ear
- Rinne test should be positive (AC>BC)

Conductive Hearing Loss

Associated Conditions

Associated with external or middle ear problems that prevent normal sound transmission. Otoscopic examination is essential for detecting cerumen impaction, eardrum perforation, and otitis media.

DISPLAY 2-1 *Types of Hearing Losses* (Continued)

Causative Factors
- ► Congenital ear malformations
- ► Traumatic eardrum perforation
- ► Trauma disrupting the ossicles
- ► Cerumen impaction
- ► Middle ear inflammation (otitis media)
- ► Otosclerosis

Signs and Symptoms
- ► Hearing loss that may be less noticeable in a noisy environment
- ► Normal tone of voice usually observed

Hearing Tests
- ► Whisper test and watch-tick test may indicate hearing loss.
- ► Weber test usually shows sound lateralization to the affected ear because this ear is less distracted by environmental noise and is therefore more perceptive to vibration.
- ► Rinne test should be negative (BC>AC) because vibrations passing through bone bypass the obstructive process.

Mixed (Combined) Hearing Loss
Hearing losses may be secondary to ineffective conduction and sensory perception. Both air and bone sound conduction are impaired.

a. Weber test—strike tuning fork, place on top of head and ask client to indicate where sound is heard [should be equal in both ears]	*Indicates sensory perception of sound*
b. Rinne test—strike tuning fork and place on mastoid process, when client states that buzzing has stopped, place tuning fork near auditory meatus, client should still hear a soft vibrating sound.	*Shows that air conduction is greater than bone conduction*
c. Whisper test—stand behind the client and whisper numbers in one ear while client covers other ear ask client to repeat what was whispered.	*Indicates ability to hear high-frequency sounds*

Nose

1. Inspect nasal mucosa and turbinates.	*Determines presence of deviated septum, drainage, nasal obstruction, tenderness and inflammation*
2. Palpate the frontal and maxillary sinuses.	*Determines presence of swelling*

Mouth

1. Inspect lips, tongue, teeth, and buccal cavity.	*Detects evidence of oral lesions, infections, cyanosis*

2. Evaluate swallowing function.	*ecchymosis, dental caries, asymmetry, dysphagia. (Display 2-2) Detects evidence of dysphagia.*

Neck

1. Inspect and palpate the neck, thyroid, and trachea.	*Detects evidence of dysphagia, enlarged nodes, enlarged thyroid, tracheal deviation*
2. Palpate lymph nodes (see Figure 2-2).	*Detects evidence of masses, tenderness or enlargement of the lymph nodes*

DOCUMENTATION

The following should be included in the nursing note:

All abnormal clinical findings
Results of hearing tests
Results of eye test
Status of dentitition
Client's ability to swallow, put neck through full range of motion

INTERDISCIPLINARY COLLABORATION

Inform physician of abnormal findings and document actions taken

Discuss with the physician the need for possible referrals for neurology, speech-language pathology, opthalmology, audiology, denistry, nutrition support, otolaryngology, or occupational therapy

Consider need to consult with social worker to identify community resources [3, 10, 17–19, 31, 32, 37, 43]

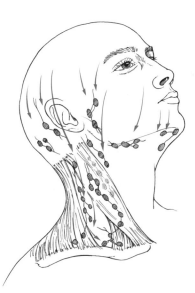

FIGURE 2-2 ▶ Distribution of lymph nodes

DISPLAY 2-2 *Oral Lesions and Conditions*

Lip Vesicles

- ► Small lesions
- ► Occur singularly or in clusters
- ► Serous, fluid-filled masses

Example:
Herpes simplex

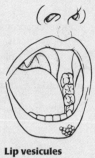

Lip vesicules

Mucocele

- ► Small, bluish, mucus-filled cyst
- ► Benign
- ► May be removed for cosmetic purposes

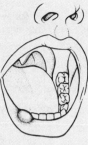

Mucocele

Lip Ulcers

- ► Necrotic loss of lip tissue

Examples:
The chancre that is the primary lesion of syphilis. A chancre ulcerates in the center and leaves a crusty residue. Pressure ulcer, such as those resulting from prolonged contact with tubes.

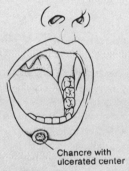

Chancre with ulcerated center

Lip ulcer

Cheilitis

- ► Inflammation and crust formation
- ► Lower lip most often affected
- ► May be chronic
- ► Cause often unknown

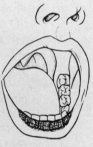

Cheilitis

Squamous Cell Carcinoma

- ► May appear as plaque, warty papule, or ulcer
- ► Nonhealing lesion
- ► Appears on lips or underside of tongue
- ► Most common form of oral cancer
- ► If not healed within 2 to 3 weeks, should be evaluated to rule out malignancy

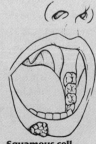

Squamous cell carcinoma

Torus Palatinus

- ► Nodular mass midline on the hard palate
- ► Benign
- ► Masses away from the midline may represent malignancies
- ► May not develop until adulthood

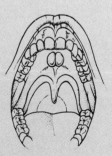

Torus palatinus

(continued)

DISPLAY 2-2 *Oral Lesions and Conditions* (Continued)

Fordyce Spots (Granules)
▶ Small yellow papules on oral mucosa
▶ Represent sebaceous glands
▶ Common benign lesion

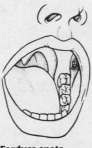

Fordyce spots

Glossitis
▶ Tongue becomes bright red, edematous, and smooth as papillae are lost
▶ Associated with stomatitis, malnutrition, chronic illness

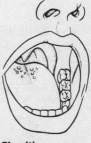

Glossitis

Aphthous Stomatitis (Canker Sore)
▶ Ulcerated lesion of oral mucosa
▶ Surrounded by white halo
▶ Tender
▶ Heals and recurs spontaneously
▶ May occur in groups

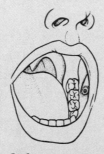

Canker sore

Hairy Tongue
▶ Hairy appearance secondary to papillae elongation
▶ Papillae dark brown or black
▶ Benign
▶ Associated with antibiotic therapy

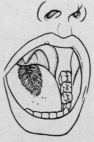

Hairy Tongue

Leukoplakia
▶ Smooth, white, paint-like patch on the oral mucosa
▶ May represent a premalignant transformation of oral mucosa
▶ Associated with oral tobacco usage

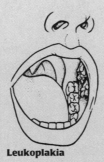

Leukoplakia

Pseudomonas Infection
▶ Necrotic ulcers
▶ Dark brown central eschar (scar)
▶ Surrounded by erythematous ring

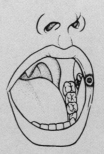

Pseudomonas infection

DISPLAY 2-2 *Oral Lesions and Conditions* (Continued)

Stomatitis

- ▶ Inflammation of the oral cavity
- ▶ Mucosa, red, dry, edematous
- ▶ Predisposes oral mucosa to ulceration
- ▶ Red demarcation line may be noted at the vermilion border
- ▶ Associated with chemotherapeutic agents, dehydration, infectious agents, and radiation

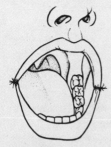

Stomatitis

Candida albicans (Yeast, Thrush, Moniliasis)

- ▶ Oral mucosa covered by white, curd-like patches
- ▶ Underlying mucosa may be bright red
- ▶ Associated with chronic illness, antibiotic therapy

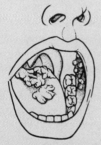

Candida albicans

Streptococcal Pharyngitis

- ▶ Posterior pharynx bright red
- ▶ Tonsils, uvula, pillars may be swollen and covered with white or yellow exudate
- ▶ Definitive diagnosis requires throat culture
- ▶ Physical findings may vary

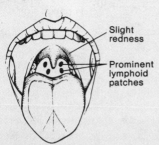

Slight redness

Prominent lymphoid patches

Streptococcal pharyngitis

Viral Pharyngitis

- ▶ Posterior pharynx red or normal in color
- ▶ Slight swelling of tonsils and uvula may occur
- ▶ Throat culture required to rule out streptococcal pharyngitis

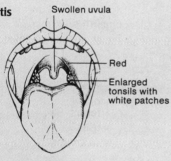

Swollen uvula

Red

Enlarged tonsils with white patches

Viral pharyngitis

PROCEDURE

Thorax and Lung Assessment

DESCRIPTION

The examination of the chest and respiratory system is made to assess the structure and function of the thoracic skeleton, organs, and muscles of respiration. The quality of lung sounds, character of sputum, use of accessory muscles, chest configuration, and percussion tones make up the components of the respiratory assessment. Evidence of cyanosis, dyspnea, and respiratory tract infections is documented, and appropriate interventions are implemented to treat underlying pathology

PURPOSE
To assess the respiratory system and determine adequacy of oxygenation

EQUIPMENT
Health Assessment Forms
Stethoscope
Watch with second hand

OUTCOMES
The client/caregiver will:

▶ Report any symptoms of respiratory compromise
▶ Demonstrate an ability to maintain a patent airway
▶ Demonstrate correct use of respiratory equipment
▶ Maintain an environment free of pollutants

ASSESSMENT DATA
Review client's history of smoking or exposure to smoke and family history of respiratory diseases
Check for evidence of upper-respiratory infection
Note evidence of shortness of breath, paroxysmal nocturnal dyspnea, dyspnea on exertion
Note results of TB and allergy skin tests
Document use of respiratory equipment
Report any previous exposure to coal, asbestos, allergens (dust, mites, dander)

RELATED NURSING DIAGNOSES
Impaired gas exchange
At risk for infection
Ineffective airway clearance
Alteration in comfort
Knowledge deficit
Anxiety
Ineffective breathing patterns

SPECIAL CONSIDERATIONS
Detailed assessments will need to be made on the initial visit and for all acutely ill clients
In life-threatening situations, body assessment areas will need to prioritized

TRANSCULTURAL CONSIDERATIONS
An interpreter will be needed for clients unable to speak or understand English
Darker skin pigmentation may obscure clinical findings in persons of color
For some cultures smoking or exposure to smoke may be an integral component of certain cere-
monial activities performed during religious functions.
Consider use of the AT&T Language Line.
See Culturological Assessment procedure for general overview of cultural considerations.

▶ INTERVENTIONS

1. Wash hands.   *Prevents transmission of mi-*
                                                         crobes

2. Explain procedure.   *Allays anxiety*

Anatomical Structure

1. In a sitting position, locate the anterior landmarks (suprasternal notch, Angle of Louis first rib and intercostal space, manubrium, mid-clavicular lines) and compare findings bilaterally.

Detects structural irregularities

2. Locate posterior landmarks (C7 to T1).

Detects structural irregularities

3. Visually outline the location of the posterior and lateral lung fields.

Permits the examiner to establish an approximate location of the posterior and lateral lobes of the lung

Inspection

1. Inspect chest configuration.

Detects abnormality in the anteroposterior and transverse diameters

2. Determine chest symmetry.

Determines presence of scoliosis, kyphosis, lordosis

3. Note color of lips, nail beds, mucous membranes.

Indicates presence of cyanosis

4. Assess pattern of respiration.

Indicates presence of alteration in rhythm of breathing

5. Note use of accessory muscles.

Indicates presence of dyspnea

6. Observe for evidence of activity intolerance.

Suggests possible inablity to perform ADLs

Palpation

1. Determine symmetric chest expansion.

Assesses client's effort to ventilate

2. Palpate for tactile fremitus.

Detects obstruction in the transmission of vibrations

3. Palpate chest wall noting lumps, tenderness, skin temperature, and moisture.

Determines presence of lesions or masses

Percussion

1. Percuss all lung fields systematically.

Uses an organized approach to detect changes in percussion tones

2. Identify percussion tones elicited.

Detects presence of dullness, resonance and hyperresonance

Auscultation

1. Note quality of breath sounds.

Screens for presence of airway obstruction, atelectasis, fluid and consolidation

2. Find normal locations for the three types of breath sounds (vesicular, bronchial, and bronchovesicular).

Screens for presence of airway obstruction, atelectasis, fluid and consolidation

3. Note presence of adventitious sounds (crackles or wheezes).

Screens for presence of airway obstruction, atelectasis, fluid and consolidation

DOCUMENTATION
The following should be included in the nursing note:

All abnormal clinical findings and follow-up action taken
Client/caregiver's ability to:
    assess for signs of respiratory distress and appropriately intervene
    maintain an environment free of allergens
    correctly use all respiratory equipment
    correctly implement ordered treatment plan

INTERDISCIPLINARY COLLABORATION
Inform physician of abnormal findings and suggest possible need for referrals for consulation with the respiratory therapist, pulmonologist, physical or occupational therapist. Consult with social worker to assist in locating community resources for client education programs regarding smoking cessation, cystic fibrosis, asthma, etc. Consider need for home health aide to assist with ADLs [3, 10, 17–19, 31, 32, 37, 43]

PROCEDURE
Breast and Axillary Assessment

DESCRIPTION
The examination of the breast and axilla of both the male and female client is performed to assess structure and shape to detect the presence of masses or lesions, and to note evidence of nipple discharge. Breast self examination (BSE) should be performed regularly by both the male and female client. BSE is considered an appropriate screening activity when used in conjunction with clinical breast examination and mammography.

PURPOSE
To determine presence of lesions, discharge, masses, or tenderness of the breast tissue

EQUIPMENT
Health Assessment Forms
Rolled towel

OUTCOMES
The client/caregiver will:

Report any changes in breast or nipple shape, discharge, or evidence of tenderness or lumps
Demonstrate ability to perform BSE
Maintain regular screening activities (mammography, clinical breast examination)

ASSESSMENT DATA

Review client/family history of breast cancer or fibrocystic disease
Check for node enlargement; change in breast size; pain; discharge, retraction or scaling of nipple
Determine if client is taking hormonal medications, oral contraceptives or is postmenopausal
Note client's knowledge of and ability to perform breast self examination (BSE)

RELATED NURSING DIAGNOSES

Impaired skin integrity
At risk for infection
Altered body image
Alteration in comfort
Knowledge deficit
Anxiety

SPECIAL CONSIDERATIONS

Detailed assessments will need to be made on the initial visit and for all acutely ill clients.

In life-threatening situations body assessment areas will need to prioritized. While the child-bearing female client will be instructed to perform BSE 2 to 3 days after the end of the menstrual cycle, the post-menopausal and male client will be instructed to perform BSE every 30 days.

The male breast examination follows the same format used for the female breast examination. The size and shape of male breast tissue will vary according to fat distribution, body weight, and body structure. Enlarged male breast tissue that is glandular, or the presence of gynecomastia, should be documented and reported for follow-up.

TRANSCULTURAL CONSIDERATIONS

An interpreter will be needed for clients unable to speak or understand English
Darker skin pigmentation may obscure clinical findings in persons of color
For some cultures, adolescents, and elderly clients, exposure of the breasts may be considered in-
   trusive or a violation of cultural practices. During the assessment it may be appropriate to
   have another member of the family or significant other present.
Consider use of AT&T Language Line.
See the Culturological Assessment procedure for a general overview of cultural considerations.

▶ INTERVENTIONS

1. Wash hands.	*Prevents transmission of microbes*
2. Explain procedure.	*Allays anxiety*

Breast Assessment

1. In a sitting or standing position note breast contour, size and symmetry, and observe the skin for any abnormality (see Figure 2-3).	*Detects presence of irregular shape, masses, or lesions (see Display 2-3).*
2. Direct client through maneuvers to identify dimpling.	*Detects presence of irregular shape, masses, or lesions.*
3. Position towel under scapula on the side of the breast being examined.	*Detects presence of irregular shape, masses, or lesions.*
4. In a supine position palpate the breast in in a systematic manner (see Figure 2-4).	

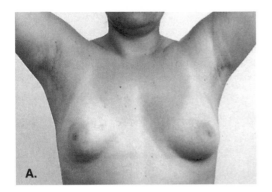

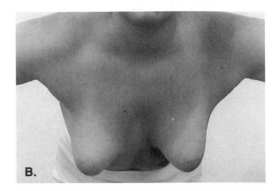

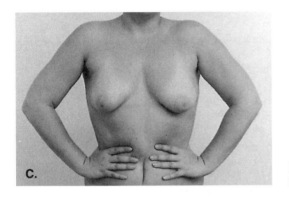

FIGURE 2-3 ▶ Breast examinations: **A.** Arms over head; **B.** Leaning over; **C.** Pressing hands onto hips

    a. clock method—with the nipple as the center mark, compare the breast tissue to the face of a clock (see Figure 2-5a). Identify positions of lesions or other abnormalities according to the time on the face of the clock, e.g., 1 o'clock position.

    b. quadrant method—divide the breast into four quadrants: upper inner, upper outer, lower inner, lower outer (see Figure 2-5b). The horizontal and vertical lines should intersect at the nipple. Palpate and identify findings in each quadrant.

Detects presence of irregular shape, masses, or lesions

5. Palpate the nipple.

Detects presence of abnormal discharges, pain, or inversion

Axillary Assessment

1. Inspect axillary area.

Determines presence of masses or lesions

2. Palpate for node enlargement (see Figure 2-6).

Determines presence of masses or lesions

DISPLAY 2-3 *Deviations from Normal Breast Findings.* (Continued)

Retraction Signs

▶ Signs include skin dimpling, creasing, or changes in the contour of the breast or nipple

▶ Secondary to fibrosis or scar tissue formation in the breast

▶ Retractions signs may appear only with position changes or with breast palpation.

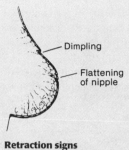

Dimpling

Flattening of nipple

Retraction signs

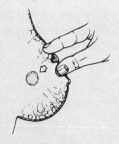

Retraction with compression

Breast Cancer Mass (Malignant Tumor)

(See Chapter 5 for risk factors)

▶ Usually occurs as a single mass (lump) in one breast

▶ Usually nontender

▶ Irregular shape

▶ Firm, hard, embedded in surrounding tissue

▶ Referral and biopsy indicated for definitive diagnosis

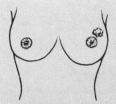

Breast cancer mass

Breast Cyst (Benign Mass of Fibrocystic Disease)

▶ Occur as single or multiple lumps in one or both breasts

▶ Usually tender (omitting caffeine reduces tenderness); tenderness increases during premenstrual period

▶ Round shape

▶ Soft or firm, mobile

▶ Referral and biopsy indicated for definitive diagnosis, especially for first mass; later masses may be evaluated over time by a specialist

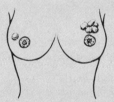

Breast cysts

Fibroadenoma (Benign Breast Lump)

▶ Usually occurs as a single mass in women aged 15–35 years

▶ Usually nontender

▶ May be round or lobular

▶ Firm, mobile, and not fixed to breast tissue or chest wall

▶ No premenstrual changes

▶ Referral and biopsy indicated for definitive diagnosis

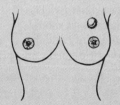

Fibroadenoma

(continued)

Deviations from Normal Breast Findings. *(Continued)*

Increased Venous Prominence

- ▶ Associated with breast cancer if unilateral
- ▶ Unilateral localized increase in venous pattern associated with malignant tumors
- ▶ Normal with breast enlargement associated with pregnancy and lactation if bilateral and bilateral symmetry

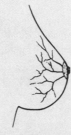

Increased venous prominence

Peau d'Orange (Edema)

- ▶ Associated with breast cancer
- ▶ Caused by interference with lymphatic drainage
- ▶ Breast skin has "orange peel" appearance
- ▶ Skin pores enlarge
- ▶ May be noted on the areola
- ▶ Skin becomes thick, hard, immobile
- ▶ Skin discoloration may occur

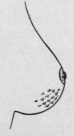

Peau d'orange

Nipple Inversion

- ▶ Considered normal if long-standing
- ▶ Associated with fibrosis and malignancy if recent development

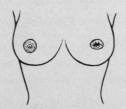

Nipple inversion

Acute Mastitis (Inflammation of the Breasts)

- ▶ Associated with lactation but may occur at any age
- ▶ Nipple cracks or abrasions noted
- ▶ Breast skin reddened and warm to touch
- ▶ Tenderness
- ▶ Systemic signs include fever and increased pulse

Paget's Disease (Malignancy of Mammary Ducts)

- ▶ Early signs: Erythema of nipple and areola
- ▶ Late signs: Thickening, scaling, and erosion of the nipple and areola

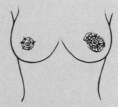

Paget's disease

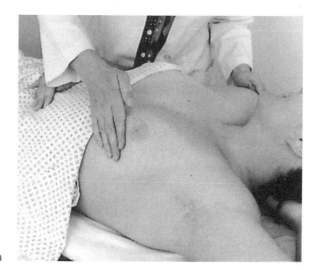

FIGURE 2-4 ▶ Breast palpation: Supine position

Breast Self Examination (BSE)

1. Give directions to the client for self breast examination (see Display 2-4).
2. Have client perform BSE.

Instills concepts of health promotion/disease prevention
Enables evaluation of client's ability to perform BSE

DOCUMENTATION
The following should be included in the nursing note:

All abnormal clinical findings and follow-up action taken
The client's ability to perform BSE

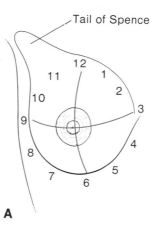

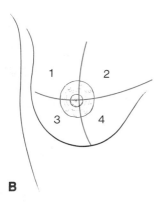

FIGURE 2-5 ▶ Breast examination landmarks. **A.** Breast clock landmarks, including Tail of Spence; **B.** Breast quadrants.

Breast Self Examination

Screening Recommendations

The American Cancer Society recommends monthly BSE for women over age 20. About 90% of all breast lumps are found by women or their significant others.

Procedure

1. Examine the breasts in the tub or shower when skin is wet and hands move easily over breast tissue (*A, B*). Use the right hand to examine the left breast as you raise the left arm over the head to expose more breast tissue.

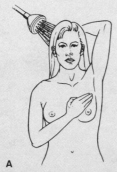

A

B

2. Examine the breasts in front of a mirror to detect unusual contours or changes in the skin appearance, such as puckering, dimpling, or retraction of the nipple. Note the appearance of the breasts in three different positions: arms at the sides (*C*), arms over the head (*D*), and hands on the hips while flexing the chest muscle (*E*).

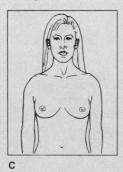 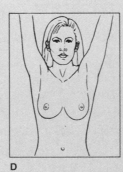 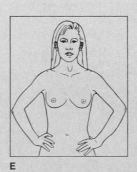

C

D

E

3. Examine the breasts lying down. Place a small pillow or blanket under your shoulder on the side being examined, to expose more breast tissue (*F*). Use the right hand to examine the left breast. Be thorough, proceeding in a circular pattern from the center of the breast outward. Feel the breast tissues that extend to the armpit. Squeeze the nipple to detect any discharge. (*G*). Any hard lumps, clear or bloody nipple discharge, or skin changes should be reported to a health professional.

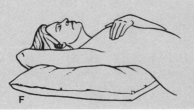 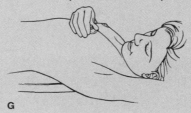

F

G

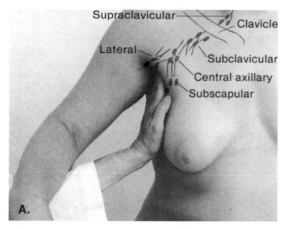
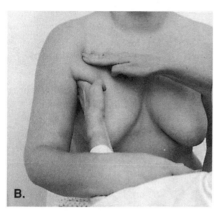

FIGURE 2-6 ▶ Axillae palpation:. **A.** Axillae nodes; **B.** Seated position

Any history of breast surgery or disease
Currently prescribed hormonal medications

INTERDISCIPLINARY
Inform physician of abnormal findings, and discuss need to obtain referral for gynecologist. Consult with social worker to assist in locating community support groups (breast cancer survival and lactation support groups) [3, 10, 17–19, 31, 32, 42].

PROCEDURE
Cardiovascular Assessment

DESCRIPTION
The cardiovascular examination is performed to assess the precordium, heart, and neck vessels. The examination includes an evaluation of heart sounds, cardiac rate and rhythm, jugular vein and carotid artery, blood pressure reading, and evidence of thoracic and/or abdominal heaves/thrills. This examination is a standard component of every home bound assessment.

PURPOSE
To examine the heart and neck vessels

EQUIPMENT
Health Assessment Forms
Stethoscope
Watch with second hand
Sphygmomanometer

OUTCOMES
The client/caregiver will:

▶ Report any symptoms of cardiovascular distress
▶ Demonstrate an ability to perform cardiopulmonary resuscitation

▶ Demonstrate correct use of cardiovascular equipment
▶ Follow the plan of treatment

ASSESSMENT DATA

Review client's history of smoking or exposure to smoke, drug or alcohol abuse, heart murmur, rheumatic fever

Review family history of heart disease, elevated cholesterol, hypertension, diabetes, obesity, varicosity

Note evidence of shortness of breath, paroxysmal nocturnal dyspnea, or dyspnea on exertion

Note results of ECG, echocardiogram, phonocardiogram, chest x-ray

RELATED NURSING DIAGNOSES

Activity intolerance
Altered cardiac output
Altered tissue perfusion
Alteration in comfort
Knowledge deficit
Anxiety
Self-care deficit

SPECIAL CONSIDERATIONS

Detailed assessments will need to be made on the initial visit and for all acutely ill clients

In life-threatening situations body assessment areas will need to prioritized

TRANSCULTURAL CONSIDERATIONS

An interpreter will be needed for clients unable to speak or understand English

Darker skin pigmentation may obscure clinical findings in persons of color, e.g., assess the mucus membranes for evidence of cyanosis.

Heart disease is more prevalent among the nation's medically underserved populations.

Consider use of AT&T Language Line.

See Culturological Assessment procedure for a general overview of cultural considerations

▶ INTERVENTIONS

1. Wash hands.	*Prevents transmission of microbes*
2. Explain procedure.	*Allays anxiety*

Anatomical Structure

1. In a sitting position, locate the thoracic landmarks (suprasternal notch, pulmonic area aortic area, tricuspid area, mitral area [PMI], Erb's point, epigastric area) (see Figure 2-7).	*Correctly locates areas for auscultation*
Identify location of jugular vein and carotid artery.	*These vessels reflect the efficiency of cardiac function*

Inspection

1. In the semi-Fowler's position note jugular venus pulsation.	*Detects presence of jugular vein distension*

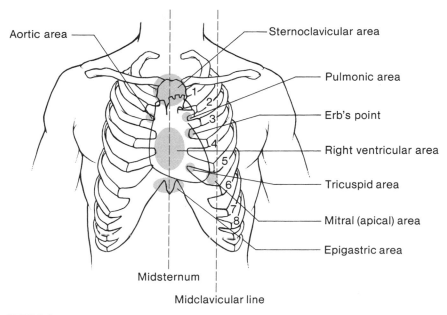

Aortic area — Sternoclavicular area

— Pulmonic area

— Erb's point

— Right ventricular area

— Tricuspid area

— Mitral (apical) area

— Epigastric area

Midsternum

Midclavicular line

FIGURE 2-7 ▶ Precordial landmarks

2. Inspect the anterior chest.

3. Note color of lips, nail beds, and mucous membranes.

Determines visibility of the apical impulse and the presence of abnormal pulsations

Detects alteration in tissue perfusion

Palpation

1. Determine location of the PMI.

2. Palpate the carotid artery.
3. Palpate across the precordium.

Detects displacement of the cardiac apex

Detects stroke volume

Determines presence of heaves or thrills

Percussion

1. Percuss the anterior chest.

Notes normal borders of cardiac dullness

Auscultation

1. Place the stethoscope over the carotid artery at three levels: angle of jaw, midcervical area, base of neck.
2. Listen at four standard areas of the chest (aortic, pulmonic, tricuspid, mitral) (see Figure 2-8).

Detects abnormal presence of bruit

Detects normal and abnormal heart sounds

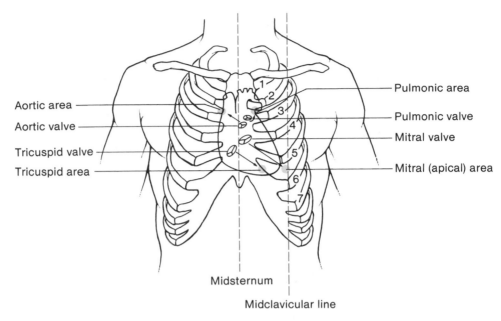

Aortic area
Aortic valve
Tricuspid valve
Tricuspid area

Pulmonic area
Pulmonic valve
Mitral valve
Mitral (apical) area

Midsternum
Midclavicular line

FIGURE 2-8 ▶ Four standard areas of the chest (aortic, pulmonic, tricuspid, mitral)

3. Identify first and second heart sounds.

These sounds occur during the systolic phase of the cardiac cycle and indicate the closing of the heart valves

4. Note presence of third and/or fourth heart sound.

Consistent with clinical findings of heart failure, coronary artery disease, aortic stenosis

5. Note splitting of the second heart sound (physiological, paradoxical, fixed).

Detects normal/abnormal aortic and pulmonic valve closure

6. Note presence of pericardial friction rub.

Consistent with clinical finding of pericarditis

7. Note presence of murmur (timing, grading, quality, location, pitch).

Detects valvular abnormalities

8. Determine apical rate and rhythm.

Detects presence of bradycardia, tachycardia and dysrhythmia

9. Obtain blood pressure reading.
   a. bladder width of sphygmomanometer should be 1/3 to 1/2 circumference of limb
   b. bladder length should be @ 80% of the circumference of the extremity

Measures the pressure of the blood against the blood vessels

c. in the obese client, the cuff should be wrapped around the forearm, and the stethoscope should be placed over the radial artery

d. when use of the upper extremities is countraindicated, wrap the cuff around the thigh and auscultate the popliteal artery, or wrap the cuff around the lower leg and auscultate the pedal artery.

DOCUMENTATION
The following should be included in the nursing note:

All abnormal clinical findings and follow-up actions taken
The client/caregiver's ability to:
 correctly follow the treatment plan
 perform CPR
 identify untoward cardiovascular changes
 correctly use all cardiovascular equipment (self–blood-pressure apparatus, cardiac monitoring device, etc)

INTERDISCIPLINARY COLLABORATION
Inform physician of abnormal findings and discuss the need for possible referrals for a cardiologist, or physical therapist for strengthening exercises
Consult with social worker for assistance in locating community client education programs for cardiac rehabilitation, low impact cardiovascular workout exercises, smoking cessation, stress management
Consider need for nutrition counseling for low sodium, low cholesterol, low fat diets, etc
Consider need for home health aide to assist with ADLs [3, 10, 17–19, 31, 32, 37, 43]

PROCEDURE
Peripheral Vascular Assessment

DESCRIPTION
The examination of the peripheral vascular system includes an assessment of the arterial and venous blood flow to the upper and lower extremities. During the examination, a general assessment is made of the venous patterns and skin temperature. Bilateral comparisons are made of the quality and strength of the peripheral pulses. The amplitude of the pulses and the degree of peripheral edema are graded and recorded. A Doppler ultrasound blood flow detector is used when the pulse is faint or weak on palpation.

PURPOSE
To evaluate vascular circulation in the upper and lower extremities

EQUIPMENT
Health Assessment Forms
Stethoscope
Doppler ultrasound blood flow detector, if needed

OUTCOMES

The client/caregiver will:

▶ Report any symptoms of impaired circulation
▶ Demonstrate ability to monitor pulse rate
▶ Follow the plan of treatment

ASSESSMENT DATA

Review client's history of smoking or exposure to smoke, substance abuse
Review family history of heart disease, elevated cholesterol, hypertension, diabetes, obesity, varicosity
Check for evidence of intermittent claudication, edema, numbness, tingling or coldness in extremities
Note results of doppler studies
Document recent weight gain
Grade quality of peripheral pulse and degree of peripheral edema

RELATED NURSING DIAGNOSES

Activity intolerance
Altered cardiac output
Altered tissue perfusion
Alteration in comfort
Knowledge deficit
Anxiety
Self-care deficit

SPECIAL CONSIDERATIONS

Detailed assessments will need to be made on the initial visit and for all acutely ill clients
In life-threatening situations body assessment areas will need to prioritized

TRANSCULTURAL CONSIDERATIONS

An interpreter will be needed for clients unable to speak or understand English
Darker skin pigmentation may obscure clinical findings in persons of color.
Consider use of the AT&T Language Line.
See Culturological Assessment procedure for general overview of cultural considerations

▶ INTERVENTIONS

1. Wash hands.	*Prevents transmission of microbes*
2. Explain procedure.	*Allays anxiety*

General Assessment

1. Inspect all skin surfaces (note color, texture, hair distribution rashes, pigmentation, scars).	*Detects any abnormality in circulation*
2. Inspect venous patterns.	*Detects the presence of venous engorgement or varicosity*
3. Palpate for overall skin temperature, tenderness.	*Detects any abnormality in circulation*

4. Compare radial and apical pulses.

Determines presence of pulse deficit

5. Assess amplitude of pulsations and grade on a scale of 0–4
   0 = absent
   +1 = diminished, thready, easily obliterated
   +2 = normal, not easily obliterated
   +3 = increased, full volume
   +4 = bounding

Evaluates quality of pulse

Upper Extremities

1. Palpate radial pulse.

Non-palpable pulses may indicate cessation of blood flow

2. Palpate ulnar pulse.

Non-palpable pulses may indicate cessation of blood flow

3. Palpate brachial pulse.

Non-palpable pulses may indicate cessation of blood flow

4. Note characteristic of pulse (rate, rhythm, amplitude, symmetry).

Identifies weak, absent, thready, bounding, or irregular pulses

5. Perform Allen Test:
   a. occlude the radial artery while client makes a fist
   b. have client open the fist and note the return of color to the hand, repeat occluding ulnar artery

Determines patency of ulnar and radial arteries

6. Teach client/caregiver to obtain pulse rate and permit return demonstration.

Documents client/caregiver's ability to perform task

Lower Extremities

1. Palpate femoral pulse.

Nonpalpable pulses denote cessation of blood flow

2. Palpate popliteal pulse.

Nonpalpable pulses denote cessation of blood flow

3. Palpate dorsalis pedal pulse.

Nonpalpable pulses denote cessation of blood flow

4. Palpate posterior pedal pulse.

Nonpalpable pulses denote cessation of blood flow

5. Test for Homan's sign.
   flex the knee and gently dorsiflex the ankle, observe for pain in calf

May indicate presence of deep vein thrombosis

6. Observe for edema (see Display 2-5).
   grade on a scale of 1 to 4
         1+ = 2 mm indentation
         2+ = 4 mm indentation
         3+ = 6 mm indentation
         4+ = 8 mm indentation
   brawny = tissue is hard, fluid can no longer be displaced, skin is shiny warm and moist

Indicative of poor circulation and fluid accumulation

DISPLAY 2-5 *Grading Edema*

1+ Pitting Edema
- ▶ Slight indentation (2 mm)
- ▶ Normal contours
- ▶ Associated with interstitial fluid volume 30% above normal

2+ Pitting Edema
- ▶ Deeper pit after pressing (4 mm)
- ▶ Lasts longer than 1+
- ▶ Fairly normal contour

3+ Pitting Edema
- ▶ Deep it (6 mm)
- ▶ Remains several seconds after pressing
- ▶ Skin swelling obvious by general inspection

4+ Pitting Edema
- ▶ Deep pit (8 mm)
- ▶ Remains for a prolonged time after pressing, possibly minutes
- ▶ Frank swelling

Brawny Edema
- ▶ Fluid can no longer be displaced secondary to excessive interstitial fluid accumulation
- ▶ No pitting
- ▶ Tissue palpates as firm or hard
- ▶ Skin surface shiny, warm, moist

Doppler Ultrasound Measurement

This device is used to magnify sound in weak or hard to hear peripheral pulses

1. Clean tip of the probe with antiseptic solution per agency protocol
2. Apply gel to probe
3. Place probe on skin over pulse point
4. Turn power on and regulate volume of sound
5. Slowly move the probe in concentric circles until achieving the best sound transmission
6. Count the pulse beats for 60 seconds
7. Record pulse rate
8. Cleanse the probe

DOCUMENTATION

The following information should be included in the nursing note:

All abnormal clinical findings and follow-up action taken
The client/caregiver's ability to:

accurately obtain pulse rate
verbalize knowledge of symptoms of poor perfusion and when to call physician/nurse
follow the plan of treatment

INTERDISCIPLINARY COLLABORATION

Inform physician of abnormal findings. Discuss with the physician possible need for referral to podiatrist for foot care, physical therapist for evaluation of strength and gait training and need
for mobility assistive devices.
Consider need for home health aide to assist with ADLs [3, 10, 17–19, 31, 32, 37, 43].

PROCEDURE

Abdominal Assessment and Evaluation of Nutritional Status

DESCRIPTION

The abdominal cavity contains several of the body's vital organs: kidneys, ureters and bladder, alimentary canal, adrenal glands, gallbladder, liver, pancreas, spleen and internal gonads. The alimentary canal is a long tube approximately 27 feet in length in the adult, extending from the
mouth to the anus, and includes the esophagus, stomach, small and large intestines. Its function is
to ingest and digest food; absorb nutrients, electrolytes and water; and, excrete waste products.
The liver metabolizes carbohydrates, fats and proteins, and the adrenals produce corticosteroids
(glucocorticiods, mineralcorticoids, and androgens). The gallbladder stores bile used to emulsify
fats. The pancreas produces insulin for the utilization of glucose, and digestive juices for the breakdown of proteins, fats, and carbohydrates. The spleen serves as a filter for the reticulendothelial
system. The kidneys are responsible for the removal of water soluble waste products, and the production of renin, erythropoietin, and Vitamin D. The gonads consist of the internal and external
male and female reproductive organs (see Genitourinary Assessment).

PURPOSE

To assess the organs located in the abdominal cavity and to evaluate the client's nutritional status

EQUIPMENT

Health Assessment Forms
Stethoscope
Weight log

OUTCOMES

The client/caregiver will:

▶ report any signs of abdominal distress (indigestion, pain, vomiting, diarrhea, constipation, incontinence, dysuria)
▶ record dietary intake
▶ maintain adequate bowel/bladder function
▶ maintain weight log

ASSESSMENT DATA

Review client's history of gastrointestinal disorder, abdominal surgeries, patterns of bowel and
bladder elimination
Evaluate muscle mass and subcutaneous fat stores
Note nutritional intake, change in taste/swallowing
Document use of parenteral/enteral nutritional support
Evaluate status of dentition
Record date of last bowel movement

Review family history of gastrointestinal illnesses
Check for recent weight gain or loss, edema and ascites
Determine if client is currently pregnant
Note evidence of abdominal pain
Measure and record abdominal girth
Note results of stool hemacult, endoscopy, sigmoidoscopy, barium enema
Evaluate relevant laboratory data: iron, albumin, transferrin, retinol-binding protein, lymphocyte
    count, hemoglobin, hematocrit, cholesterol, glucose, folate, triglycerides
Observe for evidence of vitamin/mineral deficiency: dermatitis, fissures of lips and mouth, glossitis,
    neuromuscular irritability, hair loss

RELATED NURSING DIAGNOSES

Altered elimination
Altered nutrition
Alteration in comfort
Knowledge deficit
Anxiety
Constipation/Diarrhea
Incontinence
Fluid volume deficit

SPECIAL CONSIDERATIONS

Detailed assessments will need to be made on the initial visit and for all acutely ill clients. Document use of enteral/parenteral feeding formulae. Assess enteral tube placement or intravenous access site as appropriate. Evaluate functional status of feeding pumps/equipment. Evaluate client's feeding tolerance. Review weight log at each visit. Obtain relevant serum specimens for blood analyses as ordered.

TRANSCULTURAL CONSIDERATION

An interpreter will be needed for clients unable to speak or understand English
Darker skin pigmentation may obscure clinical findings in persons of color
Cultural food sanctions and restrictions will need to be considered in planning dietary modifica-
    tions
Consider use of the AT&T Language Line
See Culturological Assessment procedure for general overview of cultural considerations

▶ INTERVENTIONS

1. Wash hands.

Prevents transmission of microbes

2. Explain procedure.

Allays anxiety

Nutritional Assessment

1. Have client relate 24-hour food intake.

Indicates client's adequacy of nutritional intake

2. Use Food Guide Pyramid.
    bread-cereal: 6–11 servings daily
    fats: use sparingly
    vegetable: 3–4 servings daily

When using the Food Guide Pyramid be aware that no one food group contains all of the essential nutrients for

milk-cheese: 2–3 servings daily
meat-poulty-fish-beans: 2–3 servings daily
fruit: 2–4 servings daily

each category. Note that choices and amounts may be contraindicated for some therapeutic diets

2. Compute client's body mass index (BMI), divide body weight in kg by height in meters squared
    a. normal BMI
        women   = 19.1–27.3
        men   = 20.7–27.8
        children = not yet established

Objective assessment to determine presence of cachexia or obesity

Inspection

In the supine position, note contour, skin, symmetry, umbilicus, pulsations.

Detects presence of hernia (see Fig. 2-9), masses, jaundice, lesions, rashes, marked pulsations, peristalsis, cachexia, obesity, distension, scars, ostomies

Auscultation

1. Divide the abdomen into four quadrants.

To describe location of findings, the abdomen is divided into four sections by imaginery vertical and horizontal lines intersecting at the umbilicus

2. Systematically place the stethscope over each of the four areas listening for absence or presence of bowel sounds, move in clockwise direction (see Figure 2-10).

Assesses peristaltic activity

3. Listen for 2 to 5 minutes at each area.

Assesses peristaltic activity

4. Determine quality of bowel sounds (present, absent, hyperactive, hypoactive, borborygmi).

Assesses peristaltic activity

5. If aortic bruit is heard, discontinue assessing and notify physician immediately.

May indicate presence of abdominal aortic aneurysm

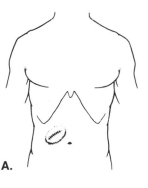

FIGURE 2-9 ▸ Hernia:. **A.** incisional; **B.** umbilical **A.**   **B.**

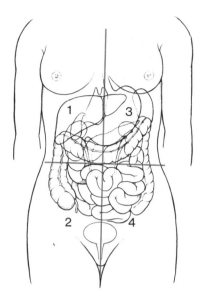

FIGURE 2-10 ▶ Four-region abdominal map: (1) right upper quadrant, (2) right lower quadrant, (3) left upper quadrant, (4) left lower quadrant.

Percussion

1. Percuss the abdomen in each of the four quadrants systematically moving in clockwise direction.

Notes normal tympanic sounds

2. Note areas of tympany and dullness.

Tympanic sounds indicate the presence of air, and dull sounds may indicate the presence of fluid, masses, or adipose tissue

3. Percuss the liver border.

An enlarge liver span indicates hepatomegaly

Palpation

1. Lightly palpate the abdomen in all four quadrants systematically moving in clockwise direction.

Detects presence of masses, organ enlargement, pain

2. Follow with deep palpation in all 4 quadrants.

Detects presence of masses, organ enlargement, pain

3. Observe for tenderness, masses, guarding.

Detects presence of masses, organ enlargement, pain

4. If tenderness is observed, press slowly and deeply into the area, let go quickly (perform at the end of the abdominal assessment).

Tests for rebound tenderness

5. Assess liver by having client take a deep breath while examiner places left hand under the client's back and right hand on the RUQ.

Normally the liver edge may be palpable or absent

6. Assess the spleen by having the client take a deep breath while examiner places left hand under the left side and the right hand on the LUQ.

Normally the spleen is not palpable

7. Percuss the costovertebral angle for evidence of kidney tenderness.

Normally the kidney area will not be tender

DOCUMENTATION
The following should be included in the nursing note:

All abnormal clinical findings and all follow-up action taken
The client/caregiver's ability to:
    plan and prepare a therapeutic diet as ordered
    maintain adequate bowel/bladder function
    report any symptoms of abdominal distress
    maintain oral hygiene
    monitor weight gain/loss
    correctly use all nutritional infusion devices and demonstrate ability to troubleshoot

INTERDISCIPLINARY COLLABORATION
Inform physician of abnormal findings and discuss need for possible referral for a gastroenterologist, or nutritionist. Consult with social worker to locate community client education programs for bulimia/anorexia, stress management, nutrition counseling, etc. [3, 10, 17–19, 20, 31, 32, 37, 41, 43].

PROCEDURE
Musculoskeletal Assessment

DESCRIPTION
The examination of the musculoskeletal system includes assessing the joints, long bones, spine, and gait. To evaluate structure and function, each joint is put through full range of motion, being careful to discontinue any action which results in joint pain. Any evidence of inflammation, irritation, contracture, or deformity is documented. An assessment of gait is performed to evaluate client's ability to ambulate safely and to determine the need for assistive devices.

PURPOSE
To examine the long bones, joints, spine, and client's ability to ambulate

EQUIPMENT
Health Assessment Forms
Tape measure

OUTCOMES
The client/caregiver will:

▶ Report any symptoms of pain or discomfort
▶ Demonstrate ability to ambulate safely and correctly use assistive devices
▶ Follow the treatment plan

ASSESSMENT DATA
Review client's history of bone or joint disease
Assess client's ability to function independently in ADLs

Check for evidence of osteoporosis
Determine extent of pain or discomfort, and note deformities and crepitation
Evaluate structural symmetry and alignment
Determine muscle strength and tone
Observe skin appearance over joints
Document use of assistive devices (walkers, canes, crutches, wheelchairs, scooters, etc.)

RELATED NURSING DIAGNOSES
Activity intolerance
Altered mobility
At risk for injury
Alteration in comfort
Knowledge deficit
Anxiety
Self-care deficit

SPECIAL CONSIDERATIONS
Detailed assessments will need to be made on the initial visit and for all acutely ill clients
In life-threatening situations body assessment areas will need to prioritized

TRANSCULTURAL CONSIDERATIONS
An interpreter will be needed for clients unable to speak or understand English
Darker skin pigmentation may obscure clinical findings in persons of color
Bone density varies among minority ethnic population, may be more dense in blacks and less dense in Asians
Consider use of AT&T Language Line.
See Culturological Assessment procedure for general overview of cultural considerations

▶ INTERVENTIONS

Intervention	Rationale
1. Wash hands.	*Prevents transmission of microbes*
2. Explain procedure.	*Allays anxiety*
3. If limb inequalities are noted: a. measure the arm from the acromion process to the tip of the second finger b. measure the leg from the anterosuperior iliacspine to the tibial malleolus	*Accurate measurements are necessary to enable comparison of findings over time*
4. Grade muscle strength. On a scale of 0–5: 0 = no detectable muscle contraction 1 = barely detectable contraction 2 = complete ROM with gravity eliminated 3 = complete ROM against gravity 4 = complete ROM against gravity and with some resistance 5 = complete ROM against gravity with full resistance	*Accurate measurements are necessary to enable comparison of findings over time*

Shoulder Assessment

1. Inspect and compare right and left joints (note redness, atrophy, deformity or rashes, pigmentation, scars).
2. Palpate the joint (note tenderness, swelling, heat, or masses).

3. Put joint through full range of motion (elevation, depression, flexion, extension, abduction, adduction, internal/external rotation). See Figure 2-11.
4. Observe for crepitus.

5. Have client shrug shoulders against resistance.

Shows any evidence of deformity

Indicates presence of inflammation, tumor formation

Indicates presence of contracture, bursitis, fracture

Occurs when articular joint surfaces are roughened as in arthritis

Assesses shoulder strength

Elbow Assessment

1. Inspect and compare right and left joints (note redness, atrophy, deformity or swelling rashes, pigmentation, scars).
2. Palpate the joint (note tenderness, swelling, heat, or masses).

Shows any evidence of deformity

Indicates presence of inflammation, tumor formation, irritation

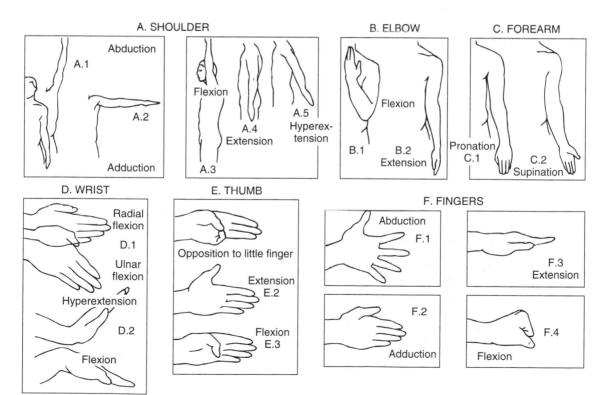

FIGURE 2-11 ▶ Upper extremities range of motion

3. Put joint through full range of motion (flexion, extension, pronation, supination). See Figure 2-11.	*Indicates presence of contracture, deformity*
4. Observe for crepitus.	*Occurs when articular joint surfaces are roughened as in arthritis*
5. Have client resist attempt to extend arm at elbow.	*Assesses arm strength*

Wrist and Hand Assessment

1. Inspect and compare joints of right and left hands (note redness, atrophy, deformity or swelling rashes, pigmentation, scars).	*Shows any evidence of deformity*
2. Palpate the joint (note tenderness, swelling, heat, or masses).	*Indicates presence of inflammation, tumor formation, irritation*
3. Put joint through full range of motion (flexion, extension, abduction, adduction, pronation, supination) See Figure 2-11.	*Indicates presence of contracture, nodules, deformity ulnar deviation, ankylosis, carpal tunnel syndrome*
4. Observe for crepitus.	*Occurs when articular joint surfaces are roughened as in arthritis*
5. Have client squeeze examiner's hand.	*Assesses hand strength*

Hip Assessment

1. Inspect and compare right and left joints (note redness, atrophy, deformity or swelling rashes, pigmentation, scars).	*Shows any evidence of deformity*
2. Palpate the joint (note tenderness, swelling, heat, or masses).	*Indicates presence of inflammation, tumor formation, irritation*
3. Put joint through full range of motion (flexion, extension, hyperflexion, abduction, adduction, internal/external rotation). See Figure 2-12.	*Indicates presence of contracture, deformity motion dysfunction*
4. Observe for crepitus.	*Occurs when articular joint surfaces are roughened as in arthritis*
5. Have client lift thigh against resistance.	*Assesses hip strength*

Knee Assessment

1. Inspect and compare right and left joints (note redness, atrophy, deformity or swelling rashes, pigmentation, scars).	*Shows any evidence of deformity*
2. Palpate the joint (note tenderness, swelling, heat, or masses).	*Indicates presence of inflammation, tumor formation, irritation*
3. Put joint through full range of motion (flexion, extension). See Figure 2-12.	*Indicates presence of contracture, fluid, deformity, injury, torn ligament*

A. LEGS

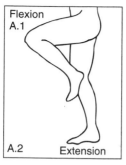

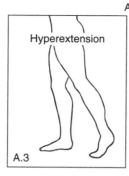

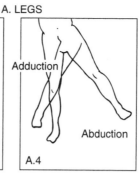

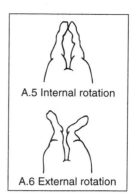

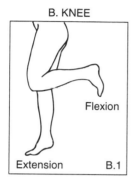

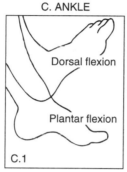

FIGURE 2-12 ▶ Lower extremities range of motion

4. Observe for crepitus.	*Occurs when articular joint surfaces are roughened in arthritis*
5. Have client resist extension of lower leg.	*Assesses leg strength*

Ankle and Foot Assessment

1. Inspect and compare right and left joints (note redness, atrophy, deformity or swelling rashes, pigmentation, scars).	*Shows any evidence of deformity*
2. Palpate the joint (note tenderness, swelling, heat or masses).	*Indicates presence of inflammation, tumor formation, irritation*
3. Put joint through full range of motion (internal/external rotation, eversion, inversion). See Figure 2-12.	*Indicates presence of contracture, bunion, deformity*
4. Have client plantar and dorsiflex foot.	*Assesses ankle strength against resistance*

Spinal Assessment

1. In standing position, inspect spinal curvatures (cervical, thoracic, lumbar, sacral).	*Shows any evidence of scoliosis, kyphosis, or lordosis (See Figure 2-13)*

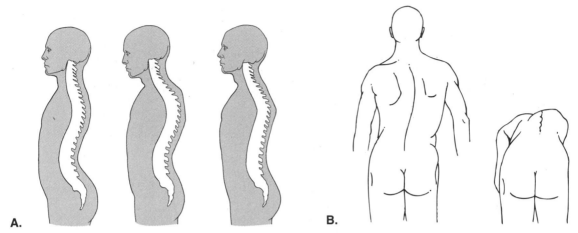

FIGURE 2-13 ▶ **A.** Spinal deformities: (left) lordosis; (center) kyphosis; (right) gibbus. **B.** scoliosis

2. Palpate the spinal processes (note tenderness, swelling, heat, or masses).

Indicates presence of inflammation, tumor formation, irritation

3. Put spine through full range of motion (hyperextension, rotation, lateral bending).

Indicates presence of injury, disc disease, deformity

4. Observe ability to walk a straight line note use of assistive devices.

Detects problems with ambulation (see Display 2-6)

DOCUMENTATION

The following should be included in the nursing note:

All abnormal clinical findings and follow up action taken
The client/caregiver's ability to:
    report evidence of joint discomfort, immobility
    demonstrate safe use of assistive devices
    observe for bone fracture
    perform mobility exercises as ordered
    follow the treatment plan

INTERDISCIPLINARY COLLABORATION

Inform physician of abnormal findings, and discuss with physician need to obtain consults for orthopedic specialist or physical therapist
Consider need to provide services of home health aide to assist with ADLs
Consult with social worker to determine eligibility for finanical assistance to purchase assistive devices
Contact DME supplier to order assistive devices [3, 10, 17–19, 31, 32, 37, 43]

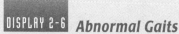

Abnormal Gaits

Ataxic Gait

The foot is raised high and strikes the ground suddenly with the entire sole. The person may stagger or fall to one side. Occurs with cerebellar disorders; alcohol or barbiturate toxicity.

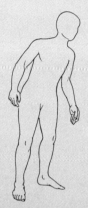

Ataxic gait

Parkinsonian Gait (Festinating)

Body bends forward, rigid, with flexion of elbows, wrists, hips, and knees. Steps are short and shuffling with feet barely leaving the ground. May walk on toes as though pushed. Starts slowly and gradually accelerates Sudden forward movement (propulsion) may continue until person can grasp some object for support. Occurs with Parkinson's disease and other basal ganglia defects.

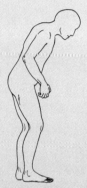

Parkinsonian gait

Hemiplegic Gait

One leg is paralyzed. The paralyzed leg is abducted and swung around so that the foot comes forward and to the front, or the paralyzed leg may be dragged forward in a semicircle. Occurs with unilateral upper motor neuron disorder, as in stroke.

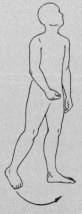

Hemiplegic gait

Scissors Gait

Legs cross of the thighs or knees with each step. Takes short steps. Very slow and awkward leg movements. Occurs with upper motor neuron disorders, as in stroke.

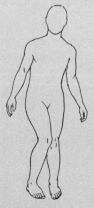

Scissors gait

(continued)

DISPLAY 2-6 *Abnormal Gaits* (Continued)

Steppage Gait

Foot and toes lifted high with knees flexed. Foot brought to ground suddenly, heel first, with slapping noise. Person watches ground to know where to place foot. Occurs with peripheral neuritis, late stages of diabetes, alcoholism, and chronic arsenic poisoning.

Waddling Gait

Feet wide apart, and stride resembles that of a duck. Regular steps. Occurs with congenital hip displacement with lordosis, muscular dystrophy.

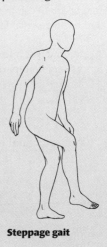

Steppage gait

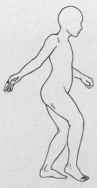

Waddling gait

PROCEDURE

Neurological Assessment

DESCRIPTION

The examination of the neurological system includes assessing the system's central and peripheral divisions. Because of the complexity of this body system, the nurse may need to complete this assessment in more than one home visit. The cranial nerves and motor and sensory systems are evaluated for any evidence of abnormality. The neurological assessment is performed together with the mental status, developmental, musculoskeletal, and head and neck assessments to complete a full evaluation of the motor, sensory, autonomic, cognitive, and behavioral elements of the physical examination.

PURPOSE

To examine the nervous system

EQUIPMENT

Health Assessment Forms
Opthalmoscope
Broken tongue blade
Cotton ball

Reflex hammer
Vials containing aromatic spices
Snellen eye chart

OUTCOMES
The client/caregiver will:

▶ Report any symptoms of sensory or motor impairment or changes in sensorium
▶ Demonstrate correct use of assistive devices (eyeglasses, hearing aids, crutches, canes, etc.)
▶ Maintain safety when ambulating
▶ Follow the plan of treatment

ASSESSMENT DATA
▶ Determine if client is taking any analgesics, central nervous system depressants, antipsychotics
▶ Screen for headaches, seizures, vertigo, syncope, visual disturbance, hemiparesis, dypsphagia or sensory-perceptual impairment
▶ Note changes in sensorium
▶ Observe motor function
▶ Determine need for hearing or visual aids
▶ Document findings of home safety assessment (throw rugs, stairs, structural integrity, etc.)

RELATED NURSING DIAGNOSES
At risk for injury
Impaired mobility
Self-care deficit
Altered sensory perception
Altered thought process

SPECIAL CONSIDERATIONS
Detailed assessments will need to be made on the initial visit and for all acutely ill clients
In life-threatening situations, body assessment areas will need to prioritized

TRANSCULTURAL CONSIDERATIONS
An interpreter will be needed for clients unable to speak or understand English
Consider use of AT&T Language Line
See Culturological Assessment procedure for general overview of cultural considerations

▶ INTERVENTIONS

1. Wash hands.	*Prevents transmission of microbes*
2. Explain procedure.	*Allays anxiety*

Cranial Nerve Assessment

1. Have client identify familiar odors.	*Determines function of CN 1 Olfactory Nerve*
2. Test visual fields and visual acuity.	*Determines function of CN 2 Optic Nerve*

3. Locate optic discs, evaluate cup margins.	*The width of the cup should not exceed one-half of the disc diameter*
4. Assess extraocular movements.	*Determines function of CN 3 Oculomotor Nerve*
5. Test pupillary reaction to light and accommodation.	*Detects pupillary response*
6. Inspect the eyelids for drooping.	*Determines function of CN 4 Trochlear Nerve*
7. Assess facial symmetry.	*Determines function of CN 5 Trigeminal Nerve*
8. Lightly stroke face with wisp of cotton.	*Determines function of CN 5 Trigeminal Nerve*
9. Assess direction of gaze.	*Determines function of CN 6 Abducens Nerve*
10. Observe for nystagmus.	*Detects the presence of sustained involuntary rhythmic movements of the eye*
11. Assess symmetrical movement of face.	*Determines function of CN 7 Facial Nerve*
12. Assess client's ability to identify salty or sweet taste on tip of tongue.	*Determines function of CN 7 Facial Nerve.*
13. Perform hearing tests.	*Determines function of CN 8 Acoustic Nerve*
14. Assess client's ability to identify salty or sweet taste at back of tongue.	*Determines function of CN 9 Glossopharyngeal Nerve*
15. Elicit gag reflex.	*Determines function of CN 10 Vagus Nerve*
16. Note hoarsenss of voice.	*Determines function of CN 10 Vagus Nerve*
17. Note symmetry of uvula and soft palate.	*Determines function of CN 10 Vagus Nerve*
18. Have client shrug shoulders and turn head against resistance.	*Determines function of CN 11 Spinal Accessory Nerve*
19. Have client protrude tongue and move from side to side.	*Determines function of CN 12 Hypoglossal*

Motor System Assessment

1. Observe gait (see musculoskeletal system).	*Detects abnormality of cerebellar function, upper motor neuron disorders, basal ganglia defects, peripheral neuritis, alcoholism, muscular dystrophy, congenital hip displacement*
2. Check coordination (finger to nose, rapid finger to thumb, heel down shin).	*Assesses fine motor skills*
3. Check reflexes (see Display 2-7 for scoring & recording reflexes).	*Detects presence of motor neuron disorders*

DISPLAY 2-7 *Documenting Reflexes*

Grading Deep Tendon Reflexes

Deep tendon reflexes are graded on a scale of 0 to 4:

0 No response
1+ Diminished (hypoactive)
2+ Normal
3+ Increased (may be interpreted as normal)
4+ Hyperactive (hyperreflexia)

The deep tendon responses and plantar reflexes are commonly recorded on stick figures. The arrow points downward if the plantar response is normal and upward if the response is abnormal.

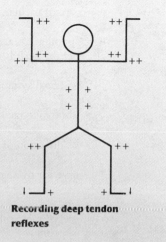

Recording deep tendon reflexes

a. biceps—flex the arm at the elbow 45 degrees with the reflex hammer strike the antecubital fossa, observe for flexion of the elbow (see Figure 2-14)
b. triceps—flex the arm at the elbow 90 degrees with the reflex hammar strike the strike the triceps tendon and observe for extension of the elbow (see Figure 2-15)
c. brachioradialis—with the arm resting comfortably on the leg strike the brachioradialis tendon
d. patellar—flex the knee 90 degrees, with the reflex hammer strike the patellar tendon just below the knee, observe for extension of the lower leg (see Figure 2-16)
e. achilles—flex the knee 90 degrees, support foot with hand and with the reflex hammer strike the the achilles tendon and observe for plantar flexion of the foot (see Figure 2-17)

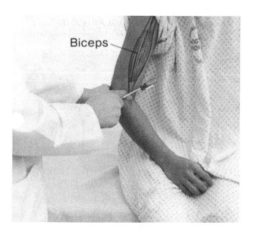

FIGURE 2-14 ▶ Biceps reflex testing

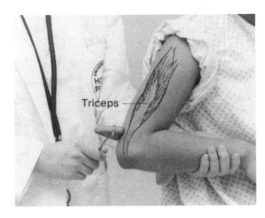

FIGURE 2-15 ▶ Triceps reflex testing

e. ankle clonus—flex the knee, dorsiflex the foot and
hold in the flexed position. Observe for the absence of
rhythmic oscillating movements between dorsiflexion
and plantar flexion

4. Perform Romberg Test— have client stand with feet
together and eyes closed. Client should maintain
equilibrium.

Evaluates ability to maintain balance

Sensory System Assessment

Check sharp and dull sensation of extremities.
  a. use a wisp of cotton to elicit dull sensation
  b. use broken edge of tongue blade to elicit sharp sensation

Detects presence of upper or lower neuron disease

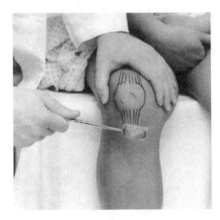

FIGURE 2-16 ▶ Patellar reflex testing

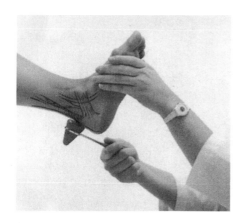

FIGURE 2-17 ▶ Achilles reflex testing

DOCUMENTATION

The following should be included in the nursing note:

All abnormal clinical findings and follow-up action taken
The client's motor and sensory function
The client/caregiver's ability to:
    maintain a safe environment
    report any symptoms of impaired cognitive, motor, or sensory impairment
    demonstrate correct use of assistive devices
    perform therapeutic exercises as ordered
    follow the treatment plan

INTERDISCIPLINARY COLLABORATION

Inform physician of abnormal findings, and discuss with the physician the need to obtain consults for speech-language pathology and audiology; neurology; physical or occupational therapy. Consult with social worker to assist in determining eligibility for financial assistance and in locating community resources. Contact DME supplier to order assistive devices and support mattresses. Consider need to order home health aide to assist in ADLs [3, 10, 17–19, 31, 32, 37, 43]

PROCEDURE
Integumentary Assessment

DESCRIPTION

The integumentary assessment is performed to examine skin surfaces and mucus membranes. The examination includes an assessment of the skin, hair, and nails. The skin is evaluated for evidence of infection, infestation, irritation, erosion, and loss of integrity. Alteration in skin integrity compromises the skin's ability to protect against microbial invasion and fluid loss, regulate body temperature, produce vitamin D, repair wounds, excrete certain body toxins, and act as a specialized receptor for sensory perception. The chapter on Complex Wound Management describes the procedures for wound staging, application of dressings, assessment of healing, and removal of staples and sutures.

PURPOSE
To examine all body skin surfaces and to identify normal and abnormal findings

EQUIPMENT
Health assessment forms
Gloves

OUTCOMES
The client/caregiver will:

► Report any symptoms of altered skin integrity
► Demonstrate ability to maintain cleanliness of the skin
► Follow the plan of treatment

ASSESSMENT DATA
Observe and document skin color, pigmentation, temperature, texture, turgor, hygiene, lesions, and masses
Describe all wounds and exudates
Report any evidence of infection, infestation, or inflammation
Evaluate skin surfaces over all bony prominences
Record shape and configuration of nails and nailbed color
Monitor nutritional status, oxygenation, circulation, complications of debilitating disease, responses to radiation therapy, and physiological changes associated with advanced age

RELATED NURSING DIAGNOSES
Altered skin integrity
At risk for infection
Altered tissue perfusion
Altered nutrition
Altered self-care deficit
Altered self-esteem
Altered body image

SPECIAL CONSIDERATIONS
Examination of the skin is performed as a head-to-toe assessment. At-risk skin surfaces are those covering bony prominences and areas in direct contact with tubes. In addition to evaluating the skin for evidence of erosion, infection, infestation, and injury, an assessment will also need to be made of all injuries where abuse may be suspected. The nurse should carefully assess hidden areas such as the axillae, soles of the feet, palms of the hands, inner thighs and buttocks, observing for bruising, burns, abrasions, or tenderness. Bruising that shows evidence of various stages of healing may indicate abuse. Examine the client in a private, quiet area of the home and be sensitive to the psychosocial issues associated with abuse. If abuse is suspected a report must be filed. Follow agency protocol in the reporting and follow-up of such findings. Young children, the elderly, and disabled clients will be more at risk for injury secondary to falls.

Infant/child—The skin surface of the infant and child is smoother than that of the adult. The skin of the newborn will flake and shed and may be covered with lanugo. The underlying subcutaneous layer is poorly developed in the neonate, and the hair on the head sheds at about 2 to 3 months of age and is replaced by more premanent hair. Mongolian spots, flat pink areas on the back of the neck, and a papular rash may be evident for the first few days of life.

Adolescent—The sweat glands become more active during adolescence producing an increase in sweating, and increasing hormone levels cause an oily appearance to the skin which may lead to the development of acne.

Pregnancy—The pregnant client may demonstrate a hyperpigmentation of the face, nipples, areolae, axillae, and vulva. More fat may be deposited under the dermal layer, and the skin will thicken. The sweat glands may accelerate activity and vasodilation may occur in response to increased metabolism. Striae gravidarum may appear on the abdomen, thigh, and breasts.

Elderly—The skin of the older client will appear drier, thinner, and less elastic. Subcutaneous tissue decreases producing a more angular appearance. The hair will grey and pubic and axillary hair will decrease in density and distribution. Hair distribution on extremities may decrease secondary to the development of peripheral vascular disease. Nail growth slows and the nails become thicker, brittle, and yellow in color.

TRANSCULTURAL CONSIDERATIONS

Color changes in the dark-skinned client are best noted in the sclera, conjunctiva, oral cavity, lips, nailbeds, palms of the hands, and soles of the feet. Freckling of the oral cavity may be evident, and the sclera may naturally have a yellow-brownish coloration. The lips and gums of some dark-skinned clients may have a bluish hue, which can be mistaken for cyanosis.

Some Asian cultures may perform a home remedy known as "coining," a traditional healing practice which involves placing a heated coin onto the skin. A burn on the skin in the shape of the coin may be produced, and may be mistakenly identified as evidence of abuse.

Consider use of AT&T Language Line. See Culturological Assessment procedure for general overview of cultural considerations.

▌ INTERVENTIONS

1. Wash hands.	*Prevents transmission of microbes*
2. Explain procedure.	*Allays anxiety*

Skin

Inspection

1. Observe all skin surfaces and evaluate for the following characteristics.
   Hygiene
   Color: jaundice, erythema, pallor, cyanosis
   Pigmentation: color distribution
   Bleeding: ecchymosis, petecchiae, purpura
   Thickness
   Symmetry
2. Examine skin for presence of lesions, measure and record characteristics (see Display 2-8).
   Measure width, depth, length in cm
   Note location and pattern of distribution
   Describe exudate, color, blanching, and texture
3. Note characteristics of any skin alterations, and describe. Measure width, depth, length, and diameter in cm and note pattern of distribution.

Documents baseline findings of skin assessment

Documents abnormal physical findings

Provides basis for comparison over time

Palpation

1. Feel skin for evidence of moisture.

Minimal oiliness and perspiration should be present

DISPLAY 2-8 *Skin Changes Associated with Malignancy*

► sores that do not heal
► persistent lump or swelling
► newly formed or change in nevi (moles)

2. Note skin temperature.	*Skin temperature will range from cool to warm to touch and will be affected by environmental conditions and pathophysiological states*
3. Feel the skin for evidence of smoothness.	*Extensive skin roughness may be evidence of hyperkeratoses or callous formation*
4. Assess turgor by rolling skin on forearm between thumb and forefinger.	*Evaluates skin resilience*
5. Assess for evidence of edema and score (see Peripheral Vascular Assessment).	*Evaluate degree of fluid volume excess*

Hair

Inspection and Palpation

1. Evaluate color and texture.	*Hair should be shiny, smooth and resilient with color variation from blond to black to grey*
2. Note quantity and distribution.	*Hair loss may be generalized or localized*

Nails

Inspection and Palpation

1. Observe the shape and configuration.	*Nail should be smooth and flat and slightly convex*
2. Note color.	*Nailbed color should be variations of pink, with pigment bands in dark-skinned clients*
3. Determine capillary refill.	*Assesses tissue perfusion*
4. Inspect nail folds for evidence of redness, swelling, pain, exudate, warts, cysts, tumors.	*Provides evidence growths, infection, trauma*
5. Palpate nail plate for texture, firmness, thickness, uniformity, adherence.	*Evaluates presence of infection, trauma, ischemia*

DOCUMENTATION
The following should be included in the nursing note:

Date and time of interview
Condition of all skin surfaces
Nutritional status
Oxygenation
Circulatory status
Evidence of exudate, lesions, inflammation, masses
Wound measurement
Use of support surfaces/mattresses
Stage of healing surgical wounds
Stage of decubitus ulcers
Prescribed dressing change protocol
Ability of client/caregiver to follow the treatment plan

INTERDISCIPLINARY COLLABORATION
Depending on the clinical findings, the nurse will discuss with the client's physician the need to consult with the physical therapist; WOC nurse; nutritionist; or other health discipline in meeting the client's needs

Consult with the social worker to determine client eligibility for reimbursement for air flotation devices or support surfaces and complex wound dressings.

Contact DME supplier for support mattresses and/or surfaces, complex dressing supplies for wound management

Obtain orders for home health aide to assist with activities of daily living, if needed [3, 10, 17–19, 31, 32, 37, 43]

PROCEDURE
Genitourinary Assessment

DESCRIPTION
The genitourinary assessment is performed to evaluate the urinary and reproductive systems of the male and female. The examination includes assessing the rectum, urinary elimination, the internal structures of the female reproductive system, and the inguinal areas and external structures of the male reproductive system

PURPOSE
To determine normal and abnormal clinical findings of the reproductive and urinary systems

EQUIPMENT
Health Assessment Forms
Gloves
Speculum
Light source
Lubricant
Specimen containers

OUTCOMES

The client/caregiver will:

Verbalize understanding of purpose of the examination
Report any abnormal clinical findings
Ventilate feelings of concern

ASSESSMENT DATA

Determine onset of menarche or menopause
Record obstetrical history
Ascertain history of infection: sexually transmitted disease (STD) or HIV
Note evidence of abnormal bleeding, discharge, or presence of masses
Assess use of contraceptive devices, medications, or surgical intervention (vasectomy/tubal ligation)
Obtain history of cancer, diabetes, thyroid or adrenal disorders
Document any changes in urination or renal disorders
Determine if female client performs breast self examination (BSE) or if male client performs testicular self examination (TSE)
Note maternal use of diethylstilbesterol (DES)

RELATED NURSING DIAGNOSES

At risk for infection
Rape trauma syndrome
Altered sexual pattern
Sexual dysfunction
Knowledge deficit
Altered urinary elimination

SPECIAL CONSIDERATIONS

A detailed male and female genitourinary assessment is not routinely performed in the home setting. An invasive genitourinary assessment must have clear medical orders and must be performed by nurses with advanced training.

The female genital structures are evaluated by inspection and palpation, using a vaginal speculum to inspect the internal structures. Many women will express concerns regarding the procedure. Time should be taken to answer all questions, to explain the procedure, and to respect issues related to cultural considerations and need to maintain modesty. The presence of a significant other or family member may be requested to provide support. The lithotomy position may not be possible for women with skeletal deformity, advanced age, or some musculoskeletal disorders.

The male genitalia are examined by inspection and palpation. The client should stand facing the examiner to faciliate the examination of the inguinal areas. As with the female client, time should be taken to answer all questions, to explain the procedure, and to respect cultural issues. During the examination, the male client may experience an erection. Should this occur, the nurse should reassure the client and proceed with the examination. The presence of a significant other or family member may be requested to provide support.

TRANSCULTURAL CONSIDERATIONS

An interpreter will be needed for clients unable to speak or understand English
Darker skin pigmentation may obscure clinical findings in persons of color. Observe for color changes in mucus membranes, conjunctiva, sclera, nailbeds, or palmar surfaces of the hands and feet.

Some cultures may not support exposure of genital structures, especially for the female client. Care will need to be taken to ensure proper draping and maintainence of modesty.

Consider use of the AT&T Language Line.

See Culturological Assessment procedure for general overview of cultural considerations.

▶ INTERVENTIONS

1. Wash hands.	*Prevents transmission of microbes*
2. Explain all procedures.	*Allays anxiety*

Female Examination

1. Instruct client to empty her bladder.	*Client will be less likely to feel the urge to void during examination.*
obtain urine specimen for analysis or culture as indicated by symptomatology	*Laboratory findings will document presence of infection or renal dysfunction*
2. Assist the client to assume lithotomy position.	*Permits visualization of external structures and facilitates the intravaginal assessment*
3. Drape client.	*Prevents unnecessary exposure*
4. Inspect the external genitals.	*Observe for excoriation, rashes, or lesions which may suggest inflammatory or infectious processes.*
spread the labia majora and observe clitoris, urinary meatus, and vaginal os (see Figure 2-18)	*Watch for bulging of the labia which may suggest a hernia*
5. Palpate Skene's Glands (see Figure 2-19). a. insert index finger into vaginal opening b. move finger from inside to outside of the vagina to evaluate anterior vaginal wall	*Observe for cystic nodules suggestive of sebaceous cysts. Note presence of warts, ulcers, or lesions.* *Observe for discharge or tenderness which may indicate presence of infection*
6. Palpate Bartholin's Glands (see Figure 2-20). a. insert index finger into lower lateral aspect of the vagina and place thumb opposite the labia majora b. squeeze the skin between the thumb and index finger	*Observe for presence of Bartholin cyst, infection, masses, or tenderness*
7. Evaluate vaginal musculature (see Figure 2-21). a. insert index finger 2–4 cm into the vaginal os b. instruct client to squeeze the vaginal opening close c. instruct the client to bear down	*Note presence of swelling or discharge caused by trauma. Observe for lesions, masses, or fissures Observe for bulging of the vaginal wall and urinary incontinence suggestive of cystocele, and for protrusion of the cervix indicating uterine prolapse*
8. Insert speculum (see Figure 2-22).	*The size of the speculum used*

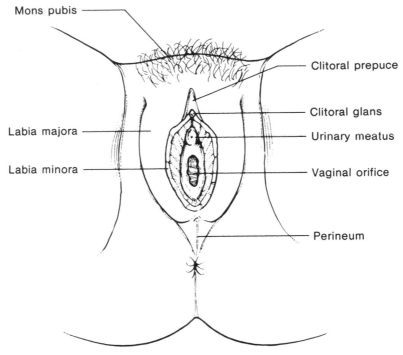

FIGURE 2-18 ▶ External female genitals

a. warm speculum under running water
b. insert index and middle finger into the vagina and press down
c. direct the speculum over the finger into the vagina at a 45–60 degree angle
d. remove finger and rotate the blade into position

will be determined by age of the woman and size of the vagina. Typically, the Graves speculum will be used in most adult women and the Pederson speculum

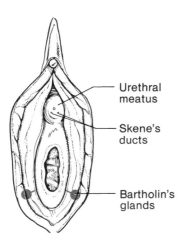

FIGURE 2-19 ▶ Location of Skene's ducts and Bartholin's glands

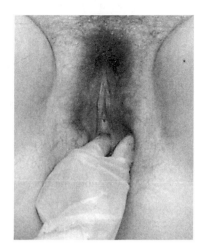

FIGURE 2-20 ▶ Bartholin's gland palpation

Note: If cultures or smears are to be obtained, do not use water or gel to lubricate the speculum

9. Inspect the cervix (see Figure 2-23).
   a. open the blade and inspect the cervix
   b. lock blades in the open position
   c. observe for lesions, tears, drainage
10. Obtain a culture.
    a. use a sterile cotton-tipped applicator to collect a specimen from the vagina and/or cervix
    b. spread the specimen onto an agar plate or place in a culture medium to send to the lab

will be used for the adolescent, geriatric, or female adult who has never delivered

Projection or deviation of the cervix may indicate a pelvic or uterine mass. Lacerations may indicate trauma.

Screens for presence of infectious organisms

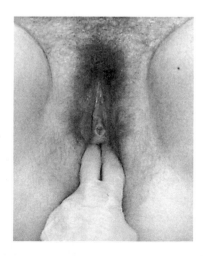

FIGURE 2-21 ▶ Evaluating vaginal musculature

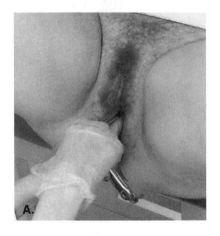

A.

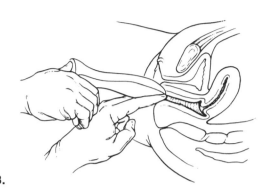

B.

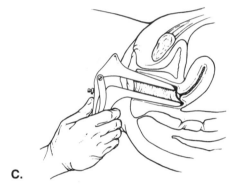

C.

FIGURE 2-22 ▶ **A.** Insert the vaginal speculum;. **B.** vaginal speculum insertion; **C.** vaginal speculum in place

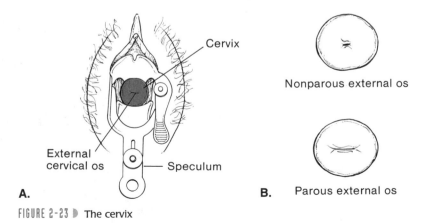

Cervix

Nonparous external os

External cervical os

Speculum

Parous external os

A.

B.

FIGURE 2-23 ▶ The cervix

THE PAP SMEAR IS NOT TYPICALLY PERFORMED IN THE HOME SETTING. IF ORDERED, HOWEVER, ONLY A SPECIALLY TRAINED ADVANCED PRACTICE NURSE SHOULD OBTAIN THE SPECIMEN FOLLOWING AGENCY POLICY AND GUIDELINES.

11. To obtain a Papanicolaou (PAP) smear from the vaginal pool:
    a. use a cotton-tipped applicator to obtain cells from the vaginal mucosa below the cervix
    b. smear the specimen onto a slide and spray with fixative

The PAP smear screens for cervical cancer. The client should be instructed to not douche, tub bathe, engage in intercourse, or insert vaginal medications for 24 hours prior to the examination.

12. To obtain a PAP smear from cervical cells:
    a. use a spatula to obtain a specimen from the cervical os rotating 360 degrees in one direction.
    b. smear the specimen onto a slide and spray with fixative

13. Inspect the vaginal wall.
    a. while slowly removing the speculum, inspect the vaginal walls
    b. keep the speculum open until the cervix is no longer visible
    c. allow the blades to close slowly
    d. remove the speculum with the blades in the completely closed position

A bluish coloration of the vaginal mucosa may indicate pregnancy. Anemia may be associated with a paleness in color of the vaginal wall.

14. Palpate the vagina and cervix.
    a. lubricate and insert gloved index and middle finger of the dominant hand into the vagina (see Figure 2-24)
    b. flex fingers to palpate vaginal wall
    c. note presence of nodules, masses or tenderness
    d. place the nondominant hand on the client's abdomen and press to push the pelvic organs in place for the intravaginal hand to palpate.
    e. determine the version of the uterus (see Figure 2-25)
    f. determine the mobility of the uterus

15. Perform rectal examination.
    a. change gloves
    b. insert gloved lubricated index finger into the rectum

The bimanual pelvic examination is performed to assess the uterus, determine the presence of pain, nodules, or tumors

The uterus may be retroverted or retroflexed

The uterus should bounce freely between the abdominal and intravaginal han

Screens for evidence of masses or tenderness

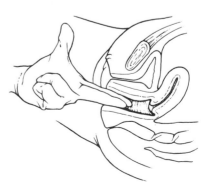

FIGURE 2-24 ▶ Vaginal palpation

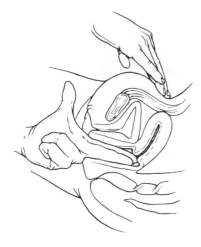

FIGURE 2-25 ▶ Bimanual palpation: Uterus

   c. palpate the anal canal
   d. palpate the cervix
16. Complete the examination.
   a. remover fingers and wipe lubricant from external structures
   b. assist client to sitting position
   c. provide privacy for client to redress
   d. remove gloves wash hands

Maintain modesty and client comfort

Male Examination

1. Instruct client to empty his bladder.
   obtain urine specimen for analysis or culture as indicated by symptomatology

Client will be less likely to feel the urge to void during examination.

Laboratory findings will document presence of infection or renal dysfunction

2. Inspect and palpate the penis.
   a. retract the foreskin of the uncircumscribed male
   b. observe the glans
   c. inspect the external urinary meatus by compressing the glans anteriorly and posteriorly between the thumb and forefinger. (see Figure 2-26)

Note presence of phimosis (fixed foreskin), paraphimosis (foreskin fixed in retracted position), hypospadias (ventrally located meatus), or epispadias (dorsally located meatus). The penis should feel firm, smooth, and non-tender, and should have no discharge.

3. Inspect and palpate the scrotum
   a. displace the penis to the side to observe the scrotal sac.
   b. lift the sac to observe the posterior aspect
   c. if the scrotum is enlarged, place a flashlight under the sac to observe for transillumination of the scrotum

Examination of the scrotum is performed to assess for the presence of undescended or absent testes, edema nodules, hydrocele, spermatocele, or varicocele

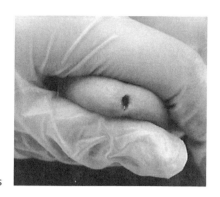

FIGURE 2-26 ▶ Inspecting the urinary meatus

d. inspect one testicle at a time by grasping between thumb and forefinger gently squeeze to detect the testicle (see Figure 2-27)
e. palpate the epididymis by feeling posteriorly for a comma-like structure (see Figure 2-28)
f. palpate for the vas deferens by moving anteriorly from the epididymis to the vas deferens
4. Observe for evidence of hernia.
    a. have client bear down while observing for bulging in the abdomen
    b. insert gloved finger into the inguinal canal and have client cough while feeling for presence of viscus against finger (see Figure 2-29)
    c. palpate scrotum as above

5. Instruct the client in self testicular examination (TSE). See Display 2-10.
    a. have the client examine his testicles each month
    b. usually performed in the shower
    c. hold the scrotum in the palm of the hand and use the thumb and first two fingers to feel for an egg-

In the male client there are three common types of hernias: indirect inguinal, direct inguinal, and femoral (see Display 2-9)

Bulging that increases with straining indicates presence of hernia

Clients from 13 years to adulthood should be encouraged to perform TSE. Testicular cancers are highest in young men between 15 and 34 years of age.

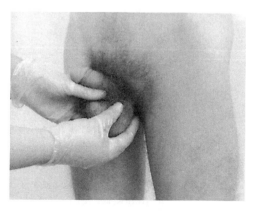

FIGURE 2-27 ▶ Scrotal palpation

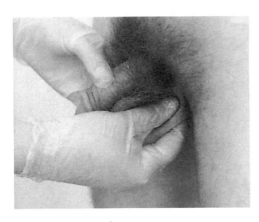

FIGURE 2-28 ▶ Palpating the epididymis

DISPLAY 2-9 *Inguinal and Femoral Hernia!*

Indirect Inguinal Hernias

An indirect inguinal hernia is a herniation through the inguinal canal. The hernia may be felt with the fingertip as a bulge in the canal or may extend beyond the canal into the scrotum. Indirect inguinal hernias may be detected by inserting your index finger into the inguinal canal.

Direct Inguinal Hernia

A direct inguinal hernia does not travel through the inguinal canal; rather, the hernia sac protrudes anteriorly through the abdominal wall. During inguinal canal palpation, the hernia displaces the examining finger forward.

Alternatively, a direct hernia may be felt as a bulge between the thumb and forefinger when palpating the skin around the external canal as the person bears down. Direct inguinal hernias rarely descend into the scrotum.

Femoral Hernia

A femoral hernia may be detected below the inguinal ligament and medial to the femoral pulse as a visible or palpable bulge. Femoral hernias are more common in women.

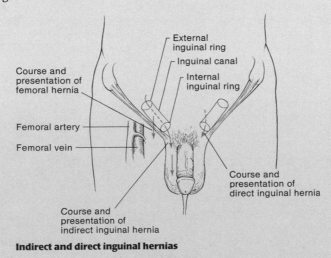

Indirect and direct inguinal hernias

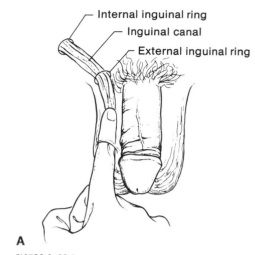

Internal inguinal ring
Inguinal canal
External inguinal ring

A

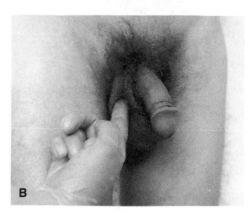

B

FIGURE 2-29 ▶ Inquinal renal palpation

shaped and movable organ that is non-tender to touch. The epididymis should feel slightly softer to the touch.

6. Insert a gloved, lubricated index finger into the rectum
   a. help the client to assume a sims position or to bend over at the waist.
   b. palpate the anterior rectal wall for the two-lobed structure of the posterior prostate gland

7. Complete the examination
   a. wipe lubricant from external structures
   b. assist client to sitting position
   c. provide privacy for client to redress
   d. remove gloves, wash hands

Early detection improves prognosis.

The prostate may be enlarged indicating benign prostatic hypertrophy or tender indicating prostatits, or hard and irregular indicating cancer
Maintain modesty and client comfort

DOCUMENTATION
The following should be included in the nursing note:

Document any abnormal clinical findings (penile, vaginal/urethral discharge, pain, masses, lesions, hernias, hemorrhoids) and report measures taken to follow-up
Document client's ability to perform BSE/TSE
Record use of contraceptive devices, medications, or surgeries

INTERDISCIPLINARY COLLABORATION
Inform physician of abnormal findings
Consider need to consult gynecologist, protologist, or urologist.
Locate community client education programs for HIV, and breast/uterine/testicular cancer awareness programs or support groups [3, 10, 17–19, 32, 37]

Testicular Self-Examination

Screening Recommendations

Monthly testicular self-examination (TSE) is recommended by the American Cancer Society for early detection and cure of testicular cancer.

Characteristics of Testicular Tumors

An established testicular tumor is palpable as an irregular, non-tender, fixed mass. A dragging sensation or heaviness may be reported. Nearby lymph node enlargement is rarely noted because the scrotal lymphatics drain deep within the abdominal cavity.

Procedure

1. TSE is performed as a 3-minute examination, preferably after a warm bath or shower when the scrotal skin is relaxed and easy to manipulate.
2. Examine each testicle along a horizontal plane by rolling the skin between the thumb and forefinger of each hand (A).
3. Repeat the procedure by feeling for lumps or other abnormalities along the vertical plane (B). Perform this examination on each testis. It is normal to find one testis larger than the other. Any hard lumps or nodules should be reported to a health professional.

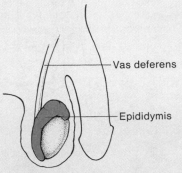

Vas deferens

Epididymis

Normal anatomy

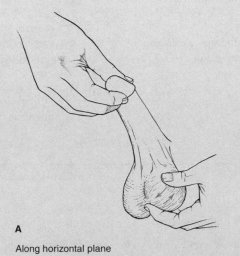

A

Along horizontal plane

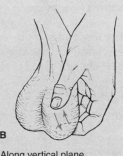

B

Along vertical plane

Antepartal Assessment

DESCRIPTION
The antepartal assessment is performed to evaluate the status of the mother and fetus. At-risk antepartal homecare clients must be monitored for the development of potential complications. The examination includes a head-to-toe physical assessment of the mother, fetal height measurement, auscultation of fetal heart tones, and performance of Leopold's Manuevers. The mother's psychosocial orientation is also assessed and supportive interventions are implemented, to allow client opportunity to ventilate concerns, and to network with others who may be undergoing or who have had similiar experiences.

PURPOSE
To assess maternal and fetal well being and the progression of the pregnancy and to evaluate fetal development.

EQUIPMENT
Fetoscope/doppler
Thermometer
Sphygmomanometer
Stethoscope
Measuring tape
Health Assessment Forms

OUTCOMES
The client/caregiver will:

▶ Follow prescribed therapeutic diet
▶ Demonstrate normal weight gain and physiological changes of pregnancy
▶ Verbalize knowledge of untoward symptoms and appropriate measures to follow as prescribed
▶ Ventilate feelings of concern

ASSESSMENT DATA
Document date of last menstrual period (LMP) and expected date of confinement (EDC)
Maternal vital signs
Fetal heart tones and fetal kick counts (after the 12th week)
Determine gestational age in weeks
Note any evidence of vaginal bleeding or discharge, uterine pain/contractions, edema, epigastric pain, visual changes, headache
Determine client's psychosocial adjustment to the current pregnancy
Obtain history of previous deliveries
Document physical assessment findings
Obtain and record laboratory data as ordered: hematology, cytology, biochemistries, microbiology, virology
Note effects of prescribed regimen on family dynamics
Ascertain any history of infection (sexually transmitted disease, HIV)
Assess client support systems, environment, social issues

RELATED NURSING DIAGNOSES
At risk for altered nutrition
Fatigue
At risk for altered family process

At risk for altered parenting
At risk for spiritual distress
At risk for altered sexual patterns

SPECIAL CONSIDERATIONS

The perinatal client can be referred to homecare from the hospital, physician office, or the client's home. To maintain modesty, the homecare environment must contain a private area in which to perform the antepartal assessment. Prior to positioning the client, the nurse will need to assess the client's ability to assume the supine and semi-Fowler's positions. The internal vaginal/rectal examination (see Genitourinary Assessment) of the pregnant client will be performed only by the physician, or by the nurse with advanced training and certification (nurse practitioner or nurse midwife).

Normal Physiological Changes in the Pregnant Client

Integumentary—Hyperpigmentation may be noted over the cheeks and forehead, and a dark brown line may extend from the umbilicus to the pubic bone. Spider nevi may appear on the face, chest and abdomen, and stretch marks may appear on the breasts, abdomen and thighs. Increased venous pressure in the lower extremities may result in the development of benign, localized edema of the the ankles

Genitourinary—Development of hemorrhoids may occur during the latter part of the pregnancy. If present, the nurse should observe the hemorrhoids for size, extent, location, pain, bleeding or infection. Hyperpigmentation of the labia and vulva may be noted. The vaginal wall will take on a bluish hue and become slightly edematous. The cervix will develop a bluish color, and the uterus will enlarge, soften, and flex at the junction.

Breasts—Nipple and breast engorgement will occur during the second month through to term and lactation. Week 16 through term, colostrum may be secreted from the nipples.

Musculoskeletal—A waddling gait will be noted when the client ambulates. The normal spinal curvature will change and lumbar lordosis will be evident as a result of the enlarging uterus.

Cardiovascular—The heart rate, diastolic blood pressure and respiratory rate will all slightly increase. After the seventh month, thoracic breathing will replace abdominal breathing. A soft systolic (grade II/IV) murmur may be heard during the third trimester, and the PMI may be laterally displaced by 1 cm.

Gastrointestinal—The client may complain of mild nausea during the first trimester, and may complain of constipation through to term. Stools may be dark in color due to the intake of prescribed iron medication.

TRANSCULTURAL CONSIDERATIONS

An interpreter will be needed for clients unable to speak or understand English. Consider use of AT&T Language Line. See the Culturological Assessment procedure for a general overview of cultural considerations.

▶ INTERVENTIONS

1. Wash hands.

   Prevents transmission of microbes

2. Explain procedure.

   Allays anxiety

3. Allow client to ventilate concerns.

   Provides emotional support

4. Observe interactions with family members and significant others.

   Assesses family dynamics

Fundal Height Measurement

1. Have the client empty her bladder.

2. Assist client to assume position of comfort (supine or semi-Fowler's).

3. Use finger breadths to determine relationship of the fundus to the umbilicus (one or two fingers above/below the umbilicus).

4. When the fundus extends above the umbilicus, the uterus can be measured with a tape measure (see Figure 2-31).
   a. place the end of the tape at the symphysis pubis
   b. identify height of fundus
   c. measure the distance in centimeters from the symphysis pubis to the top of the fundus
5. Assist the client to a sitting position. Observe for orthopnea, syncope, vertigo.

A full bladder will cause dis comfort during the examination

This position allows for an accurate abdominal assessment

The fundus normally increases in size at a rate of 1 cm per week until the client reaches term (see Figure 2-30).

A decrease in fundal height at the end of pregnancy signals the onset of pelvic engagement of the presenting part.

The fundal height in cm should coincide with the gestational age of the fetus. Notify MD if a difference of more than 2cm/2weeks is noted.

A shift in blood pressure can occur resulting from weight and position changes of the uterus on the vena cava

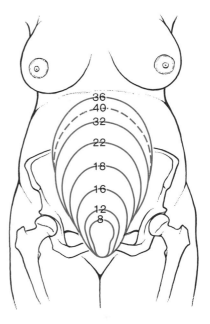

FIGURE 2-30 ▶ Fundal height and gestational age.

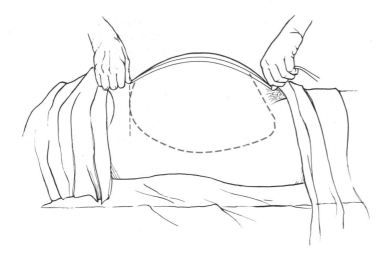

FIGURE 2-31 ▷ Fundal height measurement

Auscultation of Fetal Heart Tones (FHT)

1. Assist the client to assume a semi-Fowler's position.

   The semi-Fowler's position allows the nurse to assess the entire abdomen.

2. Apply contact gel and place the fetoscope or Doppler over the area between the symphysis pubis and the umbilicus. (see Figure 2-32).

   The Doppler will detect FHTs at the 10th - 12th week of gestation.

   The fetoscope will detect FHTs at the 18th to 20th week of gestation

3. Count FHT for 60 seconds.

   Normal FHTs are regular and range from 120–160 beats/minute

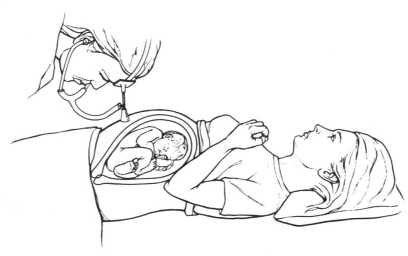

FIGURE 2-32 ▷ Fetal heart ascultation

4. If FHT <100 BPM take the pulse of the mother.

5. Contact MD immediately if FHT are less than 110/min or greater than 160/min.

Differentiates between uterine souffle and FHTs
Slow or increased rate indicates fetal compromise

Leopold's Manuevers

1. Assist client to position of comfort supine with knees flexed on pillow or semi-Fowler's position.
   a. First manuever: fundal palpation- using both hands, gently but firmly palpate the abdomen for uterine position/firmness palpate the midline and right and left quadrants (see Figure 2-33). [Prior to 13 weeks gestation the uterus will only be palpable using the bimanual pelvic examination, a procedure which is performed by the physician or advanced practice nurse]
   b. Second manuever: lateral palpation—use both hands to assess the sides of the abdomen, using one hand to palpate and the other to support one side of the abdomen (see Figure 2-34).
   c. Third manuever: Pawlik palpation—place hand above the symphysis pubis and gently grab skin between thumb and third finger (see Figure 2-35).
   d. Fourth manuever: Deep Pelvic Palpation—place both hands over the pelvic inlet and, on exhalation, apply pressure to each side of the pelvic inlet (see Figure 2-36).

Maintains client comfort during this phase of the assessment
Determines which fetal part occupies the fundus. A change in tissue consistency from soft to firm is noted when the fundus has been palpated.
Determines the position of the fetal spine
Determines which fetal part lies over the pelvic inlet. Non-engaged part will be moveable
Determines the position of the head One hand will descend deeper in the abdominal cavity if the presenting part is engaged.

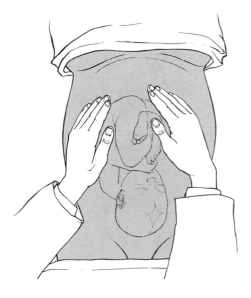

FIGURE 2-33 ▶ First Leopold's maneuver: Fundal palpation

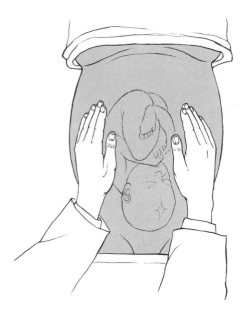

FIGURE 2-34 ▶ Second Leopold's maneuver: Lateral palpation

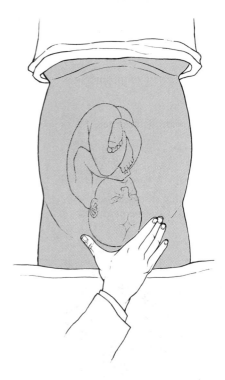

FIGURE 2-35 ▶ Third Leopold's maneuver: Pawlick palpation

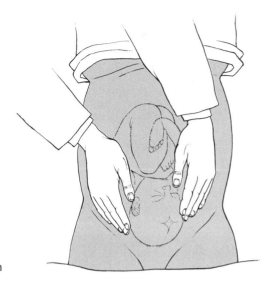

FIGURE 2-36 ▶ Fourth Leopold's maneuver: Deep pelvic palpation

2. Assist the client to a sitting position. Observe for orthopnea, syncope, vertigo

A shift in blood pressure can occur resulting from weight and position changes of the uterus on the vena cava.

DOCUMENTATION
The following information should be included in the nursing note:

Document and report immediately any signs of fetal distress or maternal compromise
Record fundal height measurement and fetal heart tones
Record history of previous pregnancies and deliveries
Observe and document psychosocial interactions with family and significant others
Note and record normal physiological changes

INTERDISCIPLINARY COLLABORATION
Inform physician of any abnormal findings
Consider need to consult social work for evaluation of socioeconomic status and/or referral to appropriate community resources (Bedrest Hotline, Sidelines, and Confinement Lines) [3, 5, 10, 16, 18, 32, 37]

PROCEDURE
Pediatric Assessment

DESCRIPTION
The pediatric assessment includes an examination of the physical development of the child from birth to adolescence. Significant physical changes serve as developmental benchmarks in the infant, toddler, child, and adolescent. This chapter presents a general overview highlighting the physical

changes associated with each age group. The pediatric assessment, in combination with the developmental assessment, completes the evaluation of the growing child's ability to achieve age-appropriate milestones.

PURPOSE
To evaluate the presence of normal and abnormal clinical findings in the developing infant, child, and adolescent

EQUIPMENT
Scale
Tape measure
Stethscope
Otoscope
Opthalmoscope
Health assessment forms
Age-appropriate Snellen Chart
Sphygmomanometer

OUTCOMES
The client/caregiver will:

Demonstrate an ability to recognize age-appropriate physical changes
Report symptoms of growth or developmental delay
Be referred to other members of the multidisciplinary health team, as appropriate, to assist in meeting age-appropriate growth and development

ASSESSMENT DATA
Assess and document growth and development levels attained for each body system
Obtain and record baseline vital signs and physical findings
Identify possible risks
Record use of technologic equipment
Determine need for assistive devices
Evaluate client's ability to perform age-appropriate tasks

RELATED NURSING DIAGNOSES
At risk for injury
At risk for sensory-perceptual deficit
Altered body image
Altered parenting
Altered family process
Altered self esteem
Altered growth and development

SPECIAL CONSIDERATIONS

Neonate

A complete assessment of the newborn is performed within the first 24 hours of life and at 4 weeks of age. Have the parent/caregiver hold the child maintaining warmth while the head-to-toe assessment is made. Observe the cardiopulmonary system while the child is quiet, and save all intrusive procedures for last. Use the time during the assessment to instruct the parent/caregiver in normal growth and developmental changes.

Infant

After age 6 months, the baby may be more fearful of strangers and feel anxious when separated from the parent/caregiver. To create a less threatening environment, have the parent/caregiver hold the child during the assessment. For the older infant perform the DDST2 first, creating a game-like environment. The infant should be assessed at 2, 4, 6, 9, and 12 months of age. At each assessment remind the parent/caregiver of the need to maintain the child's age-appropriate vaccine schedule.

Toddler

The child ages 1 to 5 will be difficult to assess because of his fear of strangers, injury and separation anxiety. Try to engage the child during the examination, creating a playful atmosphere. Allay the child's fears by explaining all procedures and have the parent/caregiver assist with the examination. Use a doll to demonstrate procedures before doing and allow the child to assist once trust has been established. Evaluate the neurological system by watching the child at play during the DDST2 examination. If it is necessary to restrain the child, have the child sit in the parent/caregiver's lap with arms and legs secured (see Figure 2-37). At each assessment remind the parent/caregiver of the need to maintain the child's age-appropriate vaccine schedule.

Child/Adolescent

The older child and adolescent are generally more cooperative and can be assessed in the same manner as used for the adult. Allow the school-aged child to participate in the examination by explaining all procedures, and by allowing him/her to listen to heart sounds or lung sounds. The

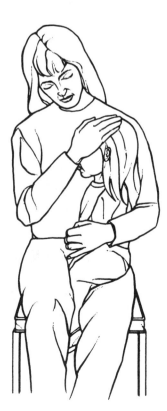

FIGURE 2-37 ▶ Restraining the young child during the physical examination

older child or adolescent may or may not wish to have the parent/caregiver present. Remember to respect his privacy, and be sensitive to the need to discuss issues related to sexual molestation and development. Use the time to teach the child/adolescent about normal body changes and expectations. At each assessment remind the parent/caregiver of the need to maintain the child's age-appropriate vaccine schedule.

TRANSCULTURAL CONSIDERATIONS

An interpreter will be needed for the child's caregivers who are unable to speak or understand English

Consider use of AT&T Language Line

See Culturological Assessment procedure for general overview of cultural considerations

▶ INTERVENTIONS

1. Wash hands.

2. Explain procedure.

Prevents transmission of microbes
Allays anxiety

Anthropometric Measurements

Neonate/Infant

1. Measure the head and chest circumference (see Figure 2-38).

The head circumference should be no greater than 3 cm greater than the chest circumference at birth, and should increase by 1.5 cm each month for the first 6 months and by 0.5 cm/month for the next 6 months. By one year the

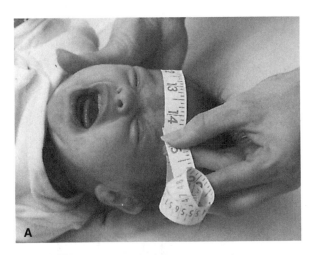 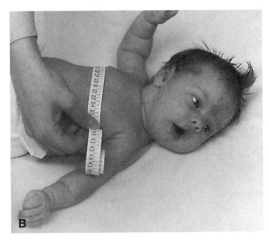

FIGURE 2-38 ▶ Measuring head circumference (a) and chest circumference (b)

2. Measure height and weight and compare against growth chart

head and chest circumference should be equal
Birth weight should double 6 months and should triple by 9–12 months. Height should increase 50% by 1 year of age

Toddler

Measure height and weight.

Weight should be proportional for height. See Appendix 2-6 for appropriate growth chart

Child/Adolescent

Measure height and weight.

Observe for rapid weight changes. Excessive weight loss or gain may be a sign of anorexia nervosa, bulimia, or endocrine disorder

Head and Neck Assessment

Neonate/Infant

1. Inspect and palpate the scalp.

2. Palpate the fontanelles (see Figure 2-39).

Detects presence of deformities, lesions, or masses
The posterior fontanelles should close by 2 months.

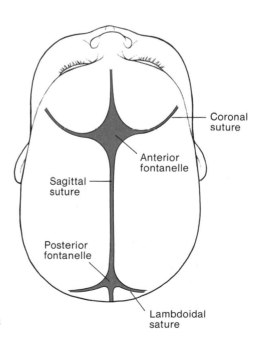

FIGURE 2-39 ▶ Palpating fontanelles

The anterior fontanelles should close by 18 months. Sunken fontanelles are indicative of dehydration. Bulging fontanelles are indicative of increased ICP.

Toddler/Child/Adolescent

Perform head and neck exam using same technique as in the adult. [see Adult Head and Neck Assessment]

Eye Assessment

Neonate/Infant

1. Perform eye assessment.
   a. determine visual acuity

   Infants should be able to focus on objects 3 feet or more away.
   Visual acuity = 20/100

   b. perform fundoscopic examination if infant is cooperative

   Internal eye structures are small. The macular area will not be visible until 1 year of age

   c. assess eye color

   Light-skinned newborns typically have gray or dark blue eyes, and dark skinned newborns have brown eyes. Permanent eye color is established at 6 to 12 months of age. Lack of eye color is indicative of albinism

   d. evaluate external eye structures

   Tearing should occur at 1–2 months of age

Toddler

1. Elicit corneal light reflex

   A brilliant uniform red reflex is observed when no abnormalities are present

2. Assess for visual acuity—use modified Snellen Chart, child may not be able to cooperate until after the age of 3 years.

   Strabismus may be noted.
   Visual acuity at 4 yrs = 20/40.
   Visual acuity at 5 yrs = 20/30

Child/Adolescent

Perform eye examination using same technique as for the adult. [see Adult Eye Assessment]

1. Assess need for corrective lens.

   Visual acuity at 9 or 10 yrs = 20/20

2. Encourage regular eye examinations.

   Routine screenings foster health promotion and disease prevention

Ear Assessment

Neonate/Infant/Toddler

Perform ear examination.
   a. inspect external ear structures
   b. pull the auricle down and back
   c. use a small speculum to evaluate the tympanic
      membrane

Ear findings are same as those for the adult. Observe for evidence of ear infections. Note any history of hearing deficit.

Child/Adolescent

Perform ear exam same as for adult—test hearing acuity.

Ear findings are same as those for adult

Oral Assessment

Neonate/Infant

Assess the oral cavity.
   a. use a tongue blade to elicit gag reflex
   b. evaluate tongue, palate, teeth, gums, tonsils and
      oral mucosa

By 6 months the first teeth to erupt should be the lower central incisors, and by 12 months the upper central incisors and the lateral upper and lower incisors should have appeared. The molars and cuspids should have erupted by the second year of life

Toddler

1. Children may be uncooperative, if so, try holding
   nose until mouth opens then make quick assessment
   of the oral cavity.

Observe for evidence of respiratory tract infections. Observe for enlarged tonsils

Child/Adolescent

For oral exam use same techniques as in the adult.
[see Adult Oral Assessment]
Encourage regular dental examinations.

Routine screenings foster health promotion and disease prevention

Cardiopulmonary Assessment

Neonate/Infant

1. Use stethoscope with smaller attachments, auscultate
   heart sounds.
2. Use a doppler to obtain blood pressure reading.

The heart rate should range from 80–160 BPM
The rhythm may be slightly irregular. A normal S3 may be heard. Murmurs may be innocent but must be evaluated. The normal systolic blood pressure is 70–80 mmHg.

3. Observe patterns of respiration.

Observe for clear bronchovesicular sounds

4. Auscultate lung sounds.

Observe for clear bronchovesicular sounds between the scapula and over the upper third of the sternum, vesicular sounds over the lung periphery, and bronchial sounds over the trachea and larynx

Toddler

1. Auscultate heart sounds.

Heart rate at 2 years = 80–130 BPM.
Heart rate at 3–5 years = 80–120 BPM.
Sinus dysrhythmia is normal in children

2. Percuss chest.

Percussion note is slightly more resonant than in adult

3. Measure blood pressure.

Blood pressure at < 5 years = 110–116/70–76

4. Evaluation peripheral pulses.

Pulse quality = 3+ on 4 point scale

Child/Adolescent

1. Cardiopulmonary assessment is same as for adult.

Heart rate at 6 years = 75–115 BPM
Heart rate at 7 years to young teen = 70–110 BPM
Heart rate in older teen = 60–100 BPM

2. Assess breathing pattern.

Abdominal breathing will be evident in all male age groups and in girl children until age 7 years, then becomes thoracic in girls

3. Measure blood pressure.

Blood pressure at 6–9 years = 110–122/70–78
Blood pressure at 10–13 years = < 130/80
Blood pressure in girls at 16–20 years < 140/85
Blood pressure in boys at 14–19 years = < 128/84

Breast and Axillary Assessment

Adolescent

Breast exam in adolescent girl same as for adult.

The maturing female breast development begins during

preadolescence and reaches maturity at 14–16 years

Abdominal Assessment

Neonate/Infant

1. Inspect the abdomen, note presence of hernias.

The umbilicus should appear dry and inverted by two weeks of age

2. Auscultate bowel sounds.

Bowel sounds should be audible every 10–30 seconds

3. Percuss the abdomen to identify presence of air.

Percussion tones should be tympanic

Toddler

1. Observe contour of abdomen while child is standing.

Child's abdomen has rounded appearance. Umbilical hernias should resolve in light-skinned children by 2 yrs, and in dark-skinned children by 6–7 years

2. Percuss liver using one hand to palpate.

Liver may be palpable 1–2 cm below costal margin

Child/Adolescent

Abdominal assessment is same as for adult.

School-aged child—Liver may extend 0–2 cm below costal margin

Adolescent—same findings as for adult

Genitourinary Assessment

Neonate/Infant

1. Female
   a. Part the legs and inspect labia, vaginal and urethral orifices
   b. Internal assessment is not typically performed

The labia minora will be more prominent than the labia majora. Redness or swelling may indicate infection or molestation.

2. Male
   a. Inspect the penis

Frequent erections are common during infancy

   b. Inspect and palpate the scrotum

The testes will freely move from the inguinal canal to the scrotal sac

Toddler

1. Assist the child to sit in frog-leg position with back supported.

Facilitates the examiner's ability to directly observe the external genital structures

	Findings are same as in infancy
	Observe for continuous descending of the testes in the male child > 4 years. If not observed, refer to physician for treatment and follow-up
2. Drape appropriately.	*Maintain modesty*

Child/Adolescent

1. Assist school-aged child to assume frog-leg position.	*Facilitates the examiner's ability to directly observe the external genital structures*
2. Perform hernia assessment of older male adolescent same as for adult.	*Screens for bulging in the inguinal and femoral areas*
3. Inspect pubic hair growth and external genitalia of female.	*Determines the sex maturity rating and physical sexual development*
4. Inspect pubic hair growth, penis, and scrotal sac of male.	*Determines the sex maturity rating and physical sexual development*

Musculoskeletal Assessment

Neonate/Infant

1. Assess upper extremities.	*The hand grasp should be strong and equal. Note the manner by which the infant uses the hands and fingers*
2. Assess lower extremities.	*Assess the hip joint for evidence of dislocation*
3. Perform Ortolani's Test—flex the knees and abduct the thighs (see Figure 2-40).	*There should be no click or slipping of the femoral head which would indicate hip dislocation*

4. Perform Barlow's Test (See Figure 2-41)
  a. stabilize the pelvis with one hand and grasp the thigh with the other
  b. put the hip through full ROM
	Note presence of any slipping movements

Toddler

1. Musculoskeletal function can be evaluated during the DDST2 examination.	*Bow-legged appearance of infancy will disappear by 3 years. Knock-kneed appearance may be evident until 2–4 years. Arch of feet should develop by 3 years*
2. Observe child at play.	*Permits assessment of the child's diversional activity and process of socialization*
3. Routinely examine hips and lower extremities.	*Detects presence of deformity*

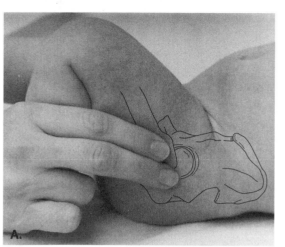
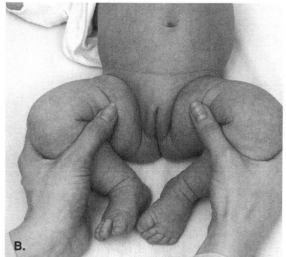

FIGURE 2-40 ▶ Ortolani's test for congenital hip displasia. **A.** Placement of examiner's hands. **B.** Abduction of infant's displasia.

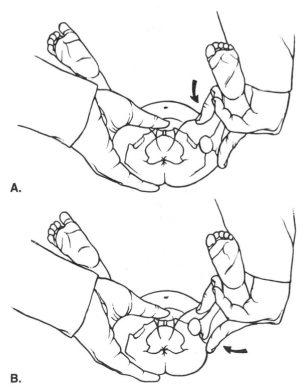

FIGURE 2-41 ▶ Barlow's test for congenital hip displasia. **B.**

Child/Adolescent

Perform musculoskeletal assessment using same technique as for the adult.
[see Adult Musculoskeletal Assessment]
Screen for scoliosis.

Scoliosis is commonly noted during and after growth spurts.

Neurological Assessment

Neonate/Infant

Test age-appropriate reflexes.

a. Moro

Arms should abduct with hands open, then clasp together

b. *Startle*

Arms should abduct with hands clenched

c. Tonic neck

Note extension of extremities on side to which head is turned and flexion of extremities on opposite side

d. Stepping

Legs should move up and down in a walking motion

e. Palmar grasping

Fingers curl tightly around object placed in hand

f. Plantar grasping

Toes should curl when examiner's thumb is placed on ball of foot

g. Babinski

Fanning of toes when lateral aspect of foot is stroked from heel to toe

h. Rooting

Mouth opens and head turns toward stimulus when cheek is stroked

i. Sucking

Sucking movement occurs when lips are touched

j. Blinking

Eyes closed when exposed to bright light

k. Accoustic blinking

Eyes close in response to loud noise

l. Parachuting

Arms and fingers extend in protective motion when body is suddenly lowered head first

m. Neck righting

When head is turned the side, body will follow in same direction

n. Body righting

When hips or shoulders are turned other body parts will turn in same direction

o. Landau

With body held prone and head is raised, legs and spine will extend

Toddler

The young child will typically not be able to cooperate
   to obtain accurate neurological assessment.
If appropriate, have the caregiver assist the examiner
   or directly observe the child at play.

Child/Adolescent

Perform the neurological assessment for the young
   child and adolescent using the same technique as in
   the adult
[See The Adult Neurological Assessment]

DOCUMENTATION

The following information should be included in the nursing note:

Date and time of the interview
Name and relationship of the person assisting with the assessment
Identification of the presence of any communication barriers
Identification of all technologic equipment
Documentation of all clinical findings
A report of all abnormal findings, information for the physician, and document-related interven-
   tions
Modifications needed and approaches taken to ensure client safety
Consultations and referrals made to other disciplines and agencies
Client's/caregiver's ability to maintain a safe environment
Availability and willingness of caregiver to follow the plan of care

INTERDISCIPLINARY COLLABORATION

Depending on the findings associated with each body system, the nurse will discuss with the
client's physician the need to consult with the social worker; physical or occupational therapist;
WOC nurse; nutritionist; or other health discipline in meeting the client's needs

   Identify and contact community resources needed for social support, transportation, meal
preparation, schooling, etc.

   Obtain orders for home health aide to assist with activities of daily living, if needed [3, 4, 10,
18, 31, 37, 42]

PROCEDURE
Gerontological Assessment

DESCRIPTION

The gerontological examination includes an assessment of the normal physiological changes associated with aging. In general, the aging adult becomes shorter in stature, demonstrates decreased kidney function, a loss of calcium, a decrease in liver mass, a loss of blood volume, a decrease in albu-

min levels, a loss of elasticity of the cardiopulmonary system, and an increase in the proportion of fat to muscle mass.

PURPOSE
To determine normal and abnormal physiological changes in the elderly client

EQUIPMENT
Scale
Tape measure
Stethoscope
Otoscope
Opthalmoscope
Health assessment forms

OUTCOMES
The client/caregiver will:

► Demonstrate an ability to recognize age-appropriate physical changes
► Report symptoms of abnormal physical changes
► Follow the plan of treatment for all disorders
► Be referred to other members of the multidisciplinary health team, as appropriate, to assist in meeting the goals of therapy

ASSESSMENT DATA
Assess age-related physiological changes
Determine functional and mental status
Determine lifestyle factors which may contribute to illness states: tobacco/alcohol abuse, occupational or environmental hazards, etc.
Differentiate between findings associated with physiologic aging and pathologic process
Review the client's medication profile and note and document any indication of polypharmacy
Assess the client's support system and availability/willingness of caregiver

RELATED NURSING DIAGNOSES
At risk for injury
At risk for altered skin integrity
At risk for altered nutrition
At risk for sleep pattern disturbance
At risk for impaired mobility
Knowledge deficit

SPECIAL CONSIDERATIONS
Detailed assessments will need to be made on the initial visit and for all acutely ill clients
In life-threatening situations, body assessment areas will need to prioritized
The elderly client may fatigue easily, have difficulty assuming certain positions for the complete examination, have decreased sensation, have hearing or visual loss, or may feel chilled without a blanket or light covering.

TRANSCULTURAL CONSIDERATIONS
An interpreter will be needed for clients unable to speak or understand English. Some elderly clients may feel the need to have other members of the family present during the assessment, may be reluctant to disclose or discuss intimate subject matters, or may feel uncomfortable exposing the

body for examination. The nurse should be respectful of such feelings, and should allow the client to ventilate concerns. Consider use of the AT&T Language Line. See Culturological Assessment procedure for general overview of cultural considerations.

▶ INTERVENTIONS

1. Wash hands.

Prevents transmission of microbes

2. Explain procedure.

Allays anxiety

Anthropometric Measurements

1. Obtain height and weight.

Variable weight loss may be seen in persons above 80 years of age. A shortening in stature may be related to osteoporosis.

Head and Neck Assessment

1. Perform eye assessment—note changes associated with aging.

Pupillary response slows with aging. Arcus senilis may be noted surrounding the cornea. Farsightedness increases with aging, and near-sightedness lessens. Peripheral vision, ability to distinguish pastel shades, ability to adapt to changes in light intensity, and abilty to accommodate to near objects diminishes with age

2. Perform ear examination—note chages associated with aging.

The pinna increases in size, cerumen becomes drier, and hair growth increases around the external structures. Hearing loss for high-pitched sounds decreases with age

3. Assess the oral cavity.
   a. note changes associated with aging

Mucus membranes will appear pale as a result of decreased capillary blood flow associated with aging. The gum line will recede and the loss of tooth enamel will cause a yellow discoloration of the teeth. The sensation of taste may be diminished

   b. review care of dentures

Reinforces learned information

4. Examine the nose—note changes associated with aging.

The nose will elongate with aging

Peripheral Vascular Assessment

Assess peripheral circulation.

Findings should be the same as in the normal adult

Cardiovascular Assessment

Auscultate heart sounds.

S1 and S2 may be less intense with aging. An S4 may be heard as a result of decreased ventricular compliance. An S, may indicate CHF.

Respiratory Assessment

1. Observe patterns of respiration.

Detects abnormalities in rhythm of breathing

2. Auscultate lung sounds.

Lung percussion tones will be hyperresonant secondary to an increase in residual lung volume. Costal calcification will result in a decrease in the transverse-thoracic diameter, and a decrease in ventilatory air flow will result in a decrease in breath sounds

Abdominal Assessment

1. Inspect the abdomen.

Detects presence of scars, ostomies, heaves, thrills, or pulsations

2. Auscultate bowel sounds.

Bowel sounds become less frequent and bladder capacity decreases with aging

3. Percuss/palpate the abdomen to identify organs.

The lower liver border may extend past the costal margin as a result of increased lung distension

Genitourinary Assessment

1. Examine the female genitalia—use a left-lateral sims position if it is uncomfortable for the client to flex the knees.
   a. part the legs and inspect labia, vaginal and urethral orifices

Estrogen depletion results in thinning and graying of the pubic hair. The labia will appear wrinkled and the clitoris will decrease in size

b. internal assessment is not typically performed in the home setting
2. Examine the male gentalia.
   a. inspect the penis
   b. inspect and palpate the scrotum

A decrease in the sex hormones results in a decrease in the size of the penis and testes. The scrotal sac becomes less firm and more pendulus, and the pubic hairs become thinner and grayer

Musculoskeletal Assessment

Assess upper and lower extremities.

The lumbar spine will flatten and kyphosis may be evident. Muscle strength will decrease bilaterally.

Breast and Axillary Assessment

Perform a breast examination.

The breast will flatten and elongate with aging in the female. The male may demonstrate gynecomastia secondary to hormone alteration. Masses and tenderness are abnormal findings.

Neurological Assessment

Examine the cranial nerves and motor and sensory sys
-tems.

Findings should be the same as for the normal adult

DOCUMENTATION

The following information should be included in the nursing note:

Date and time of the interview
Name and relationship of the person present during the assessment
Identify presence of any communication barriers
Identify all technologic equipment
Document all clinical findings
Report all abnormal findings, inform the physician and document related interventions
Modifications needed and approaches taken to ensure client safety
Consultations and referrals made to other disciplines and agencies
Client's/caregiver's ability to maintain a safe environment
Availability and willingness of caregiver to follow the plan of care
Client/caregiver's ability to correctly administer medications
Functional and mental status of the client

INTERDISCIPLINARY COLLABORATION

Depending on the findings associated with each body system, the nurse will discuss with the client's physician the need to consult with the social worker; physical or occupational therapist; WOC nurse; nutritionist; optometrist, dentist, or other health discipline in meeting the client's needs. Identify and contact community resources needed for social support, transportation, meal preparation, etc. Obtain orders for home health aide to assist with activities of daily living, if needed [3, 10, 18, 20, 31, 32, 38].

REFERENCES

1. AAN. Expert panel report: culturally competent health care. *Nursing Outlook* 40:277, 1992
2. Ahmann, E. *Home care for the high risk infant: A family centered approach.* Gaithersburg, MD: An Aspen Publication, 1996
3. Carpenito, LJ. *Nursing Diagnosis: Application to clinical practice,* 7th edition. Philadelphia: Lippincott, 1997
4. Chestnut, MA. *High-risk newborn home care manual.* Philadelphia: Lippincott-Raven. 1998
5. Chestnut, MA. High-risk *perinatal* Home Care manual. Philadelphia: Lippincott-Raven, 1998
6. Clark, MJ. *Nursing in the community,* 2nd edition. Standford CT: Appleton & Lange, 1996
7. Clemen-Stone, S, Eigati, DG, & McGuire, SL. *Comprehensive community health nursing: Family aggregate and community practice,* 4th edition. St. Louis, MO: Mosby Inc, 1995
8. Cook L, Petit de Mange, B. Gaining access to Native American cultures by non-Native American nursing researchers. *Nursing Forum* 30:5, 1995
9. Epstein A. 'English-only' can be fighting words. *The Philadelphia Inquirer* C4, 1994, June 5
10. Fuller, J & Schaller-Ayers, J. *Health assessment: a nursing approach.* 2nd edition. Philadelphia, PA: Lippincott. 1994
11. Geissler, EM. Transcultural nursing and nursing diagnoses. *Nursing & Health Care* 12:190, 1991
12. Gonzalez, E. Mental health of culturally diverse clients. *Journal of Cultural Diversity* 2:39, 1995
13. Green, K. *Home care survival guide.* Philadelphia, PA: Lippincott. 1998
14. Haffner, L. Translation is not enough: Interpretation in a medical setting. *The Western Journal of Medicine* 157:255, 1992
15. Hanson, MA & Boyd, ST. *Family health care nursing: Theory, practice and research.* Philadelphia: FA Davis. 1996
16. Heaman, M. Anterpartum home care for high-risk pregnant women. *AACN Clinical Issues.* 9:362. 1998
17. Jaffe, MS & Skidmore-Roth, L. *Home health nursing assessment and planning.* St Louis: Mosby. 1997
18. Jarvis, C. *Pocket companion for physical examination and health assessment.* Philadelphia, PA: W.B. Saunders Company, 1996
19. Johnson, JY, Smith-Temple, J, Carr P. *Nurses' guide to home procedures.* Philadelphia, PA: Lippincott, 1998
20. LeMone, P & Burke KM. *Medical surgical nursing: critical thinking in client care.* Menlo Park, CA: Addison Wesley Publishers, 1996
21. Leininger, MM. The transcultural nurse specialist: Imperative in today's world. *Nursing & Health Care* 10:251, 1989
22. Leininger, MM. *Culture care diversity and universality: A theory of nursing.* New York, NY: National League for Nursing Press, 1991
23. Leininger, MM. Transcultural nursing education: A worldwide imperative. *Nursing & Health Care* 15:254, 1994
24. Marrelli, TM. *Handbook of home health standards and documentation guidelines for reimbursement,* 3rd edition. St Louis, MO: Mosby, 1998
25. McGoldrick, M, Pearce J, Giordano J. *Ethnicity and family therapy.* New York, NY: Guilford Press, 1982
26. McNeal, GJ, Gonzalez, EW, Petit de Mange, E, Perez, I. Multiculturally diverse clients. In Rothrock, J (ed). *Perioperative Nursing Care Planning,* 2nd edition. St Louis, MO: Mosby, 1996
27. McNeal, GJ, Doherty, A, O'Donnell, DG, Mallory, B. Culturally sensitive mobile health care services for at-risk populations. In Ferguson VD (ed). *Educating the 21st century nurse: Challenges and opportunities.* New York, New York, National League for Nursing Press, 1997
28. McNeal, GJ. Diversity Issues in Homecare. *Critical Care Nursing Clinics of North America,* 10:3, 1998
29. McNeal, GJ: High-tech home care: an expanding critical care frontier. *Critical Care Nurse* 16:51, 1996
30. Narayan, MC: Cultural assessment in home healthcare. *Home Healthcare Nurse* 15:663, 1997
31. *Nurses' Illustrated Handbook of Home Health Procedures.* Springhouse: Springhouse Corporation, 1999

32. Seidel, HM, Ball, JW, Dains, JE et al. *Mosby's Guide to Physical Examination,* 4th edition. St Louis, MO: Mosby, 1999
33. Skolnick, AS, Skolnick, JH. *Family in transition.* Glenview: Scott, Foresman and Company, 1989.
34. Spector, RE. *Cultural diversity in health and illness.* Stamford, CT: Appleton and Lange, 1996.
35. Spruhan, JB. Beyond traditional nursing care: cultural awareness and successful home healthcare nursing. *Home Healthcare Nurse* 14:445, 1996
36. Spradley, BS & Allender, JA. *Community health nursing: Concepts and practice.* Philadelphia, PA: Lippincott Raven. 1996
37. Stanhope, M & Knollmueller, RN. *Handbook of community and home health nursing.* St. Louis, MO: Mosby, 1996
38. Stanhope, M. & Lancaster, J. *Community health nursing: Promoting health of aggregates, families, and individuals,* 4th edition. St. Louis, MO: Mosby Yearbook Inc. 1996
39. Tripp-Reimer, T, Brink, P, Saunders, J. Cultural assessment: content and process. *Nursing Outlook* 32:78, 1984
40. Tripp-Reimer, T. Crossing over the boundaries. *Critical Care Nurse* 14:134, 1994
41. Trujillo, EG, Robinson, MK, & Jacobs, DO. Nutritional assessement of the critically ill. *Critical Care Nurse* 19:67, 1999
42. Wong, DL. *Wong and Whaley's Clinical Manual of Pediatric Nursing.* St. Louis, MO: Mosby, 1996
43. Zang SM & Bailey NC. *Home care manual: Making the transitition.* Philadelphia, PA: Lippincott, 1997

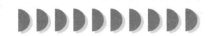

Appendices

Consent for Treatment, Release of Information, Assignment of Benefits, Notice of Client Rights

Client Name: _____

Address: _____

City: _____ State: _____ Zip: _____

I, _____ , _____ of _____ intending to be
   (custodial parent or legal guardian)   (relationship)   (minor client)

legally bound, hereby:

1. Consent to such care and treatment by _____ , and its employees and agents (collectively, the "Agency"), as prescribed by the client's physician or dictated by the client's condition.

2. Authorize the Agency to release any medical records in its possession concerning the client as may be required by law or to pay benefits on the client's behalf. I authorize the client's physicians, insurers, and hospitals to release such medical records to the Agency at the Agency's request.

3. Authorize my insurer to disclose to the Agency the terms and extent of my coverage, and the amount of payments made to me for services provided by the Agency.

4. Assign, transfer, and set over to the Agency all of my or the client's rights to insurance proceeds or other funds to which I am or the client is or will become entitled as a result of the services rendered by the Agency.

5. Consent to and authorize payment, which would otherwise be payable to me or the client, to be made directly to the Agency. The Agency may issue a receipt for such payment which shall discharge the insurance company of its obligations under the policy to the extent of such payment.

6. Agree that I remain individually responsible to pay the Agency for all charges not paid for any reason by the insurer or other third-party payor. I understand that payment in full is due upon receipt of my bill. If payment for the Agency's services is made directly to me by my insurer, I agree to endorse the check to the provider and forward it to the Agency within three days of receipt.

A photocopy of this document, if executed, shall be considered as effective and valid as the original.

The effect of this form and the Client's Rights and Responsibilities on the back of this form have been explained to me by the Agency and I understand its content and significance.

Date: _____   Signature: _____

Name: _____
(please print)

APPENDIX 2-1 ▶ Consent for Treatment, Release of Information, Assignment of Benefits, Notice of Client Rights. (*Source:* Chestnut, MA. High risk perinatal home care manual. Philadelphia: Lippincott-Raven, 1998)

Client Responsibilities

As a home health care client you have the responsibility to:

1. Give accurate and complete health information concerning your past illnesses, hospitalizations, medications, allergies, and other pertinent items.

2. Assist in developing and maintaining a safe environment.

3. Inform the Home Health Care Agency when you will not be able to keep a home health care visit.

4. Participate in the development and update of your home health care plan.

5. Adhere to your developed/updated home health care plan.

6. Request further information concerning anything you do not understand.

7. Give information regarding concerns and problems you have to Home Health Care Agency staff member.

Advance Directives

An advance directive is a written instruction, such as a living will or durable power of attorney for health care, recognized under state law, relating to the provision of health care when an individual's condition makes him/her unable to express his/her wishes. The intent of these provisions is to enhance an individual's control over medical treatment decisions.

The Agency's policy regarding implementation of a client's advance directive is to comply to the best of its ability with those instructions.

1. The client has been informed of the state living will law.   Yes _____   No _____

2. Does the client have a living will?   Yes _____   No _____

3. If so, is there a copy of the advance directive in the client's medical record?   Yes _____   No _____

Client Signature: _____   Date: _____

APPENDIX 2-2 ▶ Client Responsiblities. (*Source:* Chestnut, MA. Pediatric home care manual. Philadelphia: Lippincott-Raven, 1998)

Home Health Care Client's
Bill of Rights/Responsibilities

As a home health care client you have the right to:

1. Standard: Right to be informed and to participate in planning care and treatment (1) The client has the right to be informed in advance about the care to be furnished.

2. Be given information about your rights and responsibilities for receiving home health care services, in terms and language you can reasonably expect to understand.

3. Receive a timely response from the Home Health Care Agency regarding your request for home health care services.

4. Be given information of the Home Health Care Agency charges and policy concerning payment for services, including your eligibility for third party reimbursement.

5. Choose your home health care providers.

6. Be given appropriate and professional quality home health care services without discrimination against your race, creed, color, religion, sex, national origin, sexual preference, handicap, or age.

7. The client's family or guardian may exercise the client's rights when the client has been judged incompetent.

8. The HHA must investigate complaints made by a client or the client's family or guardian regarding treatment or care that is (or fails to be) furnished, or regarding the lack of respect for the client's property by anyone furnishing services on behalf of the HHA, and must document both the existence of the complaint and the resolution of the complaint.

9. Be treated with courtesy and respect by all who provide home health care services to you; to have your property treated with respect.

10. Before the care is initiated, the HHA must inform the client, orally and in writing, of
    a. The extent of which payment may be expected from Medicare, Medicaid, or any other federally funded or aided program known to the HHA
    b. The charges for services that will not be covered by Medicare; and
    c. The charges that the individual may have to pay
    d. The client has the right to be advised orally and in writing of any changes in payment from last financial counseling.

11. The client has the right to be advised orally and in writing of any changes in payment. The HHA must advise the client of these changes orally and in writing as soon as possible, but no later than 15 working days from the date that the HHA becomes aware of a change.

APPENDIX 2-3 ▶ Home Health Care Client's Bill of Rights/Responsibilities. (*Source:* Chestnut, MA. Pediatric home care manual. Philadelphia: Lippincott-Raven, 1998)   (continued)

12. Be given the necessary information so you will be able to give informed consent for your treatment prior to the start of any treatment.

13. Participate in the development of your home health care plan, to be informed in advance about the care to be provided and any changes in the care to be provided, including anticipated transfer of your care to another health care facility and/or termination of home health care service.

14. To be advised in advance of the disciplines that will provide care, and the frequency of visits proposed to be provided.

15. Be given data privacy and confidentiality; review your clinical record at your request.

16. Voice grievances regarding treatment or care that is (or fails to be) furnished, or regarding any lack of respect for privacy by anyone who is furnishing services on behalf of the home health care agency, without being subject to discrimination or reprisal for doing so.

    * Call _____ to voice a grievance and/or recommend changes in policies or services.
    * Medicare/Medicaid clients may also call a Hotline # (1-800-222-0989) to report grievances from 8:30 am–5:00 pm with answering service for non-business hours. This is *not* the number to reach the Home Health Care Agency or to obtain Medicare coverage/billing information.

17. Refuse all or part of your care to the extent permitted by law; to be informed of the expected consequences of such action.

18. The client's family or guardian may exercise the client's rights when the client has been judged incompetent.

APPENDIX 2-3 (CONTINUED) ▶ Home Health Care Client's Bill of Rights/Responsibilities

Newborn Universal Home Risk Assessment Form

Current Medical Profile

Client Name: _____ Date of Birth: _____

Address: _____ Phone: (   ) _____

Primary Physician: _____

Physician Address: _____ Phone: (   ) _____

Primary Diagnosis: _____ Secondary Diagnosis: _____

Allergies: _____ Functional Limitations: _____

Client's Primary Caregiver: _____ Relationship: _____ Health Status: _____

Language: _____ Race: _____ Emergency Contact: _____ Phone: _____

Insurance: _____ ID #: _____ Caseworker: _____ Phone: _____

If no Insurance, why? _____

CHILD ASSESSMENT		NORM.	ABNORM.	DESCRIBE/MEASURE/PAST MEDICAL HISTORY
SKIN	Color/Condition/Cord			
METABOLIC	TPR			
NEURO.	Sleeping/Activity reflexes/Suck			
HEENT	Fontanelles			
	Auditory/Visual Response			
CARDIOVASC.	Apical Pulse			
CHEST	Lungs			
MUSCULOSKEL.	Muscle Tone			
	Feeding Type/Amt./Freq.			
GI	Elimination			
GU	Genitalia/Anus Voiding			
NUTRITIONAL	PO/Enteral			
Status	Parenteral			
	Feeding Issues			Weight

RISK ASSESSMENT (circle risk score if applicable)

I. Life Transitions
- 2 Denial/rejection medical problem
- 1 Hx current/recent incest/rape victim
- 1 Hx infant/child chronic disability
- 1 Hx of family member death
- 1 Adoption/termination considered
- 1 Suspected domestic violence

II. Emotional Status
- 1 Hx of mental illness/mental health treat./hosp.
- 1 Unresolved grief/signif. loss
- 2 Suicidal ideation
- 1 Feels isolation/alone/inadeq. support system
- 1 Questionable coping
- 1 Hx of postpartum depression
- 1 Evidence of low self-esteem

III. Substance Abuse/Risk-Taking Behaviors
- 3 Current/recent abuse of ETOH
- 3 Current/recent abuse of street drugs
- 3 Current/recent abuse of presc. meds
- 1 Law enforcement involvement
- 1 Sexual risk-taking behaviors
- 1 Tobacco use or 2nd-hand smoke exposure

IV. Parenting issues (observed/expressed)
- 1 Teen/inexperienced parent
- 1 Develop. issues (child/fam. expectations)
- 1 Discipline issues
- 1 Relationship issues (bond/nurturing)
- 1 Hx child abuse/neglect, now resolved
- 2 Child abuse/neglect, current
- 1 3 Or more children < 6 yrs. of age

V. Educational/Cultural Factors
- 1 Low literacy/limited intellectual ability
- 1 Cognitive deficits
- 1 Language barriers
- 1 Ed. level l2th or less
- 2 Ed. level 10th or less
- 3 Ed. level 9th or less or < 17 y.o.
- 1 Culture/Beliefs

VI. Economic/Resource Needs
- 1 Insuff. income to meet basic needs
- 1 No transportation
- 2 Inadequate food
- 1 Legal needs
- 2 Chronic difficulty accessing "system"
- 1 Child care problems
- 1 Medicaid problems

APPENDIX 2-4 ▶ Newborn Universal Home Risk Assessment Form. (*Source:* Chestnut, MA. High-risk newborn home care manual. Philadelphia: Lippincott-Raven, 1998)   (continued)

VII. Medical/Nutritional Factors

2 Abnl. phys. fndgs. this assess.
3 Prenatal exp. to drugs/alcohol
2 Anemia
1 Failure to thrive in sibs., prev. or existing
2 Dx or suspected malabsorption
2 Symptoms of intolerance to formula
2 Diarrhea
2 GE reflux
3 Low birth weight infant < 1500 gm

2 Problem establishing breastfeeding
3 Inadequate prenatal. care
___ immunization over 2 mos. behing due
    to no pediatric provider visits

1 Previous hosp. of sibs. in 1 st yr.
3 Extended hospitalization
2 Medical problems
3 Low birth weight infant < 2500 gm
2 STD exp. in preg., untreated
1 Lead exposure

VIII. Environmental

1 Housing
1 Utilities
1 Refrigeration
1 Water/sewer
1 High risk/unsafe neighborhood
1 Inadeq. prep. for infant

2 STD exp. in preg., untreated

SAFETY ASSESSMENT	YES	NO	COMMENTS
Teaching: Basic Home Safety?			
CPR Training Reviewed/Reinforced?			
Reviewed plan for emergency medical situation/emergency phone numbers?			
Is "do not resuscitate" order applicable?			
Reviewed safety instruction related to equipment and care being provided?			
Physical/psychosocial environment adequate for patient care?			

Other medical personnel providing care (specify name and phone): _____

List equipment in home/specify instructions for use given: _____

Reason for visit/home care needs: _____

Nursing diagnosis(es): _____

Short-term goals(s): _____

Long-term goals(s): _____

Nursing interventions (treatment, teaching, etc.): _____

Evaluation (response to interventions): _____

Referrals: _____

Date and Nursing Care Plan for next visit: _____

Communication to physician/Agency Office/Other: _____

Change in orders/Change in medication: _____
    (specify change and attach completed physician verbal order form)

RN Signature: _____ License #: _____ Date: _____

APPENDIX 2-4 [CONTINUED] ▶ Newborn Universal Home Risk Assessment Form

GENERAL GUIDELINES FOR DENVER DEVELOPMENTAL SCREENING TEST II (DDST2)

1. Find the child's chronological age on the DDST2 form. Highlight the age line across the form (a ruler is helpful). For children who were born at least 2 weeks premature and are under age 2 years, chronologically substract the number of weeks of prematurity from the chronological age to find the appropriate testing age.
2. Discuss the test with the parents. Explain that it is not an intelligence test but rather a means of evaluating the child's current level of development and that the child is *not* expected to pass every item.
3. Provide a quiet environment without distractions for testing. It is helpful to approach the screening test as a game. Introduce only one test at a time. Keep all equipment such as blocks and ball in the kit bag until needed because these often distract the child.
4. Test the child for each item intersected by the age line. Instructions for testing each item are provided with the test. Begin with "easy" items listed to the left of the age line to promote initial success and cooperation. The items that require a response from the parent may be asked first to allow both the parent and child to become more comfortable with the surroundings and the nurse.
5. Score items by writing on the form: "P" for *pass*, "F" for *failure*, "NO" for *no opportunity* to perform this skill (can only be used for report items), "R" for *refusal*, and "C" for *caution* (a "C" is always used in combination with an "R" or "F"). Be sure to refer to the back of the form any time a number appears by the skill.
6. Score the screening test by counting the number of delays and cautions identified.

INDIVIDUAL ITEMS

Advanced: Passed an item completely to the right of the age line. The child has passed an item that most children do not pass until older.

Normal: Passed, failed, or refused an item intersected by the age line between the 25th and 75th percentile.

Caution: Failed or refused items intersected by the age line between the 75th and 90th percentile. This is used to note that the child is not performing a task that many younger children can perform.

Delay: Failed an item completely to the left of the age line; refusals to the left of the age line are delays since the refusal may be related to inability to perform the task.

FOR THE TEST WITH RECOMMENDATIONS FOR FOLLOW-UP

Normal: No delays and no more than one caution for the entire test. Repeat routine screening at next well child assessment.

Abnormal: Two or more delays for the entire test. Refer for diagnostic evaluation.

Questionable: One delay and/or two or more cautions for the entire test. Rescreen in 3 months or at next well child assessment, whichever is first. Refer for diagnostic evaluation if rescreen is questionable or abnormal.

Untestable: This interpretation is based upon the number of refusals. If the number of refusals would equal an abnormal result, the child should be rescreened in 2 or 3 weeks before interpreting the results as abnormal. If the number of refusals equals questionable results, follow-up is the same as for questionable.

APPENDIX 2-5 ▶ Denver Developmental Screening Test II and Denver Articulation Screening Examination   (continued)

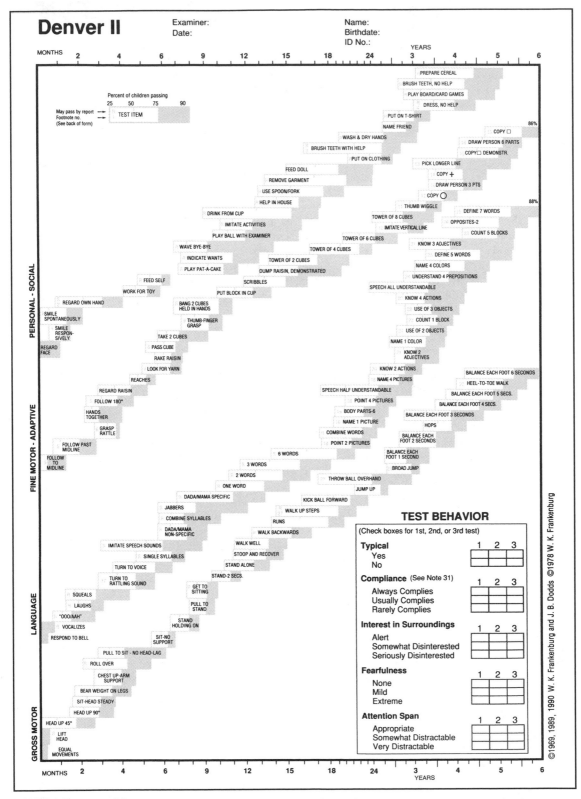

APPENDIX 2-5 (CONTINUED) ▶ Denver Developmental Screening Test II (DDST2) and Denver Articulation Screening Examination

DIRECTIONS FOR ADMINISTRATION

1. Try to get child to smile by smiling, talking or waving. Do not touch him/her.
2. Child must stare at hand several seconds.
3. Parent may help guide toothbrush and put toothpaste on brush.
4. Child does not have to be able to tie shoes or button/zip in the back.
5. Move yarn slowly in an arc from one side to the other, about 8" above child's face.
6. Pass if child grasps rattle when it is touched to the backs or tips of fingers.
7. Pass if child tries to see where yarn went. Yarn should be dropped quickly from sight from tester's hand without arm movement.
8. Child must transfer cube from hand to hand without help of body, mouth, or table.
9. Pass if child picks up raisin with any part of thumb and finger.
10. Line can vary only 30 degrees or less from tester's line.
11. Make a fist with thumb pointing upward and wiggle only the thumb. Pass if child imitates and does not move any fingers other than the thumb.

12. Pass any enclosed form. Fail continuous round motions.
13. Which line is longer? (Not bigger.) Turn paper upside down and repeat. (pass 3 of 3 or 5 of 6)
14. Pass any lines crossing near midpoint.
15. Have child copy first. If failed, demonstrate.

When giving items 12, 14, and 15, do not name the forms. Do not demonstrate 12 and 14.

16. When scoring, each pair (2 arms, 2 legs, etc.) counts as one part.
17. Place one cube in cup and shake gently near child's ear, but out of sight. Repeat for other ear.
18. Point to picture and have child name it. (No credit is given for sounds only.)
    If less than 4 pictures are named correctly, have child point to picture as each is named by tester.

19. Using doll, tell child: Show me the nose, eyes, ears, mouth, hands, feet, tummy, hair. Pass 6 of 8.
20. Using pictures, ask child: Which one flies?... says meow?... talks?... barks?... gallops? Pass 2 of 5, 4 of 5.
21. Ask child: What do you do when you are cold?... tired?... hungry? Pass 2 of 3, 3 of 3.
22. Ask child: What do you do with a cup? What is a chair used for? What is a pencil used for?
    Action words must be included in answers.
23. Pass if child correctly places and says how many blocks are on paper. (1, 5).
24. Tell child: Put block on table; under table; in front of me, behind me. Pass 4 of 4.
    (Do not help child by pointing, moving head or eyes.)
25. Ask child: What is a ball?... lake?... desk?... house?... banana?... curtain?... fence?... ceiling? Pass if defined in terms of use, shape, what it is made of, or general category (such as banana is fruit, not just yellow). Pass 5 of 8, 7 of 8.
26. Ask child: If a horse is big, a mouse is __? If fire is hot, ice is __? If the sun shines during the day, the moon shines during the __? Pass 2 of 3.
27. Child may use wall or rail only, not person. May not crawl.
28. Child must throw ball overhand 3 feet to within arm's reach of tester.
29. Child must perform standing broad jump over width of test sheet (8 1/2 inches).
30. Tell child to walk forward, 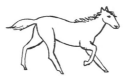 heel within 1 inch of toe. Tester may demonstrate.
    Child must walk 4 consecutive steps.
31. In the second year, half of normal children are non-compliant.

OBSERVATIONS:

APPENDIX 2-5 (CONTINUED) ▶ Denver Developmental Screening Test II (DDST2) and Denver Articulation Screening Examination (continued)

Denver Articulation Screening Examination

(For children 2.5 to 6 years of age)

Instructions: Have child repeat each word after you. Circle the underlined sounds that he or she pronounces correctly. Total number of correct sounds is the raw score. Use charts on reverse side to score results.

NAME

HOSPITAL NO.

ADDRESS

Date: _____ Child's age: _____ Examiner: _____ Raw score: _____
Percentile: _____ Intelligibility: _____ Result: _____

1. table	6. zipper	11. sock	16. wagon	21. leaf
2. shirt	7. grapes	12. vacuum	17. gum	22. carrot
3. door	8. flag	13. yarn	18. house	
4. trunk	9. thumb	14. mother	19. pencil	
5. jumping	10. toothbrush	15. twinkle	20. fish	

Intelligibility (circle one):   1. Easy to understand   3. Not understandable
                                2. Understandable half of the time   4. Cannot evaluate

Comments:

Date: _____ Child's age: _____ Examiner: _____ Raw score: _____
Percentile: _____ Intelligibility: _____ Result: _____

1. table	6. zipper	11. sock	16. wagon	21. leaf
2. shirt	7. grapes	12. vacuum	17. gum	22. carrot
3. door	8. flag	13. yarn	18. house	
4. trunk	9. thumb	14. mother	19. pencil	
5. jumping	10. toothbrush	15. twinkle	20. fish	

Intelligibility (circle one):   1. Easy to understand   3. Not understandable
                                2. Understandable half of the time   4. Cannot evaluate

Comments:

Date: _____ Child's age: _____ Examiner: _____ Raw score: _____
Percentile: _____ Intelligibility: _____ Result: _____

1. table	6. zipper	11. sock	16. wagon	21. leaf
2. shirt	7. grapes	12. vacuum	17. gum	22. carrot
3. door	8. flag	13. yarn	18. house	
4. trunk	9. thumb	14. mother	19. pencil	
5. jumping	10. toothbrush	15. twinkle	20. fish	

Intelligibility (circle one):   1. Easy to understand   3. Not understandable
                                2. Understandable half of the time   4. Cannot evaluate

Comments:

(NK Frankenburg, University of Colorado Medical Center, Denver, 1971. Copyright © 1971. Amelia F. Drumwright)

APPENDIX 2-5 [CONTINUED] ▶ Denver Developmental Screening Test II (DDST2) and Denver Articulation Screening Examination

To score DASE words: Note raw score for child's performance. Match raw score line (extreme left of chart) with column representing child's age (to the closest *previous* age group). Where raw score line and age column meet denotes percentile rank of child's performance when compared with other children that age. Percentiles above heavy line are *abnormal*, below heavy line are *normal*.

PERCENTILE RANK

Raw Score	2.5 yr	3.0 yr	3.5 yr	4.0 yr	4.5 yr	5.0 yr	5.5 yr	6 yr
2	1							
3	2							
4	5							
5	9							
6	16							
7	23							
8	31	2						
9	37	4	1					
10	42	6	2					
11	48	7	4					
12	54	9	6	1	1			
13	58	12	9	2	3	1	1	
14	62	17	11	5	4	2	2	
15	68	23	15	9	5	3	2	
16	75	31	19	12	5	4	3	
17	79	38	25	15	6	6	4	
18	83	46	31	19	8	7	4	
19	86	51	38	24	10	9	5	1
20	89	58	45	30	12	11	7	3
21	92	65	52	36	15	15	9	4
22	94	72	58	43	18	19	12	5
23	96	77	63	50	22	24	15	7
24	97	82	70	58	29	29	20	15
25	99	87	78	66	36	34	26	17
26	99	91	84	75	46	43	34	24
27		94	89	82	57	54	44	34
28		96	94	88	70	68	59	47
29		98	98	94	84	84	77	68
30		100	100	100	100	100	100	100

To score intelligibility:

		NORMAL	ABNORMAL
	2.5 years	Understandable half of the time or easy to understand	Not understandable
	3 years and older	Easy to understand	Understandable half of the time or not understandable

Test result: 1. Normal on DASE and intelligibility = *normal*
2. Abnormal on DASE or intelligibility = *abnormal**

*If abnormal on initial screening, rescreen within 2 weeks. If abnormal again, child should be referred for complete speech evaluation.

APPENDIX 2-5 [CONTINUED] ▶ Denver Developmental Screening Test II (DDST2) and Denver Articulation Screening Examination

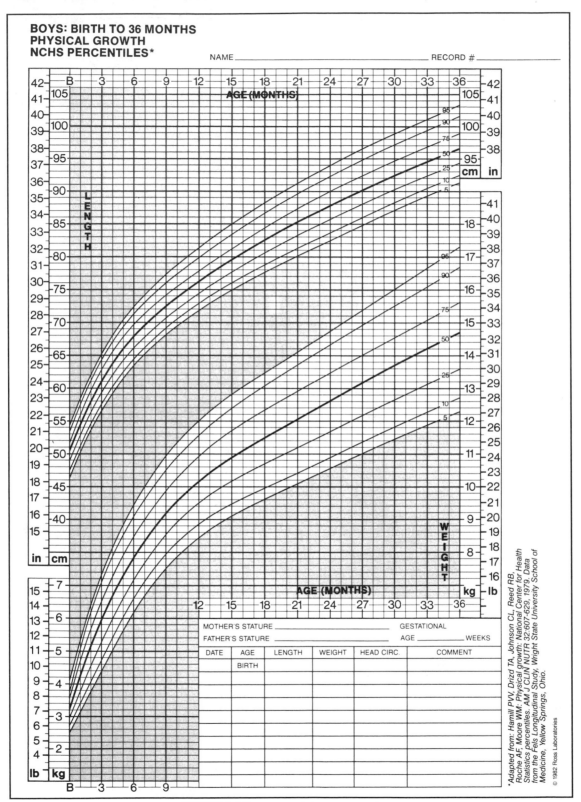

APPENDIX 2-6 ▶ Infant and Child Growth Charts

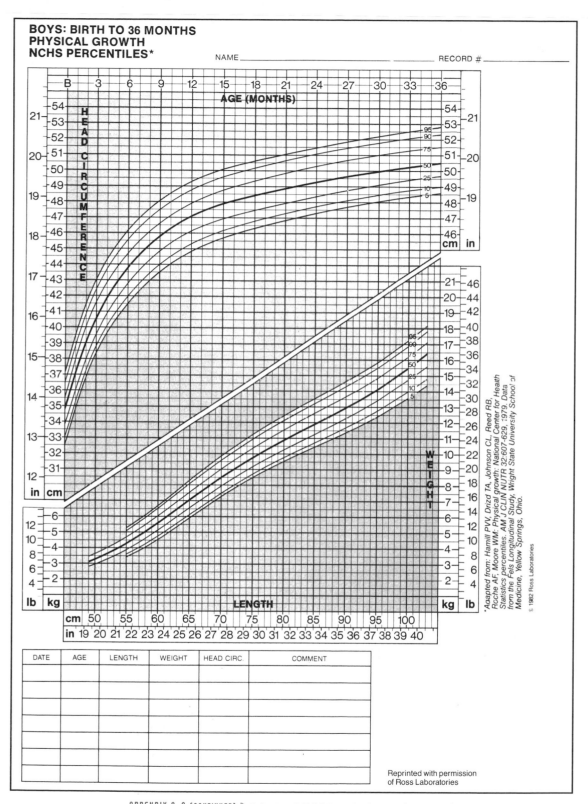

BOYS: BIRTH TO 36 MONTHS
PHYSICAL GROWTH
NCHS PERCENTILES*

NAME _____ RECORD # _____

*Adapted from: Hamill PVV, Drizd TA, Johnson CL, Reed RB, Roche AF, Moore WM: Physical growth: National Center for Health Statistics percentiles. AM J CLIN NUTR 32:607-629, 1979. Data from the Fels Longitudinal Study, Wright State University School of Medicine, Yellow Springs, Ohio.

© 1982 Ross Laboratories

DATE	AGE	LENGTH	WEIGHT	HEAD CIRC.	COMMENT

Reprinted with permission of Ross Laboratories

APPENDIX 2-6 [CONTINUED] ▶ Infant and Child Growth Charts (continued)

BOYS: 2 TO 18 YEARS
PHYSICAL GROWTH
NCHS PERCENTILES*

NAME _____ RECORD # _____

*Adapted from: Hamill PVV, Drizd TA, Johnson CL, Reed RB, Roche AF, Moore WM. Physical growth: National Center for Health Statistics percentiles. AM J CLIN NUTR 32:607-629, 1979. Data from the National Center for Health Statistics (NCHS), Hyattsville, Maryland.

© 1982 Ross Laboratories

Ross Growth & Development Program

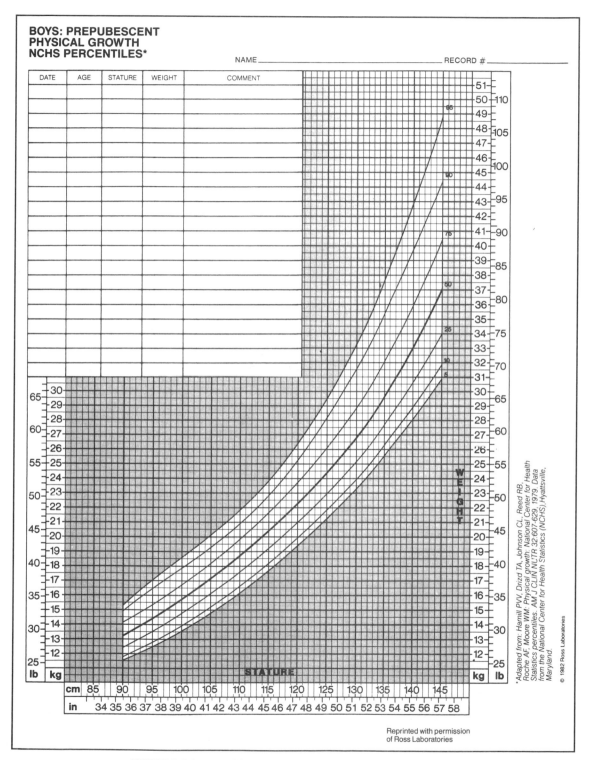

BOYS: PREPUBESCENT PHYSICAL GROWTH NCHS PERCENTILES*

Reprinted with permission of Ross Laboratories

APPENDIX 2-6 [CONTINUED] ▶ Infant and Child Growth Charts   (continued)

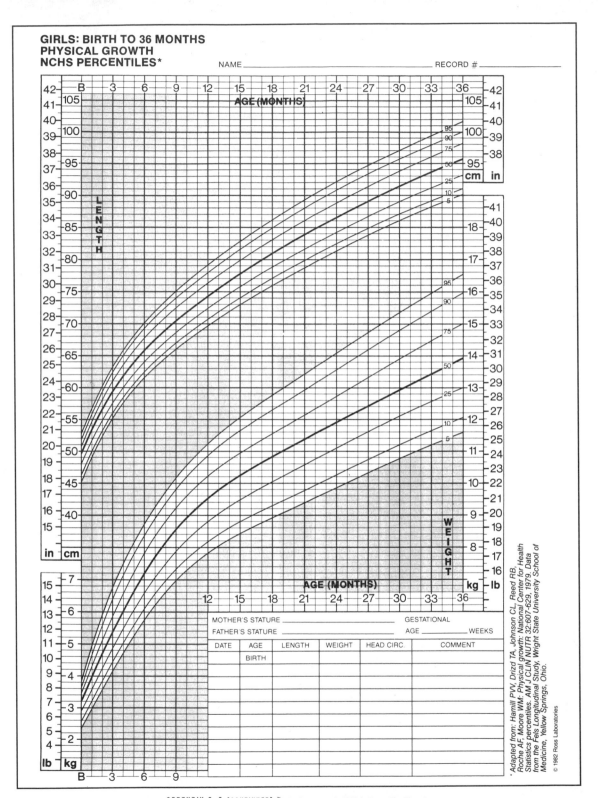

GIRLS: BIRTH TO 36 MONTHS
PHYSICAL GROWTH
NCHS PERCENTILES*

NAME _____ RECORD # _____

AGE (MONTHS)

LENGTH

WEIGHT

* Adapted from: Hamill PVV, Drizd TA, Johnson CL, Reed RB,
Roche AF, Moore WM: Physical growth: National Center for Health
Statistics percentiles. AM J CLIN NUTR 32:607-629, 1979. Data
from the Fels Longitudinal Study, Wright State University School of
Medicine, Yellow Springs, Ohio.

© 1982 Ross Laboratories

MOTHER'S STATURE _____ GESTATIONAL
FATHER'S STATURE _____ AGE _____ WEEKS

DATE	AGE	LENGTH	WEIGHT	HEAD CIRC.	COMMENT
	BIRTH				

APPENDIX 2-6 [CONTINUED] ▶ Infant and Child Growth Charts

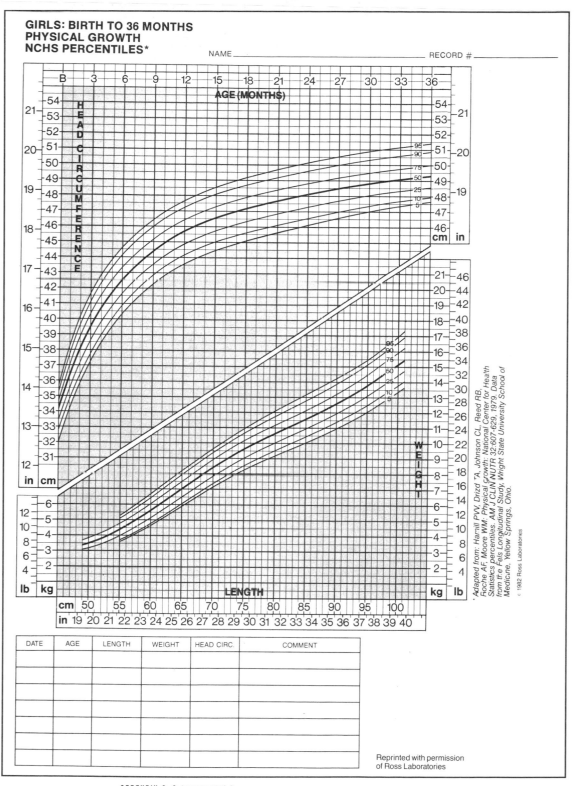

GIRLS: BIRTH TO 36 MONTHS
PHYSICAL GROWTH
NCHS PERCENTILES*

NAME _____ RECORD # _____

*Adapted from: Harrill PVV, Drizd TA, Johnson CL, Reed RB, Roche AF, Moore WM: Physical growth: National Center for Health Statistics percentiles. AM J CLIN NUTR 32:607-629, 1979. Data from the Fels Longitudinal Study, Wright State University School of Medicine, Yellow Springs, Ohio.

© 1982 Ross Laboratories

DATE	AGE	LENGTH	WEIGHT	HEAD CIRC.	COMMENT

APPENDIX 2-6 [CONTINUED] ▶ Infant and Child Growth Charts (continued)

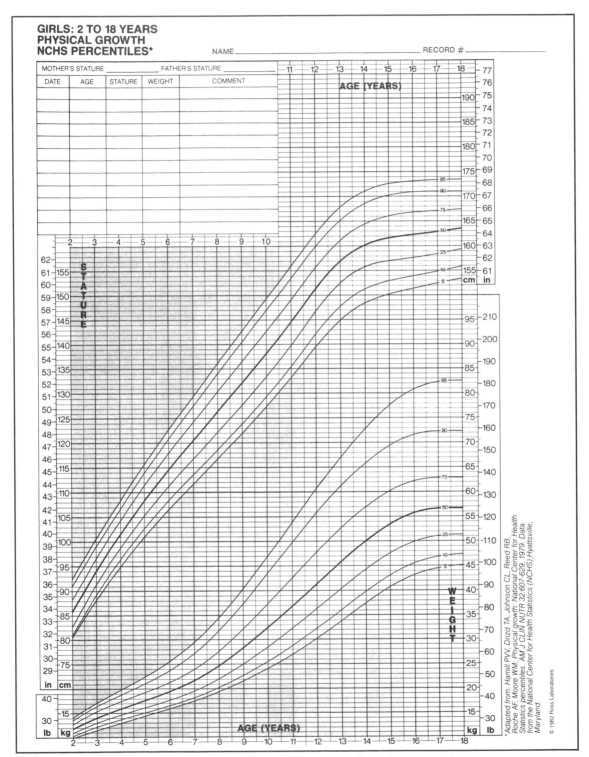

GIRLS: 2 TO 18 YEARS PHYSICAL GROWTH NCHS PERCENTILES*

APPENDIX 2-6 [CONTINUED] ▶ Infant and Child Growth Charts

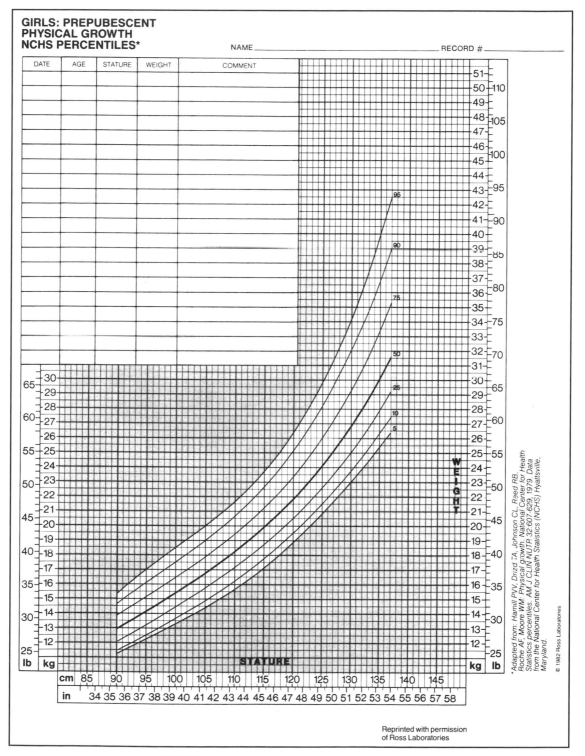

GIRLS: PREPUBESCENT PHYSICAL GROWTH NCHS PERCENTILES*

NAME _____   RECORD # _____

*Adapted from: Hamill PVV, Drizd TA, Johnson CL, Reed RB, Roche AF, Moore WM: Physical growth: National Center for Health Statistics percentiles. AM J CLIN NUTR 32:607-629, 1979. Data from the National Center for Health Statistics (NCHS) Hyattsville, Maryland.

© 1982 Ross Laboratories

APPENDIX 2-6 [CONTINUED] ▶ Infant and Child Growth Charts

Home Care Needs Assessment Tool for the Child

CLIENT

Name: _____ Client's DOB: _____ Client's Age: _____

Client's Ins. #: _____ Clients SS#: _____

Client's Race: _____ Client's Sex: _____

Current Telephone #: ( ) _____ Current Telephone #: ( ) _____

INSTITUTION: _____

_____ Home _____ Shelter _____ Homeless _____ Staying with Relatives

Address: _____
          (street)   (apt.)   (City)   (Zip)

EMERGENCY CONTACT PERSONS

Name: _____ Relationship: _____ Age: _____

Phone: _____

Address: _____
          (street)   (apt.)   (City)   (Zip)

MOTHER'S DATA

Name: _____ Phone: _____ Age: _____

Address: _____
          (street)   (apt.)   (City)   (Zip)

Best Time to Contact: _____

FATHER'S DATA

Name: _____ Phone: _____ Age: _____

Address: _____
          (street)   (apt.)   (City)   (Zip)

Best Time to Contact: _____

APPENDIX 2-7 ▶ Home Care Needs Assessment Tool for the Child. (*Source:* Chestnut, MA. High-risk newborn home care manual. Philadelphia: Lippincott-Raven, 1998)

CHILD'S DOCTOR (must use PCP if applicable)

Name: _____   Hospital: _____   Phone: _____

Address: _____
             (street)   (apt.)   (City)   (Zip)

CONSULTING DOCTORS ON CARE

1. _____   _____
        (Name)   (Phone)

2. _____   _____
        (Name)   (Phone)

3. _____   _____
        (Name)   (Phone)

OTHER CONSULTANTS

SW: _____   _____
        (Name)   (Phone)

Other: _____   _____
        (Name)   (Phone)

DIAGNOSES

1. _____   2. _____

3. _____

Exacerbating potentials: _____

I. BIRTH DATA

1. Hospital of Delivery: _____

2. History of Prenatal Care: _____

3. Gestational Age at Birth: _____   Wgt.: _____

      Problems: _____

4. Delivery: _____ Vaginal   _____ C-Section

5. Condition of Baby at Delivery/Complications

II. CURRENT STATE OF HEALTH

1. Physical

2. Mental

3. Emotional

4. Social

5. Hospitalizations/Surgeries

APPENDIX 2-7 [CONTINUED] ▶ Home Care Needs Assessment Tool for the Child   (continued)

III. CHILD'S HEALTH CARE NEEDS: (Specify with as much detail as possible)

1. Diet/Feeding Schedule:

2. Activity:

3. Physical Therapy:

4. Psychological Therapy/OT:

5. Educational Therapies:

6. Speech Therapy:

7. Equipment and use including tubes present—source of equipment—who supplies:

8. Medications—name, dose, route, freq., purpose:

9. Teaching Needed:

_____ Nutrition   _____ Community resources   _____ Respite

_____ Growth/dev.   _____ Utilities   _____ Others

_____ Formula prep and access to formula   _____ Phone

_____ Parenting education   _____ Housing

_____ Budgeting of financial resources   _____ Cooking

_____ Home safety   _____ Water

_____ Parenting

10. Referrals already made: _____

11. Referrals needed: _____

     _____ Kencrest   _____ Other

IV. FAMILY DATA/SUPPORT NETWORK

1.   Primary Caretaker of Child

     Name: _____

     Health Status: _____

     Ed. Issues: _____

     Age: _____

APPENDIX 2-7 [CONTINUED] ▶ Home Care Needs Assessment Tool for the Child

2. Siblings (Name, Age, Address, Medical Issues, Parents):

_____ no. of Siblings:

3. Other Household Members (Name, Age, Medical Issues):

4. Other Significant Others/Extended Family Members. Are they available to assist with care of child—when?

5. Summary of Household Function—Do people work together? Do they get along, who is in charge, etc.:

6. Evidence of Drug/alcohol Use:

V. HOUSING INFORMATION:

1. Current Residence: _____ permanent   _____ temporary

2. Type of Residence: _____ sngle Family   _____ apt.   _____ shelter

3. Length of Time in Current Residence: _____

4. Are there Plans for Move? _____ Yes _____ When? _____ No

   New Address: _____

5. Layout of House: _____ no. of Bedrooms   _____ no. of Bathrooms   _____ kitchen
                         _____ living Area   _____ furniture   _____ dining Area

   Condition of House: _____

6. Safety issues at House:

   Outlets: _____ 2-prong   _____ 3-prong   _____ adeq. No.'s   _____ inadeq. No.'s

   Smoke Alarms: Yes _____   No _____   no. of alarms: _____

   Stable Railings: Yes _____   No _____

   Adequate Lighting: Yes _____ No _____   Specify: _____

   Emergency No.'s Posted: Yes _____   No _____

   Sanitation: No. of Bathrooms: _____

   A. Is kitchen sanitary: Yes _____   No _____   Specify: _____

   B. Pest Control: Are the following present:

      _____ roaches   _____ rats/Mice   _____ flies

   C. Plumbing problems _____

APPENDIX 2-7 [CONTINUED] ▶ Home Care Needs Assessment Tool for the Child   (continued)

Medication storage—specify plan for storage, if refrigeration needed:

Infection control needs surrounding care:

7. Will house need modification/rearrangement for child (specify):

8. Specify space child will have to sleep, play, exercise, etc., and equipment (bed, toys) available:

VI.   FINANCIAL DATA

1. Source of income for parent/guardian   Name:

_____ DPA   Amount $ _____   _____ SSI   Amount $ _____

_____ Job   Amount $ _____

_____ Other: Specify type/amount: _____

_____ Child Support   Amount $ _____

2. Income Supplements—Program Participation

_____ WIC   _____ Food Stamps $ _____

_____ Public housing   Rent $ _____

_____ Section VIII housing   Amount $ _____ _____

_____ School lunch   _____ School breakfast

3. Expenses—Specify Amount

_____ Rent $ _____   _____ Food $ _____

_____ Utilities $ _____   _____ Meds $ _____

_____ Trans. $ _____   _____ Clothing $ _____

4. HEALTH INSURANCE:

_____ MA   _____ HMA   _____ NONE   _____ Other: _____

_____ NEEDS ASSIST—Specify:

APPENDIX 2-7 [CONTINUED] ▶ Home Care Needs Assessment Tool for the Child   (continued)

Pediatric Assessment and Care Screening for Function

Status in last 7 days, unless other time frame indicated.

Section A. Identification and Background Information

1. ASSESSMENT DATE: _____

2. CHILD'S NAME: _____

3. SS#: _____

4. Insurance type/I.D. #: _____

5. REASON FOR ASSESSMENT
   ____ initial evaluation   ____ significant change in status
   ____ hosp. reass.   ____ other
   ____ readmission assessment   ____ annual assessment

6. RESPONSIBILITY/LEGAL GUARDIAN
   ____ parent   ____ legal guardian

7. ADVANCED DIRECTIVES
   ____ living will
   ____ organ donation   ____ DNR   ____ do not hosp.
   ____ feeding restrictions   ____ autopsy request
   ____ other treatment restrictions ____ med. restrictions
   ____ none of the above

8. DISCHARGE PLANNED WITHIN 3 MONTHS
   ____ no   ____ yes
   ____ unknown, uncertain

9. PARTICIPATE IN ASSESSMENT
   child: ____ yes   ____ no
   family: ____ yes   ____ no
   guardian: ____ yes   ____ no

Section B. Cognitive Patterns

1. COMATOSE: ____ yes   ____ no

2. CHANGE IN COGNITIVE STATUS: ____ yes   ____ no
   Change in child's cognitive status, skills, or abilities in last 90 days:
   ____ no change   ____ improved   ____ deteriorated

APPENDIX 2-8 ▶ Pediatric Assessment and Care Screening for Function. (*Source:* Chestnut, MA. Pediatric home care manual. Philadelphia: Lippincott-Raven, 1998)

Section C. Communication/Hearing Patterns

1. HEARING: ____ hears and turns to sound
             ____ does not respond to sound

2. COMMUNICATION DEVICES/TECHNIQUES
   ____ hearing aid, present and used
   ____ hearing aid, present and not used
   ____ other receptive communication techniques used, e.g., lip reading
   ____ none of the above

3. MAKING SELF UNDERSTOOD
   A. All Children
      ____ communicates what he/she wants
      ____ sometimes communicates what he/she wants
      ____ rarely/never communicates what he/she wants
   B. Children < 1 year old
      ____ smiles, coos, babbles or uses other sounds
      ____ sometimes smiles, coos, babbles or uses other sounds
      ____ rarely/never smiles, coos, babbles or uses other sounds
   C. Children 2–3 years old
      ____ communicates with words so others can understand
      ____ sometimes communicates with words so others can understand
      ____ rarely/never communicates with words so others can understand

   D. Children over 3 years old
      ____ understood
      ____ usually understood—difficulty finding words or finishing thoughts
      ____ sometimes understood—ability is limited to making concrete requests
      ____ rarely/never understood

4. CHANGE IN COMMUNICATION/HEARING
   ____ child's ability to express, understand or hear information has changed over last 90 days
   ____ no change   ____ improved   ____ deteriorated

Section D. Vision Patterns

1. VISION (ability to see in adequate light and with glasses if used)
   A. Children < I year old
      ____ seems to look at things and tries to get objects that are near but beyond reach
      ____ sometimes seems to look at things and tries to get objects that are near but beyond reach
      ____ rarely/never seems to look at things or tries to get objects that are near but beyond reach
   B. Children 2 years or older
      ____ adequate—sees fine detail, including regular print in books
      ____ impaired—sees large print, but not reg. print in books
      ____ highly impaired—limited vision; not able to see newspaper headlines; appears to follow
           objects with eyes
      ____ severely impaired—no vision or appears to see only light, colors, or shapes

2. VISUAL LIMITATIONS/DIFFICULTIES
   ____ side vision problems—decreased peripheral vision (e.g., leaves food on one side of tray, difficulty
        traveling, bumps into people and objects, misjudges placement of chair when seating self)
   ____ experiences any of following: sees halos or rings around lights;
        sees flashes of light; sees "curtains" over eyes
   ____ none of the above

3. VISUAL APPLIANCES
   ____ Glasses; contact lenses; lens implant, magnifying glass: ____ yes   ____ no

APPENDIX 2-8 [CONTINUED] ▶ Pediatric Assessment and Care Screening for Function

Section E. Physical Functioning and Structural Problems

1. ADL—all children 1 year or older
   - ___ gets around the house without assistance
   - ___ does things for him/herself that he/she should do
   - ___ picks up and throws a ball or other object in intended direction
   - ___ requires the same amount of help with eating as other children his/her age

2. ADL—all children 2 years or older
   - ___ goes up and down stairs without assistance
   - ___ participates in hard exercise or play
   - ___ dresses him/herself
   - ___ gets undressed without help

3. BODY CONTROL PROBLEMS
   - ___ balance—partial or total loss of ability to balance self while standing
   - ___ bedfast all or most of the time
   - ___ contracture to arms, legs, shoulders, or hands
   - ___ hemiplegia/hemiparesis—quadriplegia
   - ___ arm—partial or total loss of voluntary movement
   - ___ hand—lack of dexterity (e.g., problem using toothbrush or adjusting hearing aid)
   - ___ leg—partial or total loss of voluntary movement
   - ___ leg—unsteady gait
   - ___ trunk—partial or total loss of ability to position, balance, or turn body
   - ___ amputation
   - ___ none of above

4. MOBILITY APPLIANCES/DEVICES
   - ___ cane/walker
   - ___ other person wheels
   - ___ none of the above
   - ___ brace/prosthesis
   - ___ lifted (manually/mechanically)
   - ___ wheels self

5. CHANGE IN ADL FUNCTION—change in ADL self-performance in last 90 days
   - ___ no change   ___ improved   ___ deteriorated

Section F. Continence Self-Control Categories

Code for Child Performance:
0. Continent—complete control appropriate for age
1. Usually continent—bladder, incontinent episodes lx/wk or less; bowel, less than weekly
2. Occasionally incontinent—bladder 2+ times a week but not daily; bowel, once a week
3. Frequently incontinent—bladder, tended to be incontinent daily, but some control present: bladder 2+ times a week but not daily; bowel 2–3 times a week
4. Incontinent—had inadequate control, bladder, multiple daily episodes; bowel, all, or almost all, of the time

- ___ BOWEL CONTINENCE—control of bowel movement, with appliance of bowel continence programs, if employed
- ___ BLADDER CONTINENCE—control of urinary bladder function (if dribbles, volume insufficient to soak through underpants), with appliances (e.g., Foley) or continence programs, if employed

INCONTINENCE-RELATED TESTING (skip if child's bladder continence code equals 0 or 1 and no catheter is used)
- ___ child has been tested for a urinary tract infection
- ___ child has been checked for presence of a fecal impaction, or there is adequate bowel elimination
- ___ none of the above

APPLIANCES AND PROGRAMS
- ___ any scheduled toileting plan
- ___ external (condom) catheter
- ___ ostomy
- ___ peds/briefs used
- ___ enemas/irrigation
- ___ did not use toilet room/ commode/urinal
- ___ indwelling catheter
- ___ intermittent catheter
- ___ none of above

CHANGE IN URINARY CONTINENCE
- ___ no change   ___ improved   ___ deteriorated

APPENDIX 2-8 [CONTINUED] ▶ Pediatric Assessment and Care Screening for Function   (continued)

Section G. Psychosocial Well Being

1. SENSE OF INITIATIVE/INVOLVEMENT
   ____ at ease interacting with others   ____ plays with other children
   ____ responds to attention

2. UNSETTLED RELATIONSHIPS
   ____ acts timid or shy   ____ acts afraid of new situations   ____ fights a lot with other children

Section H. Mood and Behavior Patterns

1. SAD OR ANXIOUS BEHAVIOR
   Demonstrated signs of mental distress
   ____ acts moody   ____ seems to feel sick and tired
   ____ seems unusually irritable or cross ____ reacts to little things by crying
   ____ seems unusually difficult   ____ acts restless and fidgety
   ____ has frequent temper tantrums

2. MOOD PERSISTENCE
   ____ sad or anxious mood intrudes daily over last 7 days
   ____ not easily altered, doesn't "cheer up"   ____ yes   ____ no

3. PROBLEM BEHAVIOR
   Code for behavior in last 7 days:
   0. Behavior not exhibited in last 7 days
   1. Behavior of this type occurred less than daily
   2. Behavior of this type occurred daily or more frequently

   ____ WANDERING (moved with no rational purpose, seemingly oblivious to needs or safety)
   ____ VERBALLY ABUSIVE (others were threatened, screamed at, cursed at)
   ____ PHYSICALLY ABUSIVE (others were hit, shoved, scratched, sexually abused)
   ____ SOCIALLY INAPPROPRIATE/DISRUPTIVE BEHAVIOR (made disrupting sounds, noisy, screams,
       self-abusive acts, sexual behavior or disrobing in public, smeared/threw food/feces)

4. CHILD RESISTS CARE (check all types of resistance that occurred in the last 7 days)
   ____ resisted taking medications/injection
   ____ resisted ADL assistance
   ____ none of the above

5. BEHAVIOR MANAGEMENT PROGRAM (Behavior problem has been addressed by clinically developed
   behavior management program. (*Note:* Do not include programs that involve only physical restraints or
   psychotropic medications in this category.)
   0. No behavior problem   1. Yes, addressed   2. No, not addressed

6. CHANGE IN MOOD (in last 90 days)
   0. No change   1. Improved   2. Deteriorated

7. CHANGE IN PROBLEM BEHAVIOR
   0. No change   1. Improved   2. Deteriorated

Section I. Activity Pursuit Patterns

1. SLEEP PATTERNS—All Children
   ____ sleeps well/through the night (if appropriate for age)
   ____ nap time and frequency appropriate for age

   Children 2 years or older
   a. During the past 2 wks did child spend all or part of the day in bed?
      ____ yes ____ no
   b. How many days did he/she stay in bed in the last 2 wks?

APPENDIX 2-8 [CONTINUED] ▶ Pediatric Assessment and Care Screening for Function

2. ACTIVITY—Children 1 year or older
    ____ concentrated or paid attention for a period of time
    ____ got involved in games or other play

3. ACTIVITY—Children 2 years or older
    ____ played games by him/herself

Section J. Disease Diagnoses

1. CURRENT ICD-9 CODES AND DIAGNOSES

    _____   _____
    _____   _____
    _____   _____
    _____   _____
    _____   _____

Section K. Health Conditions

1. PROBLEM CONDITIONS (check all that are present in last 7 days unless other time frame indicated)
    ____ constipation   ____ diarrhea
    ____ dizziness/vertigo   ____ edema
    ____ fecal impaction   ____ fever
    ____ hallucinations/delusions   ____ internal bleeding
    ____ joint pain   ____ vomiting
    ____ fainting   ____ shortness of breath
    ____ pain, daily or almost daily   ____ recurrent lung aspirations in last 90 days
    ____ none of above

2. HOSPITALIZATIONS
    ____ hospitalized in past 30 days
    ____ hospitalized in past 31–180 days
    ____ number of days hospitalized

3. STABILITY OF CONDITIONS
    ____ conditions/diseases make child's cognitive, ADL, or behavior status unstable—fluctuating, precarious, or deteriorating
    ____ child experiencing an acute episode or a flare-up of a recurrent/chronic problem
    ____ none of the above

Section L. Oral/Nutritional Status

1. ORAL PROBLEMS
    ____ chewing problem   ____ swallowing problem
    ____ mouth pain   ____ none of the above

2. HEIGHT AND WEIGHT
    ____ height   ____ weight

    Weight loss (i.e., 5% in last 30 days; or 10% in last 180 days)
    ____ yes   ____ no

APPENDIX 2-8 [CONTINUED] ▶ Pediatric Assessment and Care Screening for Function   (continued)

3. NUTRITIONAL PROBLEMS
   ___ complaints about the taste of many foods
   ___ insufficient fluid: dehydrated
   ___ did NOT consume all/almost all liquids provided during last 3 days
   ___ regular complaint of hunger
   ___ leaves 25%+ food uneaten at most meals
   ___ none of the above

4. NUTRITIONAL APPROACHES
   ___ parenteral/IV   ___ feeding tube
   ___ mechanically altered diet   ___ syringe (oral feeding)
   ___ therapeutic diet   ___ dietary supplement between meals
   ___ none of the above   ___ plaque guard, stab. built-up utensil, etc.

Section M. Oral/Dental Status

1. ORAL STATUS AND DISEASE PREVENTION
   ___ debris (soft, easily movable substances) present in mouth prior to going to bed at night
   ___ thrush
   ___ broken loose, or carious teeth
   ___ inflamed gums (gingiva); swollen or bleeding gums; oral abscesses, ulcers or rashes
   ___ daily cleaning of teeth/dentures
   ___ none of the above

Section N. Skin Condition

1. STASIS ULCER (open lesion caused by poor venous circulate to lower extremities): ___ yes   ___ no

2. PRESSURE ULCERS
   Code for highest stage of pressure ulcer:
   0. No pressure ulcers
   1. Stage I: A persistent area of skin redness (w/out a break in the skin) that does not disappear when pressure is relieved
   2. Stage 2: A partial thickness loss of skin layers that presents clinically as an abrasion, blister, or shallow crater
   3. Stage 3: A full thickness of skin is lost, exposing the subcutaneous tissues—presents as a deep crater with or w/out undermining adjacent tissue
   4. Stage 4: A full thickness of skin and subcutaneous tissue is lost, exposing muscle and/or bone

3. HISTORY OF RESOLVED/CURED PRESSURE ULCERS
   Child has had a pressure ulcer that was resolved/cured in last 90 days. ___ yes   ___ no

4. SKIN PROBLEMS/CARE
   ___ open lesions other than status or pressure ulcers (e.g., cuts)
   ___ skin desensitized to pain, pressure, discomfort
   ___ protective/preventive skin care
   ___ turning/repositioning program
   ___ pressure relieving beds, bed/chair pads (e.g., egg crate pads)
   ___ wound care/treatment (e.g., pressure ulcer care, surgical wound)
   ___ other skin care/treatment
   ___ none of the above

Section O. Medication Use

1. NUMBER OF MEDICATIONS (record # different meds used in last # days: enter 0 if none). _____

2. NEW MEDICATIONS (has child received any during the last 90 days?). ___ yes   ___ no

APPENDIX 2-8 [CONTINUED] ▶ Pediatric Assessment and Care Screening for Function

3. INJECTIONS (record # days of injections of any type received during the last # days). _____

4. DAYS RECEIVED THE FOLLOWING MEDS (record # days during last # days; enter 0 if not used; 1 if long-acting meds, used less than weekly).
____ antipsychotics   ____ antianxiety/hypnotics   ____ antidepressants

5. Previous Med Results (skip this question if child currently receiving antipsychotics, antianxiety/hypnotics, or antidepressants:

Child has previously received psychoactive medications for a mood or behavior problem, and these medications were effective (without undue adverse consequences)
0. No, drugs not used   2. Drugs were not effective
1. Drugs were effective   3. Drug effectiveness unknown

Section P. Special Treatment and Procedures

1. SPECIAL TREATMENTS AND PROCEDURES
Special Care—check treatments received during the last 14 days
____ chemotherapy   ____ radiation   ___ dialysis
____ suctioning   ____ trach care   ____ IV meds
____ transfusions   ____ O$_2$ _____ other
____ none of the above

Therapies—record the # of days each of the following therapies was administered (for at least 10 minutes during a day) in the last 7 days.
____ speech—language pathology and audiology services
____ OT   ____ PT—psychological therapy (any licensed prof)   ____ RT

2. ABNORMAL LAB VALUES
Has child had any abnormal lab values during the last 90 days?
____ yes   ____ no   ____ no tests performed

3. DEVICES AND RESTRAINT
____ 0. not used   ____ 1. used less than daily   ____ 2. used daily
____ bed rail   ____ trunk restraint   ____ limb restraint   ____ chair prevents rising

Background Information Intake at Admission

I. IDENTIFICATION INFORMATION

1. RESIDENT NAME: _____
First   Last

2. DATE OF CURRENT ADMISSION: _____

3. TYPE OF INS.: _____ INS. NO.: _____

4. FACILITY PROVIDER #: _____ _____

5. GENDER: _____   6. RACE: _____

7. DOB: _____   8. PRIMARY LANGUAGE: _____

9. MENTAL HEALTH HISTORY
Does child's record indicate any history of MH/MR, or any other mental health problem?
____ yes   ____ no

APPENDIX 2-8 [CONTINUED] ▶ Pediatric Assessment and Care Screening for Function   (continued)

10. CONDITIONS RELATED TO MR/MH STATUS (check all conditions that were manifested before age 22 and are likely to continue indefinitely)

____ Not applicable—no MR/Do (skip to item 11)

MR/Do with organic condition
____ CP   ____ Down's syndrome   ____ autism   ____ epilepsy

Other organic condition related to MR/Do
____ MR/Do with no organic condition   ____ Unknown

11. ADMITTED FROM: ____ private home or apt.   ____ hospital   ____ other

12. ADMISSION INFORMATION AMENDED (check all that apply)
____ accurate information unavailable
____ observation revealed additional information
____ child unstable at admission

II. BACKGROUND INFORMATION AT RETURN/READMISSION

1. Date of current readmission: _____
2. Admission Information amended (check all that apply)
____ accurate information unavailable earlier
____ observation revealed additional information
____ resident unstable at admission

RN Signature: _____   Date: _____

APPENDIX 2-8 [CONTINUED] ▶ Pediatric Assessment and Care Screening for Function

Section 1 Ethnicity and Race

- How does the client identify his racial affiliation?
- To what ethnic group does the client assign his membership?

Section 2 Birthplace and Place of Residence

- In which country was the client born _____
- In which country has the client resided _____ Years_____

Section 3 Communicative Competency

- Is there a written form of the client's language Y___ N___
- What is the client's native language _____
- Are health-related materials available in the client's native language? Y___ N___
    if yes, specify_____
- What is the client's English fluency level
    Mild___ Moderate___ Severe___ No difficulty with use of English ___
- Does the client require an interpreter Y___ N___
    if yes, specify_____
- List any nonverbal cues by the provider that facilitate or hinder
    communication_____
- List any nonverbal cues by the client that facilitate or hinder
    communication_____

Section 4 Food Sanctions/Restrictions

- Are religious beliefs and practices influencing factors in the client's daily diet Y___ N___
    if yes, specify_____
- Does the client's religion mandate fasting during certain times Y___ N___
    if yes, specify_____
- May certain foods be consumed during the fasting period Y___ N___
    if yes, specify_____
- Can the client identify any food sanctions or restrictions Y___ N___
    if yes, specify_____
- Are foods specially prepared Y___ N___
    if yes, specify_____
- Are any cultural meanings associated with the act of eating Y___ N___
    if yes, specify_____

Section 5 Religious and Spiritual Beliefs and Practices

- What is the client's religious affiliation
- What are the client's perceptions regarding death and dying and the grieving process
- What is the role of the client's religious representative
- Does the client's religious practices include inhalation/ingestion of substances used for sensory
- enhancement? Y___ N___
    if yes, specify_____

APPENDIX 2-9 ▶ The Culturological Assessment Guide (*Source:* McNeal GJ, Doherty A, O'Donnell DG, Mallory B: Culturally sensitive mobile health care services for at-risk populations. In Ferguson VD (ed): Educating the 21st century nurse: Challenges and Opportunities. 1997: New York, NY, National League for Nursing Press, Jones and Bartlett Publishers, Sudbury, MA. WWW.jbpub.com. Reprinted with permission)   (continued)

Section 6 Health Beliefs and Folk Practices

- What is the role of the client's beliefs and practices during health and illness

  _____

- List any folk medical/home remedies practiced by the client

  _____

- Does the client rely on lay/cultural healers Y___ N___
  if yes, specify_____

Section 7 Socioeconomic Considerations

- List the client's health insurance coverage
- Is the client employed Y___ N___
  if yes, specify_____
- What are the client's sources of financial support

  _____

- What is the client's socioeconomic level
  Upper___ Middle___ Lower ___ Below Poverty level ___
- Is there a need to consult social services Y___ N___
  if yes, specify_____

Section 8 Family structure/role and social network

- What constitutes the client's family composition
- Which members of the family serve as caregivers
- Decisionmaking in matters of health is the primary responsibility of
  the client ___ his family ___ his social support network___
- What is the composition of the client's social support network

Section 9 Educational Consideration

- What is the client's highest level of schooling completed
  1-6 years ___ 7-12 years ___ 13-16 years ___ 16+ years ___ None___
- If applicable, list the country(ies) of residence in which school was attended

  _____

- Based on the client's learning needs, behavioral learning objectives should be written in which of the
  following domains:
  Psychomotor ___ Cognitive ___ Affective___
- If the client has a learning deficit, indicate the type of deficiency and specify alternative approaches
  Cognitive ___ Perceptual ___ Sensory ___ Motor___

Section 10 Explanatory Model of Illness Causation

- From which perspective does the client view his cause of illness

  Scientific ___   Holistic ___   Magiocoreligious ___   Combination ___

APPENDIX 2-9 [CONTINUED] ▷ The Culturological Assessment Guide

Instructions for use of the Culturological Assessment Guide

The client history is obtained during the first component of the assessment phase of the nursing process. In the hightech homecare setting, the nurse and client, or caregiver, begin this phase with the interview, during which time very personal and intimate findings are shared. The culturally sensitive information so vital to the implementation of the plan of care may be obtained through the use of a culturological assessment guide. The following guide identifies ten categories under which are listed specific questions. The rationale supporting use of the related statements of inquiry is explained for each category in the following sections and will prove helpful in assisting the nurse to acquire relevant cultural information.

Section 1 *Ethnicity and Race*
The first category of the culturological guide poses questions regarding the client's ethnic and racial affiliation. Because of the importance of the client's cultural heritage, the client should be permitted to self-report his ethnic and racial affiliation, to avoid use of the often culturally insensitive approach of assuming the client's membership in one group or another.

Section 2 *Birthplace and Place of Residence*
The second category of the culturological guide presents questions that permit the client to identify his/her country of origin and current place of residence. The high-tech homecare nurse will find it helpful to know how long the client has resided in this country, which sometimes serves as an indicator of the degree to which the client may be able to adhere to the prescribed regimen, especially when the regimen differs significantly from the client's own beliefs.

Section 3 *Communicative Competency*
The third category of the culturological guide lists those questions which guide the nurse in assessing the client's language skills and use of non-verbal communication. English is a second language for 14% of the nation's diverse populations. Even when English is the primary language, choice of words, dialects, and word connotation may vary significantly from that used by members of the larger society. Further, it is important to remember that both verbal and non-verbal cues are used to effect communication. Non-verbal cues, such as gestures, touch, eye contact, and body language, help to facilitate the communication process. Because such cues are culturally related, the nurse will need to develop an awareness for their appropriate use. Both the nurse and the client may unknowingly hinder communication by demonstrating culturally inappropriate behavior. For example, it may be culturally inappropirate for some cultures to relate to questions which address the sexual history, even when such information is vital to the plan of care. The nurse will need to be sensitive to body language which indicates discomfort when initiating such dialogue and will need to be attentive to the client's cultural orientation.

In selecting a translator to assist in interpreting information, the nurse will need to be aware of the care which must be taken in choosing such assistance. Translators, while fluent in the client's language, may from the client's perspective be too young, of the wrong gender, not of the same sociocultural background, culturally forbidden to share intimate healthcare information, or unfamiliar with medical terminology.

For those with limited English reading skills, the nurse may need to develop pictorial guidelines and learning packets, and to utilize teaching method which are consistent with the client's cultural style of learning. Some cultures learn best using a hands-on (psychomotor) method of instruction. Others may require an approach which focuses more on the client's feelings and attitudes (affective). Still others may learn best when information is provided in a formal atmosphere using the teacher-learner style of instruction (cognitive).

APPENDIX 2-9 [CONTINUED] ▶ The Culturological Assessment Guide   (continued)

Section 4 *Food Sanctions/Restrictions*

Food choice and selection often holds more than just nutritive value for the client, and may be more closely related to religious practices. A nutritionist may need to be consulted to assist in developing meal plans that are consistent with the client's religious or cultural practices, as in use of herbs, organic vitamins, minerals, teas and coffee. The nurse must take into consideration the client's ability to comply with food preparation orders. Some living arrangements may not support use of familiar kitchen appliances, as for example the Native American who may live in a hogan (mud hut). Some creativity will be needed in the development of culturally sensitive therapeutic dietary regimens. The nutritionist will be helpful in assisting with the inclusion of culturally sensitive meal planning ideas.

Section 5 *Religious and Spiritual Considerations*

The hightech homecare nurse will need to determine the degree to which the client adheres to religious doctrine or spiritual beliefs. Some cultures rely on the use of spiritual healers, as, for example, the Medicine Man (Native American) and the voodoo priest (Black American). It will be important for the nurse to remember to include the religious representative in the plan of care: rabbi, priest, minister, faith healer.

At the time of the client's admission to homecare, the client will be informed of the option to select a durable power of attorney and to establish advance directives for end-of-life decisions and interventions. For most cultures these are very sensitive issues. In helping the client to relate his feelings regarding these concepts, the hightech homecare nurse will gain invaluable insight into the client's belief systems and will be better able to construct culturally relevant plans of care that address spiritual distress and the grieving process.

Section 6 *Health Beliefs and Folk Practice*

Many cultures hold views which differ significantly from those held by the larger American society. Folk remedies and practices may be very much a part of the client's healthcare regimen. The scientific approach to cure and healing makes a clear distinction between the body and the spiritual aspects of the human species. Some cultures believe in a body-mind-spirit triad which must be kept in a balanced state to maintain health. Forces within the universe or under the control of gods are believed to have the power to bring about states of health. Understanding the client's belief system will be extremely useful in developing culturally sensitive plans of care.

Section 7 *Socioeconomic Consideration*

The sources of financial support, healthcare insurance coverage, and the family's socioeconomic level are all determinants in the client's ability to access healthcare delivery options. The high-tech homecare nurse may need to consult with the medical social service worker (MSW) to assist the client to locate various financial resources. The questions posed in this section will help the nurse provide the MSW with relevant information.

Section 8 *Family Structure/Role and Social Network*

Among ethnically diverse populations nontraditional familial relationships may be more often observed. Multigenerational, multiple households, single-parent families, and unmarried cohabitants may comprise the kinship networks. Decisionmaking in some diverse families may come from a dominant authority as among the elders, or made only by the male head of household, or in still others, decisions are made by a collective community by which the client must abide. The hightech homecare nurse will need to have the client identify all relatives and related kin, and their respective roles during times of illness.

APPENDIX 2-9 (CONTINUED) ▶ The Culturological Assessment Guide

Section 9 *Educational Considerations*

In determining the client's learning ability, the high-tech homecare nurse will need to gather information regarding the client's educational level, capacity to learn, and presence of any learning deficits or developmental delays. In some cases, the client's caregiver may need to be heavily relied upon to participate in the educational process, and to be primarily responsible for the implementation of all teaching plans. Other members of the multidisciplinary team (physical, occupational and/or speech therapist) may need to be consulted to privide a more in-depth assessment and intervention.

Section 10 *Explanatory Models of Illness Causation*

Different cultures hold different views regarding the underlying cause of disease. Three different perspectives on disease states and their causative factors are recognized in the literature: scientific, holistic, and magicoreligious. Western medical healthcare practices are based on the scientific model of illness causation, which holds that all disease states have a measurable cause and effect. Nursing relies very heavily on the principles supporting the scientific model. The holistic and magicoreligious theories are more metaphysical in orientation, and are more oriented toward the achievement of a balance between the body and spiritual forces. The holistic model supports the concept that health is maintained by keeping the mind-body-spirit in balance with the universe. Among some Hispanic cultures that balance is explained by the Hot-Cold Theory, and in some Asian cultures the Yin-Yang Theory supports the concept. The magicoreligious model asserts that the supernatural forces of good and evil hold the capacity to maintain or disrupt health. Most organized religions support this theory, and use of the Medicine Man and voodoo priest in some Native American and Black American subcultures is consistent with this belief system.

It is important for the high-tech homecare nurse to remember that a combination of beliefs may be held by the client. Further it is important to note that western scientific medical practice derives some its approaches to care from each of the other two models of illness causation. Use of herbs and roots is the practice used by traditional cultural healers and root doctors; however, the essence of such plants is often the active ingredient contained in current American pharmaceutical agents. As well, nursing has long recognized the importance of incorporating holistic practice into the plan of care, as in therapeutic touch, relaxation techniques, hypnosis, biofeedback and guided imagery. It is important to note that the culturally diverse client may be quite comfortable holding a combination of beliefs [26–28].

APPENDIX 2-9 [CONTINUED] ▶ The Culturological Assessment Guide

Maximum Score	Score	
		ORIENTATION
5	( )	What is the (year), (season), (day), (month)
5	( )	Where are we: (state) (country) (town) (hospital)
3	( )	**REGISTRATION** Name 3 objects: 1 second to say each. Then ask the patient to repeat all 3 objects. Give 1 point for each correct answer. Then repeat them until all are correctly repeated. Count the trials and record. Trials _____
5	( )	**ATTENTION AND CALCULATION** Serial 7's. 1 point for each correct answer. Stop after 5 answers Alternatively spell "world" backwards [dlrow]
3	( )	**RECALL** Ask the patient to repeat the three objects named above. Give 1 point for each correct answer
9	( )	**LANGUAGE** Identify a pencil and watch [2 points]. Repeat the following "no ifs ands or buts". [1 point]. Follow a three stage command: take a paper in your right hand, fold it in half, and put it on the floor. [3 points]. Read and obey the following [1 point]:

CLOSE YOUR EYES

Write a sentence [1point]

Copy the design at the bottom of the page [1 point]

Total Score   ( )

Assess level of consciousness along a continuum

ALERT   DROWSY   STUPOR   COMA

APPENDIX 2-10A ▶ The Mini-Mental State Examination

ORIENTATION

> Ask for the date. Then specifically ask for the parts omitted. "Can you also tell me the season?" One point for each correct answer
>
> Ask in turn, "can you tell me the name of this hospital?" (town, country, etc). One point for each correct answer

REGISTRATION

> Ask the patient if you may test his memory. Then say the names of 3 unrelated objects, clearly and slowly, about one second for each. After you have said all 3 objects, ask him to repeat them. This first repetition determines his score (0 to 3) but keep saying them until he can repeat all three, up to 6 trials. If he does not eventually learn all 3, recall cannot be meaningfully tested.

ATTENTION AND CALCULATION

> Ask the patient to begin with 100 and count backwards by 7. Stop after 5 subtractions (93, 86, 79, 72, 65). Score the total number of correct answers. If the patient cannot or will not perform the task, ask him to spell the word "world" backwards. The score is the number of letters in correct order, e.g. dlrow = 5, dlorw = 3.

RECALL

> Ask the patient if he can recall the 3 objects you asked above. Score is 0 to 3.

LANGUAGE

> <u>Naming</u>: Show the patient a wrist watch and ask him to identify it. Repeat with a pencil.
> > Score 0 - 2
>
> <u>Repetition</u>: Ask the patient to repeat the sentence after you. Allow only one trial. Score 0 or 1
> <u>3-Stage Command</u>: Give the patient a piece of blank paper and repeat the command. Score 1 point for each part correctly executed
> <u>Reading</u>: On a blank piece of paper print the sentence "Close your eyes" in letters large enough for the patient to see clearly. Ask him to read it and do what it says. Socre 1 point only if he actually closes his eyes
> <u>Writing</u>: Give the patient a blank piece of paper and ask him to write a sentence for you. Do not dictate the sentence, it is to be written spontaneously. It must contain a subject and verb to be sensible. Correct grammar and punctuation are not necessary.
>
> <u>Copying</u>: On a clean piece of paper, draw intersecting pentagons, each side about 1 inch, and ask the patient to copy the design exactly as it is. all 10 angles must be present and 2 must intersect to score 1 point. Tremor and rotation are ignored.

LEVEL OF CONSCIOUSNESS

> Estimate the patient's level of sensorium along a continuum, from alert on the left to coma on the right.

(Adapted from Folstein MF, Folstein SE, and McHugh PR. Mini-mental state. J Psychiatric Res 12:189-198, 1975. Used with permission)

Action	Response	Score
Eyes open	spontaneously	4
	to speech	3
	to pain	2
	none	1
Best verbal response	oriented	5
	confused	4
	inappropriate words	3
	incomprehensible sounds	2
	none	1
Best motor response	obeys commands	6
	localizes to pain	5
	flexion withdrawal	4
	abnormal flexion	3
	abnormal extension	2
	flaccid	1
	Total Score	___

APPENDIX 2-11 ▶ The Glasgow Coma Scale

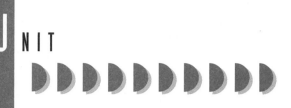

U N I T

3 *Perinatal Homecare*

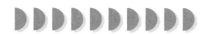

Perinatal Gastrointestinal System Procedures

1

PROCEDURE
Management of Hyperemesis Gravidarum

DESCRIPTION
Hyperemesis gravidarum is a condition characterized by excessive and pernicious vomiting occurring usually during the first trimester. As the condition persists, the client becomes lethargic, dehydrated, febrile, and demonstrates signs of jaundice and peripheral nerve involvement. As starvation develops, the urine will contain blood, bile, albumin, and ketones. Treatment includes client education, nutrition evaluation, and enteral/parenteral administration of fluids and nutrients.

PURPOSE
To prevent dehydration and malnutrition, to decrease hospital admissions, and to provide adequate nutrition for mother and fetus until mother is able to resume oral intake of food.

EQUIPMENT
Supplies for enteral or peripheral/central intravenous infusions
    (see also related adult cardiovascular and gastrointestinal system procedures)
Urine monitoring test strips (see also home urine monitoring procedure)

OUTCOMES
The client will:

▶ Achieve normal weight gain for pregnancy
▶ Maintain serum albumin > 3.5 gm/ dl
▶ Achieve positive nitrogen balance
▶ Maintain negative ketones in urine
▶ Maintain fluid and electrolyte balance
▶ Correctly administer ordered nutritional infusion
▶ Verbalize content of diet for hyperemesis & steps to take to increase oral intake
▶ Assess for signs and symptoms of complications: vaginal bleeding/spotting, leakage or gush of fluids from vagina, vomiting/diarrhea, fever/infection secondary to sexually transmitted disease or urinary tract infection
▶ Assess for fetal activity/heartones

ASSESSMENT DATA
Perform a prenatal risk assessment (see Appendix 3-1)
Document prepregnancy weight, weight history, and gestational weight gain date.
Note frequency, amount and type of emesis in 24 hours
Assess ability of client to ingest adequate amounts of fluids
If lipid infusion, monitor triglyceride for hyperlipidemia
Assess nutritional status

RELATED NURSING DIAGNOSES

Altered nutrition, less than body requirements
Fluid volume deficit
Anxiety
Powerlessness
Ineffective coping
At risk for infection
At risk for loss and grieving

SPECIAL CONSIDERATIONS

The hyperemetic client may be referred from the hospital or physician office. Often the client will be admitted to homecare service late in the day, which tends to extend the period during which the client may have been without medications or fluids. The nurse will need to coordinate the ordering of intravenous supplies with the homecare agency or DME company.

Calorie requirements are the same for orally, enterally, or parenterally fed pregnant women.

Oral supplementation and intensive nutrition counseling should be attempted before enteral nutrition support.

Clients with small amounts of emesis are the best candidates for enteral nutrition support.

The psychosocial aspects of this condition tend to be rather devastating for this client, who prior to the pregnancy was typically in excellent health. Furthermore, the debilitating nature of the condition is often not taken seriously by family and friends. Secondary depression may ensue.

If fluids are to be administered via a peripheral line, prior to the client being discharged to home, ensure that an IV access line has been placed. Often these client have veins which are difficult to access secondary to a prolonged state of dehydration and/or repeated sticks for blood draws, intravenous insertions, etc. If the client is to receive long-term intravenous therapy, arrange to have a midline or peripherally inserted catheter (PICC) placed.

The nurse should assess the client for levels of severity using the following suggested guidelines:

Mild:	sporadic vomiting with poor weight gain, nausea, and variable intolerance to solid food.
	infusion therapy is routinely not required
Moderate:	intermittent to persistent vomiting with gradual decrease in weight
	inability to tolerate solid foods or liquids.
	decreased intake and output
	routinely requires infusion therapy with or without antiemetic medication administration
	midline catheters or PICC lines should be placed for infusion therapy greater than 7 days duration
Severe:	persistent vomiting with rapid weight loss, dehydration, malnutrition leading to fluid and electrolyte imbalance
	diminished urinary output
	requires long-term parenteral hydration and/or TPN, and antiemetic medication to maintain homeostasis, the client should already have an intravenous access site: midline, PICC, or central venous access

TRANSCULTURAL CONSIDERATIONS

For clients with predominant ethnic food choices, provide appropriate list of foods with guidelines on how to incorporate these foods into the exchanges. An interpreter will be needed for the non-English speaking client. Ascertain availability of related educational materials in client's native language. Consider use of AT&T Language Line. See also the Culturological Assessment procedure in Unit 2 for general overview of cultural considerations.

▶ INTERVENTIONS

1. Wash hands.

Prevents transmission of microbes

2. Perform physical assessment.

Establishes baseline information of physiological findings

3. Obtain a nutritional assessment with dietary history and pattern of nausea and vomiting. Rate the emesis on a scale of 0 to 5 to effectively evaluate trends.

Provides baseline parameters needed to evaluate efficiency of treatment and client progress

4. Verify physician order for infusion therapy.

Reduces risk of error

5. Initiate intravenous infusion.
   a. For peripheral intravenous infusion.
      (1) Insert peripheral intravenous line and initiate intravenous infusion as ordered.

Replaces fluid losses and restores hydrational status

      (2) Administer fluid therapy as ordered.

Reverses state of dehydration

      (3) Instruct client in procedure to administer intravenous fluids/medications and assess intravenous site.

Promotes client self-sufficiency

         ▶ client changes intravenous bag using aseptic technique
            ▶ spikes bag
            ▶ primes tubing
            ▶ stops pump
            ▶ connects tubing to infusion pump
            ▶ resumes pump
         ▶ client observes intravenous site for evidence of infection, infiltration
         ▶ client administers intravenous medications as ordered
      (4) Observe client's ability to perform procedure and verbalize understanding.

Assesses client's ability to safely implement ordered procedure

   b. For total parenteral nutrition (TPN) intravenous infusion.
      (1) Verify that Hickman catheter or cental line has been placed.

Total parenteral nutrition therapy must be administered via long-term venous access lines

      (2) Administer TPN therapy as ordered.

Provides adequate nutrition to support health of mother and growth of fetus

      (3) Instruct client in procedure to administer TPN as ordered.

Promotes client self-sufficiency

         ▶ client changes intravenous bag using aseptic technique
            ▶ spikes bag
            ▶ primes tubing

▶ stops pump	
▶ connects tubing to infusion pump	
▶ resumes pump	
▶ client adds medications to TPN solution as ordered	
▶ client observes site (PICC insertion site, central venous access access site)	
▶ for evidence of infection, infiltration	
(4) Observe client's ability to perform procedure and verbalize understanding.	*Assesses client's ability to safely implement ordered procedure*
6. Instruct client to record daily intake and output.	*Monitors fluid volume and documents response to treatment*
7. Obtain pertinent serum/urine laboratory specimens as ordered.	*Monitors client response to therapy*
8. Initiate nutritional consult.	*Assesses client's nutritional status and provides instruction on ordered therapeutic dietary regimen*
9. Begin instruction on the slow introduction of foods into dietary regimen as ordered.	*Reinforces principles of diet therapy and discourages selection of inappropriate food choices*
10. Maintain log of anthropometric measurements: daily weights, pertinent serum/urinary laboratory analyses.	*Documents physiological data findings and monitors response to interventional strategies*
11. Encourage client to engage in rest and relaxation techniques.	*Restores activity tolerance*
12. Evaluate the home environment: finances, siblings, job responsibilities, support of significant other, attitudes toward pregnancy.	*Provides evidence of absent/present financial and psychosocial support systems*

DOCUMENTATION

The following should be noted in the nursing note:

Client's tolerance to the feeding
Any vomiting, abdominal distension, diarrhea, or discomfort
Client's ability to perform the procedure
Anthropometric measurements
Type of infusion, additives, volume, and method of administration
Laboratory data findings
Assessment of the home setting
All client/caregiver teaching
   Topics to include in the teaching plan:
      safe and correct equipment handling
      emergency procedures
      underlying disease pathology
      appropriate community resources and contact persons

INTERDISCIPLINARY COLLABORATION

Consult nutritionist to provide client education and to recommend dietary regimen

Report any incidence of emesis or change of status to physician and nutritionist

Collaborate with physician, pharmacist and nutritionist in ordering of appropriate
        Kcal/CHO/PRO/FAT/Vit/electrolytes, or change in antiemetic medications

Consult social worker to evaluate financial status and to identify appropriate community resources

Anticipate need to reorder supplies from DME vendor [2–4, 6, 7, 9, 11, 12]

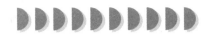

2 *Perinatal Endocrine System Procedures*

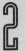

PROCEDURE

Management of Gestational Diabetes

DESCRIPTION
Gestational diabetes is defined as diabetes mellitus that develops during pregnancy as a result of hormonal changes. The condition usually subsides after delivery, although studies now show that gestational diabetics have a 40% chance of becoming diabetic for life.

PURPOSE
To prevent complications of diabetes, to reduce hospital admissions, and to assist the client to effectively manage ordered treatment modalities

EQUIPMENT
Diabetic educational materials
Blood glucose monitoring kit and record
Urine ketone strips

OUTCOMES
The client will:

▶ Maintain blood glucose and urine ketone levels as per physician order
▶ Maintain adequate nutrition to meet requirements for appropriate weight gain
▶ Administer insulin therapy as ordered
▶ Verbalize content of diet
▶ Achieve normal weight gain for pregnancy
▶ Verbalize signs and symptoms of complications

ASSESSMENT DATA
Perform a prenatal risk assessment
Document prepregnancy weight, weight history, and gestational weight gain to date
Record blood glucose monitoring, glycocylated hemoglobin, and ketone monitoring
(minimally record fasting and 2-hour postprandial glucose levels)
Document usual food intake and dietary deficiencies.
Assess for signs and symptoms of complications: vaginal bleeding/spotting, leakage or gush of flu-
    ids from vagina, vomiting/diarrhea, fever/infection secondary to sexually transmitted disease
    or urinary tract infection
Assess for fetal activity/heartones

RELATED NURSING DIAGNOSES
At risk for fluid volume deficit
Knowledge deficit
Altered nutrition
At risk for loss and grieving

SPECIAL CONSIDERATIONS
The nurse needs to consult with the nutritionist to provide any adjustment in the kcal/CHO requirements necessary to promote proper weight gain and prevention of hyperglycemia or ketonuria.

Research has shown that neonatal mobility and mortality are related to glucose levels. Although in some instances it may be acceptable for a diabetic adult to have a blood glucose level over 120 mg/dl or below 60 mg/dl, in the perinatal client these levels place the fetus at great risk. The nurse should prepare dietary teaching guides that are easy to understand, emphasize the importance of maintaining tight control of blood glucose levels, and utilize an approach to care which permits the client to rapidly apply the knowledge learned.

TRANSCULTURAL CONSIDERATIONS
For clients with predominant ethnic food choices, provide appropriate list of foods with guidelines on how to incorporate these foods into the exchanges
An interpreter will be needed for the non-English speaking client, consider use of AT&T Language Line
Ascertain availability of related educational materials in client's native language. See also the Culturological Assessment procedure in Unit 2 for a general overview of cultural considerations.

▶ INTERVENTIONS

1. Wash hands.	*Prevents transmission of microbes*
2. Perform physical assessment.	*Establishes baseline information of physiological findings*
3. Obtain a nutritional history.	*Provides basis for individualized meal planning*
4. Provide nutrition counseling.	*Enhances client awareness and acceptance of important role nutrition plays in management of diabetes*
5. Instruct client on ordered ADA diet therapy.	*Promotes client self-sufficiency*
6. Observe client's ability to plan diet according to medical regimen and to verbalize understanding.	*Documents client's ability to follow therapeutic regimen as ordered*
7. Instruct client on glucose monitoring procedure.	*Promotes client self sufficiency*
8. Observe client's ability to perform glucose monitoring procedure and verbalize understanding.	*Assesses client's ability to safely implement ordered procedure*
9. Instruct client to maintain daily log of fingerstick blood glucose readings.	*Documents physiological data findings and monitors response to interventional strategies*

10. Review physician established parameters for blood glucose levels and when to report findings.

Reinforces client learning

11. Instruct client on urine ketone-monitoring procedure.

Promotes client self sufficiency

12. Observe client's ability to perform urine ketone monitoring procedure and verbalize understanding.

Assesses client's ability to correctly implement ordered procedure

13. Review physician established parameters for urine ketone levels and when to report findings.

Reinforces client learning

14. Review signs and symptoms of hyperglycemia/ hypoglycemia.

Reinforces client learning

For Insulin Administration

1. Verify physician order for insulin therapy.

Reduces risk of error

2. Instruct client in insulin administration.

Promotes client self-sufficiency

3. Observe client's ability to administer insulin using aseptic technique.

Assesses client's ability to implement ordered procedure

4. Instruct client in possible need for changes in the insulin dosage as the pregnancy progresses.

Helps the client plan for modification in the drug regimen

DOCUMENTATION

The following will be noted in the nursing note:

Type of diet ordered and client tolerance
Need for future nutrition counseling
Laboratory data findings
Client's ability to perform procedures as ordered
Anthropometric measurements
Assessment of the home setting
All client/caregiver teaching
    Topics to include in the teaching plan:
        safe and correct equipment handling
        emergency procedures
        underlying disease pathology
        appropriate community resources and contact persons

INTERDISCIPLINARY COLLABORATION

Consult nutritionist to assist in the provision of client education and to recommend dietary regimen
Report any evidence of hyper/hypoglycemia and all abnormal laboratory findings to physician
Consult social worker to evaluate financial status or to identify community resources [1, 2, 4, 6–12]

PROCEDURE
Home Glucose Monitoring

DESCRIPTION

Self-blood glucose monitoring is a technique used to monitor blood glucose levels in the home. The technique requires use of a reflectance meter to measure blood glucose levels obtained from a drop of blood. A less precise method may be used which requires that the client place a drop of blood on a reagent strip and compare the color change with a color chart.

PURPOSE

To monitor capillary blood glucose levels in the home setting in the client with gestational diabetes

EQUIPMENT

Home monitoring unit of choice
Lancet device
Lancets
Test strip
Blood glucose log
Control solution
Cotton ball, if required by monitoring unit

OUTCOMES

The client/caregiver will:

▶ Demonstrate correct procedure for testing blood glucose
▶ Maintain a blood glucose log
▶ Perform regular cleaning of the monitoring unit in accordance with the manufacturer's recommendations
▶ Demonstrate ability to perform quality control test

ASSESSMENT DATA

Perform a prenatal risk assessment
Assess the client for signs and symptoms of hyperglycemia/hypoglycemia
Obtain diet history
Review all prescribed medications and pharmocodynamic effects on insulin or glucose production
Evaluate client's knowledge of and ability to perform procedure
Assess for signs and symptoms of complications: vaginal bleeding/spotting, leakage or gush of fluids from vagina, vomiting/diarrhea, fever/infection secondary to sexually transmitted disease or urinary tract infection
Assess for fetal activity/heartones

RELATED NURSING DIAGNOSES

Knowledge deficit
At risk for infection
Anxiety
At risk for altered skin integrity
At risk for loss and grieving

SPECIAL CONSIDERATIONS

In the adolescent population, select a monitoring unit that is simple to use. Talking glucose monitoring units are available for the visually impaired

TRANSCULTURAL CONSIDERATIONS

Several monitoring units have the capability of providing written prompts in several languages. Select appropriate monitoring units in consideration of the client's possible language barrier. Some monitoring units will convert the result from milligrams/deciliter (as used in the United States) to millimoles/liter (as used in some European countries). Consider use of AT&T Language Line. See also the Culturological Assessment procedure in Unit 2 for general overview of cultural considerations.

▶ **INTERVENTIONS**

1. Wash hands.

   Prevents transmission of microbes

2. Assemble supplies.

   Promotes efficiency and decreases error in testing

3. Explain procedure.

   Decreases anxiety and promotes cooperation

4. Don gloves.

   Serves as protective barrier

5. Select and cleanse finger for puncture.

   Rotation of sites reduces finger discomfort

6. Complete steps for testing blood glucose as per manufacturer's instructions:

   a. Obtain appropriate size blood sample

   Small sample size may alter result

   b. Apply blood to proper location on test strip

   Blood sample must cover testing area to ensure accuracy of reading

   c. Complete timing of test as per instruction

   Alteration in timing will skew results

   d. Use appropriate materials if wiping blood is required

   Rough or abrasive materials may remove color from test strip and alter results

   e. Record results in log

   Monitors response to interventional strategies

7. Instruct client on how to perform glucose monitoring procedure.

   Reinforces client learning

8. Observe client's ability to perform procedure.

   Assesses client's ability to implement ordered intervention

9. Instruct client on proper procedure for quality control testing and permit return demonstration.

   a. upon opening container, glucose solution should be dated and discarded as per manufacturer's recommendation

   Prevents outdated solution from altering results

   b. quality control testing should be performed whenever the monitoring unit has been mishandled, out of use for extended periods of time, whenever a new bottle of strips is opened

   Assures accuracy of results obtained from the monitoring unit

10. Instruct client on proper procedure for cleaning the monitoring unit and permit return demonstration.

    Cleansing should be performed when the unit becomes soiled and each time a new bottle of strips is opened

DOCUMENTATION

The following should be noted in the nursing note:

Time and date of testing
Blood glucose results

Notification of physician of abnormal results
Interventions for glucose levels exceeding ordered parameters
All client/caregiver teaching
    Topics to include in the teaching plan:
        safe and correct equipment handling
        emergency procedures
        underlying disease pathology
        appropriate community resources and contact persons

INTERDISCIPLINARY COLLABORATION

Report to the physician all results exceeding parameters
Consult the nutritionist for recommendation/reinforcement of dietary regimen
Consult social worker to assist in obtaining monitoring units for clients eligible for financial assistance [1, 8, 10]

3 *Perinatal Urinary System Procedure*

Home Urine Monitoring

DESCRIPTION

Home urine monitoring is a technique used to identify and monitor urinary levels of protein, ketone, glucose, and specific gravity. The technique requires that the client dip a reagent strip into a freshly obtained urine specimen and compare the color changes on the strip with a color chart.

PURPOSE

To monitor urinary levels of protein, ketone, glucose, and specific gravity in the home setting

EQUIPMENT

Test strip
Log
Health assessment forms

OUTCOMES

The client will:

▶ Demonstrate correct procedure for urine testing
▶ Maintain a log of urine test results
▶ Maintain blood pressure within normal limits
▶ Observe for and report symptoms of fluid volume deficit/overload, ketonuria, proteinuria, glucosuria

ASSESSMENT DATA

Perform a prenatal risk assessment
Assess the client for signs and symptoms of diabetes, fluid volume deficit/overload, hypertension, proteinuria
Review diet history and adherence to low sodium diet
Evaluate client's knowledge of and ability to perform procedure
Assess for headache, blurred vision and epigastric pain
Assess for signs and symptoms of complications: vaginal bleeding/spotting, leakage or gush of fluids from vagina, vomiting/diarrhea, fever/infection secondary to sexually transmitted disease or urinary tract infection
Assess for fetal activity/heartones

RELATED NURSING DIAGNOSES
Knowledge deficit
Altered urinary elimination
Anxiety
At risk for fluid volume overload
At risk for loss and grieving

SPECIAL CONSIDERATIONS
Color changes in the reagent strip are sometimes very subtle and difficult to detect, especially for the client who may be colorblind. Adequate lighting to see color changes and use of corrective lens will be necessary to ensure accuracy of reading.

TRANSCULTURAL CONSIDERATIONS
An interpreter will be needed for the non-English speaking client. Ascertain availability of related educational materials in client's native language. Consider use of AT&T Language Line. See also the Culturological Assessment procedure in Unit 2 for general overview of cultural considerations.

▶ INTERVENTIONS

1. Wash hands.	*Prevents transmission of microbes*
2. Assemble supplies.	*Promotes efficiency and decreases error in testing*
3. Explain procedure.	*Decreases anxiety and promotes cooperation*
4. Don gloves.	*Serves as protective barrier*
5. Have client void into clean container.	*Ensures accuracy of test results*
6. Immerse end of reagent strip into urine as per manufacturer's instructions.	*Exposes reagent to urine*
7. Remove strip from urine and tap on side of container to remove excess.	*Excess urine can dilute results*
8. Wait number of seconds as directed per manufacturer's instructions and compare color on strip with color chart.	*Ensures accuracy of results*
9. Record results in log.	*Monitors response to interventional strategies*
10. Instruct client on how to perform urine monitoring procedure.	*Reinforces client learning*
11. Instruct client on proper procedure for quality control and permit return demonstration—date and time bottle upon opening, maintain and discard per manufacturer's recommendations.	*Prevents outdated strips from altering results*
12. Observe client's ability to perform procedure.	*Assesses client's ability to implement ordered intervention*

DOCUMENTATION
The following should be noted in the nursing note:

Time and date of testing
Urine test results

Notification of physician of abnormal results

Interventions for urine test results exceeding ordered parameters

All client/caregiver teaching:

Topics to include in the teaching plan:

safe and correct equipment handling

emergency procedures

underlying disease pathology

appropriate community resources and contact persons

INTERDISCIPLINARY COLLABORATION

Report to the physician all results exceeding parameters

Consult the nutritionist for recommendation/reinforcement of dietary regimen

Consult social worker to assist in obtaining monitoring strips for clients eligible for financial assistance [2, 7, 11]

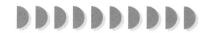

4

Perinatal Cardiovascular System Procedures

Management of Pregnancy Induced Hypertension (PIH)

DESCRIPTION

PIH is the development of hypertension after the 20th week of gestation in a previously normotensive woman without history of proteinuria. PIH has the potential to lead to preeclampsia and eclampsia, conditions that can place the mother and fetus at grave risk. The client will need to be closely monitored for a potential rapid deterioration in her health status as the pregnancy progresses.

PURPOSE

To reduce blood pressure, decrease proteinuria, prevent development of excessive edema, and decrease hospital admissions

EQUIPMENT

Sphygmomanometer
Stethoscope
Fetoscope
Doppler
Weight scale

OUTCOMES

The client will:

► Maintain blood pressure within normal limits per physician guidelines
► Demonstrate no symptoms of fluid volume overload
► Maintain urine protein levels within normal limits
► Demonstrate no signs of hyperreflexia
► Verbalize signs and symptoms of increased PIH and when to notify the physician

ASSESSMENT DATA

Perform a prenatal risk assessment
Assess for weight gain, oliguria, hypertension, hyperreflexia, vertigo, epigastric pain, and visual disturbance
Obtain gestational history
Note family history of hypertension or vascular disease
Document presence of obesity or poor nutrition
Ascertain history of PIH in previous pregnancies

Assess home and client's ability to maintain a restful environment, suggest use of significant others to manage daily household chores, care for other children in the home, etc

Assess for signs and symptoms of complications: vaginal bleeding/spotting, leakage or gush of fluids from vagina, vomiting/diarrhea, fever/infection secondary to sexually transmitted disease or urinary tract infection

Assess for fetal activity/heartones

RELATED NURSING DIAGNOSES
Fluid volume overload
At risk for altered cardiac output
Altered nutrition
Knowledge deficit
Anxiety
At risk for loss and grieving

SPECIAL CONSIDERATIONS
The client can obtain her own blood pressure measurements using digitally recording syphgmomanometers for home monitoring. Cost is a significant factor in purchasing these units. A social work consult will help to determine client's eligibility for reimbursement

TRANSCULTURAL CONSIDERATION
An interpreter will be needed for the non-English speaking client
Ascertain availability of related educational materials in client's native language
Consider use of AT&T Language Line
See also the Culturological Assessment procedure in Unit 2 for general overview of cultural considerations

▶ INTERVENTIONS

Intervention	Rationale
1. Wash hands.	*Prevents transmission of microbes*
2. Perform physical assessment.	*Establishes baseline information for physical findings*
3. Obtain blood pressure readings.	*Monitors client's response to interventional strategies*
4. Instruct caregiver in procedure to obtain blood pressure and permit return demonstration.	*Documents caregiver's ability to correctly perform procedure*
5. Instruct caregiver in procedure to test urine for protein and permit return demonstration.	*Documents caregiver's ability to correctly perform procedure*
6. Record assessment of deep tendon reflexes (DTRs).	*Evaluates presence of hyperreflexia*
7. Observe for presence of edema and record findings.	*Assesses presence of fluid volume overload*
8. Maintain bed rest with bathroom privileges lying on left side as ordered.	*Bed rest in left lateral position has been demonstrated to reduce edema and blood pressure*

9. Maintain diet regimen with recommended daily sodium intake as ordered.	*Reduces edema*
10. Instruct client and caregiver in signs and symptoms of PIH: increased edema, proteinuria, headaches, visual disturbance, increased weight gain, oliguria, hypertension.	*Reinforces client learning*
11. Instruct client to maintain daily intake and output and record daily weight.	*Reinforces client learning and monitors fluid balance*
12. Encourage rest and relaxation techniques.	*Reduces stress*
13. Perform fetal assessment.	*Monitors response of fetus*

DOCUMENTATION
The following should be noted in the nursing note:

Urine protein levels
Blood pressure readings
Neurological assessment
Weight gain
Dietary regimen
Fetal assessment
Untoward findings reported to physician
All client/caregiver teaching:
    Topics to include in the teaching plan:
        safe and correct equipment handling
        emergency procedures
        underlying disease pathology
        appropriate community resources and contact persons

INTERDISCIPLINARY COLLABORATION
Report to physician all untoward clinical findings
Consult social worker to assist in identifying appropriate community resources
Consider need to assign home health aide to assist client with ADLs [2, 7, 11]

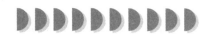

5

Perinatal Reproductive System Procedures

Management of Preterm Labor (PTL)

DESCRIPTION
Home management of preterm labor (PTL) collectively refers to clinical procedures for self-palpation, administration of tocolytic agents, and home uterine activity monitoring (HUAM). Clients eligible for initiation of PTL protocol are those with a high-antepartal risk-scoring index, history of PTL, and onset of regular uterine contraction with or without cervical dilatation.

PURPOSE
To prevent premature birth by detecting the signs of PTL before labor is well established.

EQUIPMENT
Electronic home uterine monitoring system
Fetoscope
Doppler
Stethoscope
Sphygomomanometer
Thermometer
Health Assessment forms
Educational materials
Infusion supplies

OUTCOMES
The client will:

▶ Demonstrate ability to perform home uterine activity monitoring as ordered
▶ Verbalize understanding of all treatment and emergency plans
▶ Maintain normal physiological changes of pregnancy
▶ Demonstrate ability to monitor pulse rate

ASSESSMENT DATA
Perform a prenatal risk assessment
Obtain obstetric, medical and surgical history
Assess socioeconomic status
Identify risk factors

Assess for signs and symptoms of complications: vaginal bleeding/spotting, leakage or gush of fluids from vagina, vomiting/diarrhea, fever/infection secondary to sexually transmitted disease or urinary tract infection

Assess for fetal activity/heartones

RELATED NURSING DIAGNOSES
Knowledge deficit

Anxiety

At risk for ineffective management of the therapeutic regimen

At risk for ineffective coping

At risk for loss and grieving

SPECIAL CONSIDERATIONS
In managing the client for PTL, the nurse must consider the physical environment and the availability of resources and home support systems. Noncompliance is a common challenge among clients diagnosed with this condition and results from fear, denial, knowledge deficit, frustration, depression, inadequate support systems, and the length of time required for treatment. The nurse should constantly review the plan of care (see Appendix 3-2) and assist with the identification of family and community resources to improve client compliance.

TRANSCULTURAL CONSIDERATION
An interpreter will be needed for the non-English speaking client

Ascertain availability of related educational materials in client's native language

Consider use of AT&T Language Line

See also the Culturological Assessment procedure in Unit 2 for general overview of cultural considerations

INTERVENTIONS

1. Wash hands.	*Prevents transmission of microbes*
2. Perform physical assessment.	*Establishes baseline information of physiological data findings*
3. Verify physician order.	*Reduces risk of error*

For Self-palpation

1. Position the client with pillow behind the head and tilted slightly to the left.	*Facilitates client comfort and increases placental perfusion*
2. Have client drink 1–2 cups of water, juice, or milk.	*Hydration decreases incidence of PTL*
3. Have client empty bladder.	*Full bladder inhibits accuracy of evaluation, may increase uterine irritability and increase discomfort during procedure*
4. Instruct client in self-palpation techniques.	*Promotes client self-sufficiency*

a. Place her fingertips on lower sides of abdomen and feel for tightening of abdomen

b. Time uterine contractions for 1 hour noting frequency of contraction, duration and intensity

c. Assess intensity of contraction

    mild   = feels like tip of nose

    moderate = feels like chin

    strong   = feels like forehead

d. Perform daily or as ordered

e. If contractions are above threshold standard (> 4 per hour or per physician order), the client may repeat the procedure after resting and hydrating as per physician order, if still over threshold call physician

5. Have client return demonstration.

Assesses client's ability to implement treatment modalities

6. Instruct the client to keep a daily log documenting activity, contractions (frequency, duration, and intensity), medications, pulse rate, and blood glucose levels (if applicable).

Monitors trends in client/fetal response to therapy

For Electronic Uterine Activity Monitoring

1. Initiate electronic uterine activity monitoring at 24 weeks gestation and discontinue at 36 weeks gestation.

Electronically documents uterine activity

2. Have client follow instructions provided by manufacturer to set up monitor and transmit strips to agency or physician office.

Device uses telecommunication technology to transmit electronic graphic record of uterine activity

3. Instruct client in procedure to transmit tracing twice per day or as ordered.

Establishes trends for baseline comparison

a. If contractions exceed threshold (>4 per hour or per physician order) have client lie on left lateral side, increase fluid intake and re-monitor in 1 hour

b. If contractions persist at more than 4 per hour (or as per physician order) have client notify physician

c. If symptoms indicate imminent danger or threat of delivery, direct client to call EMS team

4. Have client return demonstration.

Assesses client's ability to implement treatment modalities

For Terbutaline Subcutaneous Administration

1. Follow physician order and homecare agency protocol for the administration of continuous subcutaneous terbutaline.

Ensures accuracy of administration

2. Explain procedure.

Alleviates anxiety

3. Wash hands.

Prevents transmission of microbes

4. Don gloves.

Serves as protective barrier

5. Set up and initiate infusion per homecare agency protocol using aseptic technique.

   Prevents contamination

   a. Attach prefilled syringe to intravenous tubing and prime the line per manufacturer's recommendations. (Figure 3-1)
   b. Attach syringe to pump per manufacturer's recommendations.
   c. Prepare subcutaneous site for insertion per agency protocol.
   d. Attach subcutaneous needle and catheter sheath to intravenous line per manufacturer's recommendations.
   e. Gently pinch skin and insert the needle at a 90-degree angle into the subcutaneous tissue of the abdomen or anterior thigh per physician order. (Figure 3-2)
   f. Remove the needle leaving the catheter in place. (Figure 3-3)
   g. Apply dressing to secure catheter.
   h. turn on pump and infuse medication at ordered rate
6. Program microinfusion pump to deliver basal rate, scheduled, and demand bolus dosages as ordered

   Ensures that dosage will not exceed prescribed limits in 24-hour period
   Assesses client's ability to implement interventional strategies

7. Instruct client in management of the continuous infusion and permit return demonstration.
   a. Medication is packaged in prefilled syringes that client stores in cool dark place as per pharmacy guidelines
   b. Client checks medication for clarity and expiration date
   c. Client performs procedure to take radial pulse at least BID and prior to demand bolus (tocolytics are usually held if maternal pulse exceeds 120 BPM)
   d. Client performs syringe change
      ▶ washes hands (this is considered a clean procedure)
      ▶ stops the pump

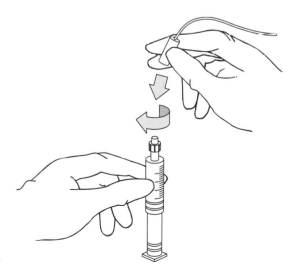

FIGURE 3-1 ▶ Connecting prefilled syringe to intravenous line.

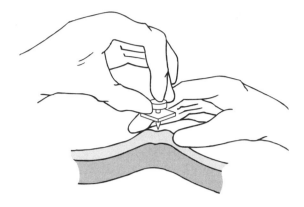

FIGURE 3-2 ▶ Inserting needle at 90-degrees into subcutaneous tissue.

- ▶ removes air bubbles from new syringe
- ▶ removes old syringe from pump chamber
- ▶ attaches new syringe and primes tubing
- ▶ places syringe in pump
- ▶ restarts pump

   e. Client performs site change
- ▶ washes hands (this is considered a clean procedure)
- ▶ stops infusion
- ▶ cleans site with alcohol and inserts introducer needle at 90 degrees
- ▶ removes needle leaving plastic catheter in place and attaches tubing
- ▶ applies dressing to secure catheter and tubing
- ▶ disposes sharps in appropriate container
- ▶ attaches pump to waistband or places in pocket
- ▶ changes site every three days or as ordered

   f. Client maintains pump
- ▶ changes batteries per recommendations of manufacturer
- ▶ calls nurse for questions regarding pump functioning
- ▶ in the event of pump failure client is instructed to take oral dose of medication *per physician order* until infusion can be resumed

   g. Client verbalizes understanding of untoward reactions and when to stop infusion

8. Have client return demonstration.

Assesses client's ability to implement treatment modalities

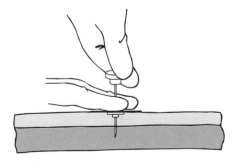

FIGURE 3-3 ▶ Removing needle, leaving catheter in place.

9. Observe for untoward reactions.
    a. Monitor uterine contractions
    b. Assess maternal and fetal heart rates
    c. Monitor blood glucose levels
    d. Record intake and output
    e. Obtain and record vital signs
    f. Auscultate lung sounds

Maintains constant assessment of client response to ordered therapy

10. Discontinue infusion as ordered.

Effect of drug is realized when uterine contractions cease

11. Review signs and symptoms of PTL with appropriate interventions as ordered.

Reinforces client learning

DOCUMENTATION

The following should be included in the nursing note:

Client's tolerance of the procedures
Client's ability to perform procedures as ordered
Physiological data findings
Untoward reactions
Notification of physician for all abnormal responses
All client/caregiver teaching:
 Topics to include in the teaching plan:
  safe and correct equipment handling
  emergency procedures
  underlying disease pathology
  appropriate community resources and contact persons

INTERDISCIPLINARY COLLABORATION

Report to physician all results exceeding parameters. Collaborate with pharmacist to obtain medications.

Consult social work to assist in obtaining monitoring units for clients eligible for financial assistance/reimbursement [2, 5, 7, 8, 11]

PROCEDURE

Management of Non-Stress Testing in the Home Setting

DESCRIPTION

The non-stress test (NST) is a procedure performed to evaluate fetal well being through an assessment of fetal heart rate (FHR) and movement. Acceleration in FHR above the baseline indicates the presence of an intact neurological system. Fetal hypoxia, the fetal sleep cycle, cigarette smoking, and use of CNS depressants are conditions that will cause an absence in FHR acceleration

PURPOSE

To evaluate fetal status through fetal heart activity and body movement assessment

EQUIPMENT

External fetal monitor
Abdominal belt
Tocodynamometer

Phono/ultrasound transducer
Aquasonic gel
Oxygen
Tocolytic medication
Intravenous infusion supplies

OUTCOMES
The client will:

▶ Maintain fetal well being
▶ Demonstrate no symptoms of fetal compromise

ASSESSMENT DATA
Perform a prenatal risk assessment
Obtain obstetrical and medical history
Determine presence of preexisting conditions: diabetes, sickle cell disease, hypertension, previous
    stillbirth, heart disease, decreased fetal movement
Perform Leopold manuevers to determine fetal placement prior to applying fetal monitor

RELATED NURSING DIAGNOSES
Altered tissue perfusion
Impaired gas exchange
Pain
Anxiety
Ineffective coping
At risk for loss and grieving

SPECIAL CONSIDERATIONS
NST should take no more than 20 minutes to perform and usually is without complication. The client is positioned on her side or in Semifowlers position to prevent hypotension. A Doppler ultrasound transducer and tocodynamometer are applied to detect FHR, uterine contractions, and fetal movement. The client is instructed to indicate fetal movement by pressing on an event marker.

TRANSCULTURAL CONSIDERATIONS
An interpreter will be needed for the non-English speaking client
Ascertain availability of related educational materials in client's native language
Consider use of AT&T Language Line
See also the Culturological Assessment procedure in Unit 2 for general overview of cultural considerations

▶ INTERVENTIONS

1. Verify physician order.	*Reduces risk of error*
2. Wash hands.	*Prevents transmission of microbes*
3. Perform physical assessment.	*Establishes baseline information of physiological data findings*
4. Explain procedure.	*Alleviates anxiety*
5. Obtain vital signs.	*Establishes baseline for comparison*
5. Apply external fetal monitor.	*Obtains monitor tracing*

6. Observe for fetal reactivity.

Test is reactive when fetal movement occurs twice during a 20-minute period and when fetal heart rate accelerates 15 beats above baseline during same 20-minute period

7. If test is nonreactive (no movement in 20 minutes), stimulate fetus.
   a. change client's position or ambulate
   b. massage or gently palpate the abdomen
   c. have client drink a cup of juice to increase fetal glucose levels

Fetal sleep cycle may last 20 minutes

8. If test is nonreactive for 40 minutes following stimulation institute the following measures immediately.
   a. Notify physician
   b. Place client on left side
   c. Insert IV per physician order
   d. Follow physician orders
   e. Call for emergency service and transport to hospital

This clinical finding constitutes a medical emergency

9. If FHR tracing is nonreassuring (FHR decelerations, decreased/absent variability, tachycardia, bradycardia) call for emergency service and transport to hospital.

This clinical finding constitutes a medical emergency

DOCUMENTATION

The following should be included in the nursing note:

Client's tolerance of the procedures
Physiological data findings
Untoward reactions
Notification of physician for all abnormal responses
All client/caregiver teaching
    Topics to include in the teaching plan:
        safe and correct equipment handling
        emergency procedures
        underlying disease pathology
        appropriate community resources and contact persons

INTERDISCIPLINARY COLLABORATION

Report all untoward reactions to the physician
Maintain emergency service on standby [2]

REFERENCES

1. Berry, R, Mohn, KR, & Hozmeister, LA. Monitoring diabetes therapy. *Home Health Care Nurse.* 13(1): 39–42
2. Chestnut, MA. *High risk perinatal home care manual.* Philadelphia, PA: Lippincott, 1998
3. *Coram healthcare corporation nursing orientation manual.* Denver, CO: The Corporation, 1995
4. *Dietetics Core Curriculum,* 2nd edition. Silver Springs, Maryland: A.S.P.E.N. 1993
5. Gorski, LA. (Ed). *High-tech home care manual.* Gaithersburg, MD: Aspen Publications, 1997

6. Gottschlich, M.M., Matarese, L.E., & Shronts, E.P., eds. *Nutrition Support Dietetics Core Curriculum,* 2nd edition. Silver Springs, Maryland: A.S.P.E.N. 1993

7. Heaman, M. Antepartum home care for high-risk pregnant women. *AACN Clinical Issues.* 9(2):362–376

8. Hodgson, B & Kizior, R. *Saunders nursing drug handbook.* Philadelphia, PA: WB Saunders, 1999

9. *Manual of clinical dietetics,* 5th edition. Chicago: The American Dietetic Association, 1996.

10. Mohn, KR. Blood Glucose Monitoring Systems. *Home health care nurse.* 13 (1): 44–47

11. O'Brien, P. High risk pregnancy and neonatal care. *Critical Care Nursing Clinics of North America.* 10(3):347–355

12. Powers, M.A., ed. *Nutrition guide for professionals: Diabetes education and meal planning.* Chicago: American Dietetic Association and Alexandria, Va: American Diabetes Association; 1988.

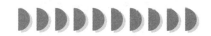

Appendices

The Prenatal Data Collection and Risk Scoring Tool
Antepartum Risk Scoring Index

Patient's Name _____

Address _____

Phone number _____ Insurance company _____

OB care provider _____ Phone number _____

Gestational date _____ Today's date _____

A score of 10 or more on this index indicates a client is at high risk.
However, in assessing your future course of action with each client, look at absolute scores instead of just the designation of low or high risk. For example, the diabetic client with no other problems rates 10 points and therefore is considered at high risk. However, the obese client (5) who has a drinking problem (5) and is a heavy smoker (5) scores 15 points; she may be at still greater risk.

Scoring Value	Condition	Actual Score of Client
Anatomical Abnormalities		
10	Uterine malformation	( )
10	Incompetent cervix	( )
10	Abnormal fetal position	( )
10	Hydramnios	( )
5	Clinically small pelvis	( )
10	Multiple pregnancy	( )
10	Vaginal spotting	( )
Miscellaneous (this pregnancy)		
5	Age 15	( )
5	Age 35	( )
5	Weight 100 lbs.	( )
5	Weight 200 lbs.	( )
1	Mild anemia, 9.0–10.9 hemoglobin	( )
5	Severe anemia, 9.0 hemoglobin	( )
10	Sickle cell disease or trait	( )
5	Rh sensitized, first time	( )
5	Positive serology	( )
5	Positive PPD	( )
3	Viral disease	( )
3	Flu syndrome	( )
3	Vaginitis	( )
5	Abnormal cervical cytology	( )
10	Pulmonary dysfunction	( )
10	Post-term (over 42 wk)	( )
10	Intrauterine growth retardation	( )
5	Emotional problems	( )
5	Smoking	( )
5	Alcohol abuse	( )
5	Excessive drug use, nonnarcotic	( )
10	Narcotic use	( )
10	No-care client (no previous medical care until late in pregnancy)	( )

(continued)

APPENDIX 3-1 ▶ The Prenatal Data Collection and Risk Scoring Tool: Antepartum Risk Scoring Index. (*Source:* Chestnut, MA. *High Risk Perinatal Home Care Manual.* Lippincott 1998.)

Scoring Value	Condition	Actual Score of Client
Cardiovascular Disorders		
10	Class I heart disease	( )
10	Severe heart disease, classes (II–IV)	( )
10	Chronic hypertension	( )
3	History of preeclampsia	( )
5	History of eclampsia	( )
5	Mild preeclampsia	( )
10	Moderate–severe preeclampsia	( )
Renal Disorders		
5	History of GU infection (including acute cystitis)	( )
10	Acute pyelonephritis	( )
10	Moderate–severe renal disease	( )
Metabolic Disorders		
3	Family history of diabetes	( )
5	Diabetes (Type II, III, IV)	( )
10	Diabetes (Type I)	( )
5	Thyroid disease	( )
3	Previous endocrine ablation	( )
History		
3	Therapeutic abortion	( )
5	Habitual abortion	( )
10	Previous stillbirth	( )
10	Previous low birth weight infant	( )
10	Previous neonatal death	( )
5	Previous infant >10 lbs	( )
3	Previous cesarean section	( )
1	Rh neg., nonsensitized	( )
10	Rh neg., sensitized	( )
5	Multiparity >5	( )
5	Epilepsy	( )
5	Previous fetal anomalies	( )
3	Drug allergy	( )

APPENDIX 3-1 [CONTINUED] ▶ The Prenatal Data Collection and Risk Scoring Tool: Antepartum Risk Scoring Index

Patient Name: _____   ID #: _____

Diagnosis(es): _____ Certification Period From: _____ To: _____

BEGIN SERVICE (Check)

( ) ASAP ( ) At _____ weeks gestation ( ) prior to discharge

Discharge from service at _____ completed weeks of gestation   Date: _____

HOME MONITORING

Monitor X60 Minutes _____ QD _____ BID and PRN

Transmit at time of scheduled nurse contact

Contraction threshold _____ (how many contractions patients is <u>allowed</u> in one hour)

Maternal pulse threshold _____ (hold Terbutaline if pulse exceeds limit)

MEDICATIONS_____

FETAL MOVEMENT (Check One)

( ) If patient is not on FKC's, notify care provider immediately if patient reports decreased fetal movement.

    Notification by   ( ) Nursing   ( ) Patient

                              OR

( ) Fetal kick counts _____ x/day.

    Notify physician if patient reports less than _____ fetal movements in _____ hour (s).

    Notification by   ( ) Nursing   ( ) Patient

    ( ) May repeat   ( ) May not repeat x1.

PHYSICAL ACTIVITY (Check One)

( ) No limits ( ) Modified Bedrest ( ) BR with BRP ( ) Strict Bedrest ( ) Other _____

If uterine activity exceeds threshold and patient is not on Terbutaline pump therapy:

( ) Instruct patient to hydrate, void and repeat session for one hour

                              OR

( ) Physician to be called by   ( ) nurse   ( ) patient

If uterine activity continues to exceed threshold on remonitor session:

( ) Physician to be called by   ( ) nurse   ( ) patient

( ) Send to L&D for further evaluation. L&D to notify physician.

TERBUTALINE PUMP THERAPY: Height _____ Weight _____ Pre-Pregnant Weight _____ Allergies ____

( ) Begin subcutaneous Terbutaline pump therapy with Terbutaline 1 mg/ml

    Basal rate _____ mg/hr (standard dose is 0.050 mg/hr; may be increased to 0.10/mg/hr)

    Bolus rate _____ mg (standard dose is 0.250 mg/hr; may be increased to .0.30 mg/hr)

    May have _____ Boluses per 24 hours (standard up to eight)

    Scheduled bolus q _____ hours

    Demand bolus _____ mg

    May have _____ demand boluses per 24 hours (standard is two)

    Current bolus schedule: _____

If uterine activity exceeds threshold:

  May give demand bolus if maternal pulse if less than pulse threshold and there is a 60 minute interval between boluses (scheduled or demand). Rest for 30 minutes, hydrate, void and remonitor for one hour.

If uterine activity continues to exceed threshold:

  May give up to _____ demand boluses once every sixty minutes. If still over threshold, notify physician.

HOME CARE

Teach patient to inspect infusion site for signs/symptoms of infection or leakage

Teach patient to change the infusion site once every 72 hours and PRN

Visit patient daily X3 then _____ weekly and PRN for assessment and teaching

( ) Lab orders _____

( ) Discontinue terbutaline pump at _____ weeks gestation

ADDITIONAL ORDERS _____

_____

_____   _____   _____   _____

Physician Signature   Date   RN Signature   Date

                            White - Site   Yellow - Physician

APPENDIX 3-2 ▶ Home Perinatal Services: Physician Orders/Plan of Treatment. (*Source:* Biomedical Systems. Perinatal Division. 314-576-6800. Used with permission.)

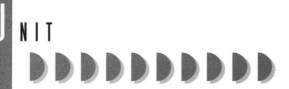

U N I T

4

Newborn Homecare

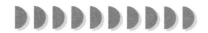

1 Newborn Cardiovascular System Procedures

Blood Sample Collection Technique

DESCRIPTION
The heel stick procedure is used in the newborn infant to obtain serum samples for laboratory analysis

PURPOSE
To obtain serum specimens for laboratory analysis

EQUIPMENT
Alcohol swabs
Sterile lancet
Blood collection tubes
2 inch by 2 inch sterile gauze pad
Labels
Gloves
Laboratory forms
Plastic bag for disposal
Biohazardous labels

OUTCOMES
The client will:

▶ Have minimal discomfort during procedure
▶ Not show signs of excessive bleeding or distress
▶ Remain free of infection at heel stick site

ASSESSMENT DATA
Obtain trending reports of laboratory data analyses
Determine presence of any contraindications for obtaining specimen from heel
Assess caregiver's ability to cope with the situation

RELATED NURSING DIAGNOSES
Pain
Altered skin integrity
At risk for infection
Anxiety

SPECIAL CONSIDERATIONS

Infant skin is sensitive to tape and easily bruised. Applying a warm compress to the area prior to the puncture helps increase circulation and promotes collection of an adequate specimen. Applying a warm compress to the bruised area after the puncture increases circulation, helps remove extravasated blood, and decreases pain.

The most common complication related to a heel stick is necrotizing osteochrondritis. To avoid this complication, perform heel punctures on the most medial aspect or the most lateral aspect of the plantar surface of the foot. Puncture no deeper than 2.4 mm. Avoid sites that have been previously used.

Bandages pose a risk of aspiration in young children; their use should be avoided. Adhesive bandages should be removed as soon as the bleeding stops.

TRANSCULTURAL CONSIDERATIONS

An interpreter will be needed for the family unable to speak or understand English. Consider use of AT&T Language Line. See also the Culturological Assessment procedure in Unit 2 for general overview of cultural considerations.

▶ INTERVENTIONS

Intervention	Rationale
1. Wash hands.	*Prevents transmission of microbes*
2. Perform physical assessment.	*Establishes baseline information of physiological data findings*
3. Explain procedure to caregiver.	*Allays anxiety*
4. Place disposable waterproof cover under extremity.	*Protects surrounding area from blood spill*
5. Select lateral aspect of infant's foot.	*Reduces risk of injury*
6. Wrap heel in warm wash cloth.	*Dilates blood vessels*
7. Don gloves.	*Serves as protective barrier*
8. Expose heel (see Figure 4-1).	*Permits direct observation of site*
9. Clean site with alcohol.	*Removes soil*
10. Puncture with sterile lancet.	*Maintains asepsis*
11. Wipe away first drop of blood with sterile gauze pad.	*Removes any contaminating fluids which may alter test results*
12. Select correct microcontainer for specimen type.	*Specific tubes are used for specific laboratory tests*
13. Touch microtainer tube to underside of drop of blood and allow blood to flow freely into collector.	*Creates wick-like effect*
14. When sample has been obtained, apply pressure to site and cover with gauze dressing, if needed.	*Stops bleeding*
15. Cap blood tube, label, and complete forms for laboratory analysis.	*Secures specimen and ensures accuracy*
16. Wrap blood tube in biohazard bag and place in designated container for transport.	*Serves as protective barrier*
17. Wash hands.	*Prevents spread of microbes*

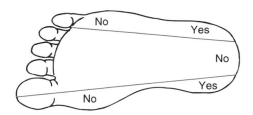

FIGURE 4-1 ▶ Locations for heel stick.

DOCUMENTATION
The following should be included in the nursing note:

Client's response to the procedure
Any untoward reactions
All caregiver instructions
Physician notification of abnormal responses
Type of specimen collected and procedure used
All caregiver teaching:
    Topics to include in the teaching plan:
        safe and correct handling of equipment/supplies
        emergency procedures
        underlying disease pathology
        appropriate community resourcs and contact persons

INTERDISCIPLINARY COLLABORATION
Coordinate with the homecare agency or the laboratory service procedure for specimen pickup or drop off
Report untoward responses and laboratory results to physician
For frequent blood draws maintain supply inventory and anticipate need to coordinate reordering with DME company [1–5]

PROCEDURE
Home Phototherapy

DESCRIPTION
Phototherapy refers to the application of intense fluorescent light on the infant's exposed skin to enhance bilirubin excretion. Through the process of photoisomerization bilirubin is structurally changed to a more soluble form. For the infant diagnosed with hyperbilirubinemia, phototherapy is used in the home to keep bilirubin levels from increasing, while allowing the family to naturally bond in the home setting. Those infants whose jaundice is physiological can usually be safely cared for at home.

PURPOSE
To reduce serum bilirubin levels

EQUIPMENT
Home phototherapy blanket
Illuminator
Fiberoptic cable and panel
Disposable panel covers

Thermometer
Blood drawing supplies
Health assessment forms
Log

OUTCOMES

Caregivers will demonstrate proper and safe use of home phototherapy equipment.
Caregivers will verbalize signs of jaundice and reasons to record infant's intake and output.
Infant will have decreased bilirubin levels.

ASSESSMENT DATA

Obtain history of infant's bilirubin levels during first 72 hours of life
Document maternal and infant blood types
Note infant's weight at birth and gestational age
Obtain infant's apgar score at birth
Assess environmental safety of home setting and ability of caregivers to perform procedure
Document infant blood levels: Coombs test, Rh sensitization, ABO incompatibility, bilirubin, H&H

RELATED NURSING DIAGNOSES

At risk for altered parenting
At risk for altered parent/infant attachment
Parental role conflict
Anxiety
Knowledge deficit
Altered health maintainence

SPECIAL CONSIDERATIONS

Most homecare agencies have a certain bilirubin level cut off to decide whether it would be prudent to do homecare. Refer to agency policy regarding safe bilirubin levels for home management.

The phototherapy equipment, usually a blanket, must be at the home prior to starting care. An electrical safety assessment must be performed. The home should have three-pronged electrical outlets.

Teaching is a major component of home phototherapy management. Caregivers must be willing to accept responsibility for safe and proper use of equipment, and must be able to assess for jaundice and dehydration.

Caregivers may be concerned about heat from the blanket. They should be told that the light from the blanket does not create heat and will not burn the infant. Because the equipment does not allow for circulation around the torso, and because parents have a tendency to swaddle the infant with blankets, caregivers will need to frequently obtain the infant's axillary temperature.

Most infants are on therapy for several days and require repeat bilirubin levels daily. Discuss this need with the parents. Most bilirubin levels should be drawn early in the morning to allow time for processing and reporting to pediatrician to decide if therapy should be changed.

When possible, having one nurse follow the infant streamlines the care and provides continuity. The regularly assigned homecare nurse will be best able to note changes from one day to the next and to note improvement or deterioration in the infant's condition.

TRANSCULTURAL CONSIDERATIONS

In some ethnic cultures, the client is not expected to actively participate in the medical treatment plan. This health belief practice can be a challenge, especially when the goal of homecare is to assist the client to achieve a state of self-sufficiency. The procedures associated with home ph+photherapy can overwhelm first-time parents causing them to question every aspect of care due to their lack of confidence, or to ignore the need for phototherapy and not maintain the infant on the equipment. Letting the family know that the nurse is available to provide support will help alleviate anxiety. Typically the homecare agency will have telephone numbers and contact persons available on a 24-hour basis to answer all questions and address concerns.

An interpreter will be needed for the non-English speaking client. Ascertain availability of related educational materials in client's native language. Consider use of AT&T Language Line. See also Culturological Assessment procedure in Unit 2 for general overview of cultural considerations.

▶ INTERVENTIONS

1. Wash hands.

   Prevents transmission of microbes

2. Assess infant, particularly, hydration and elimination patterns, weight, and waking and sleeping patterns.

   Establishes baseline information of physiological data findings

3. Verify physician orders.

   Reduces risk of error

4. Instruct caregivers on safe and proper use of phototherapy blanket and permit return demonstration.

   Documents caregivers' ability to implement interventional strategies.

   a. Place the illuminator box on a hard surface no more than 4 feet from the infant
      1) keep air vent free of blockage
      2) do not place on or near radiator
   b. Insert metal collar of fiberoptic panel into designated area of illuminator and turn clockwise one quarter turn
   c. Plug illuminator box into three-pronged electrical outlet
   d. Insert the panel into the disposable panel cover
      1) place covered panel around the infant under the arms and around the torso
      2) expose as much of the skin as possible to the light
      3) fasten the tabs using two-finger slack to assess tightness of the panel
   e. Lightly dress the infant in a T-shirt and diaper and wrap in blanket
   f. Pad the underarms to prevent irritation by rolling T-shirt up and positioning to protect skin from irritation
   g. Turn on illuminator and initiate treatment
   h. Sit in chair close to illuminator to rock, hold, cuddle or feed the infant

5. Teach caregivers how to keep track of infants' intake and output, recording wet or dry diapers.

   Monitors hydrational status

6. Teach caregivers how to obtain an axillary temperature q 8 hours.

   Monitors trends in febrile states

7. Teach caregivers to feed infant every 2–3 hours and to supplement feeding with formula as specified by physician order.

   Maintains nutritional and hydrational status

8. Teach caregivers to leave child on his or her side after eating.

   Reduces risk of aspiration

9. Teach caregivers symptoms to report to physician.

   Signals onset of complications

a. Feeding intolerance
b. Persistent febrile states
c. Fewer than five wet diapers in 24 hours
d. Pronounced change in infant's activity levels

10. Draw bilirubin by heelstick as ordered by MD, turn off phototherapy during procedure.   *Monitors bilirubin levels*

DOCUMENTATION
The following should be included in the nursing note:

Diaper counts
Bilirubin levels
Client response to procedure
Caregiver ability to perform procedure
Intake and output recordings
Notification of physician of all untoward responses
All caregiver teaching
    Topics to include in the teaching plan:
        safe and correct handling of equipment/supplies
        emergency procedures
        underlying disease pathology
        appropriate community resource and contact persons

INTERDISCIPLINARY COLLABORATION
Report all untoward findings to physician
Consider need to consult with nutritionist for symptoms of feeding intolerance
Consult with social worker to determine client's eligibility for financial assistance/reimbursement for cost of equipment
For frequent blood draws maintain supply inventory and anticipate need to coordinate reordering with DME company [2, 4]

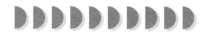

Newborn Respiratory System Procedures

2

Apnea Monitoring

DESCRIPTION
Apnea monitors are electronic devices used to maintain a constant surveillance of the infant's heart and respiratory rates. They are especially useful in preventing sudden infant death syndrome (SIDS) and are used for at-risk infants during sleep times, when episodes of apnea and/or bradycardia usually occur. In ventilator-dependent children, the apnea monitor serves as a backup for the ventilator alarm system.

PURPOSE
To signal the occurrence of episodes of apnea or bradycardia

EQUIPMENT
Apnea monitor
Electrodes
Velcro belt
Stethoscope

OUTCOMES
The caregiver will:

▶ Demonstrate ability to set up monitoring equipment
▶ Demonstrate ability to maintain monitoring equipment
▶ Verbalize procedure to follow during apneic event

ASSESSMENT DATA
Observe for evidence of cyanosis, dyspnea, impaired gas exchange
Record lung sounds
Note sputum production, record character
Assess caregiver coping skills

RELATED NURSING DIAGNOSES
Impaired gas exchange
Ineffective airway clearance
Anxiety
Parental role conflict
Altered parent/infant attachment

SPECIAL CONSIDERATIONS

Having an apnea monitor in the home can be quite stressful. Caregivers usually receive basic education, prior to discharge from the hospital, regarding methods to assess their infant's heart and respiratory rates. Parents become familiar with the apnea monitoring equipment in the hospital setting. Frequently, the infant may have had a complicated hospital stay. The parents may have received hastily provided instructions and now find themselves in the home environment expected to provide constant vigilance for their at-risk infant. Reinforcing teaching and the steps to take if and when the infant becomes apneic/bradycardic are very important. Helping the family find ways to cope and to maintain balance is a priority nursing intervention. Assisting the family to develop an emergency preparedness plan will help allay fears.

Prior to initiating this procedure, the home environment will need to be assessed for electrical safety. The monitoring unit must be properly grounded and plugged into a three-pronged electrical outlet, per manufacturer recommendations. The family should keep a charged battery ready for travel.

The home assessment should document the presence of a functioning telephone line to call for help if needed.

The nurse should be sure that notification has been sent to the local utility company, the emergency medical team, and the police and fire departments to ensure that the home is placed on priority service.

TRANSCULTURAL CONSIDERATION

Some cultures believe that direct care is provided by only the male or female head of the household. It is important to stress that all caregivers must be knowledgeable and able to intervene appropriately in caring for the infant requiring apnea monitoring. For the non-English speaking family, consider use of AT&T Language Line. See also the Culturological Assessment procedure in Unit 2 for general overview of cultural considerations.

▶ INTERVENTIONS

1. Wash hands.

2. Perform physical assessment.

3. Explain all procedures to caregiver.
4. Verify medical order.
5. Instruct caregiver in procedure to set up apnea monitoring equipment (see Figure 4-2) and permit return demonstration.
   ▶ Connect cable to monitor
   ▶ Connect lead wires to cable
   ▶ Connect lead wires to electrode
   ▶ Ensure that infant's torso, front and back, is free from oils and lotions
   ▶ Place electrode belt on a flat surface, then place infant's back on the belt, positioning belt between the infant's nipple line and bottom of rib cage
   ▶ Wrap electrode belt around the infant and secure velcro tab, leaving two-finger slack
   ▶ Turn on monitor
   ▶ When monitor alarms, perform quick assessment of the infant before hitting reset button

Prevents transmission of microbes

Establishes baseline information of physiological data findings

Allays anxiety

Reduces risk of error

Documents caregivers' ability to implement the interventional strategy ordered

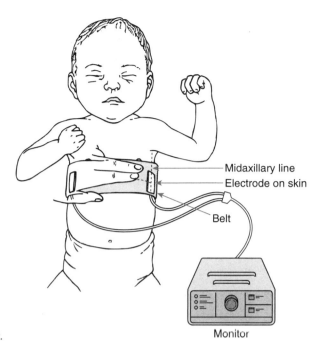

Midaxillary line
Electrode on skin
Belt
Monitor

FIGURE 4-2 ▶ Monitor properly attached to Infant.

6. Check alarm parameters and verify with physician order.	*Alarms are preset prior to delivery to the home and should not be reset without physician order*

7. Review procedure for emergency preparedness.
  a. Review CPR procedure (see pediatric unit)
  b. Review community EMS procedure
	Reinforces client learning

DOCUMENTATION
The following should be included in the nursing note:

Client's response to procedure
Caregivers' ability to implement procedure
Notification of physician for any untoward responses
All caregiver teaching
    Topics to include in the teaching plan:
        safe and correct handling of equipment/supplies
        emergency procedures
        underlying disease pathology
        appropriate community resourcs and contact persons

INTERDISCIPLINARY COLLABORATION
Report all untoward events to physician. Consult with respiratory therapist for equipment maintenance.

Consult with social worker to determine client's eligibility for financial assistance/reimbursement for cost of equipment [1, 2, 4, 5]

REFERENCES

1. Chestnut, MA. *Maternal-newborn home care manual.* Philadelphia, PA: Lippincott, 1998
2. Chestnut, MA. *High-risk newborn home care manual.* Philadelphia, PA: Lippincott, 1998
3. *Coram healthcare corporation nursing orientation manual.* Denver, CO: The Corporation, 1995
4. O'Brien, P. High risk pregnancy and neonatal care. *Critical Care Nursing Clinics of North America.* 10(3):347–355
5. Wong, D. *Wong and Whaley's Clinical Manual of Pediatric Nursing,* 4th Ed. St. Louis: Mosby 1996

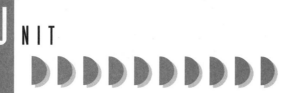

UNIT

5

Pediatric Homecare Procedures

continued

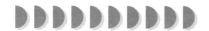

Pediatric Respiratory System Procedures

1

Tracheostomy Tube Management

DESCRIPTION

A tracheostomy is a surgical opening into the trachea made through the skin of the neck to allow for the passage of air (see Figure 5-1). This procedure is performed when an upper airway obstruction is present. The pathophysiologic conditions that require a tracheostomy are long-term ventilation, neurological conditions that disrupt the cough and swallow reflex causing an accumulation of mucus in the upper airway and lungs, and congenital upper airway anomalies.

PURPOSE

To instruct the caregiver in proper suctioning technique, care of the skin around the tracheostomy site, maintenance and changing of the tracheostomy tube, and proper feeding technique for the child with a trach.

EQUIPMENT

Health Assessment Forms
Aspirating machine
Sterile normal saline solution
Sterile gloves
Suction catheters
Tracheostomy tube
Scissors
Dressing
Twill tape or collar
Hemostat
Sterile water
Small cup
Hydrogen peroxide
Clean gloves
Adhesive backed foam if using twill tape, or other soft material
Oxygen with resuscitation bag to administer supplemental oxygen if needed
Humidifier as ordered

OUTCOMES

The caregiver will demonstrate the ability to perform:

▶ Proper skin care
▶ Suctioning of the tracheostomy tube

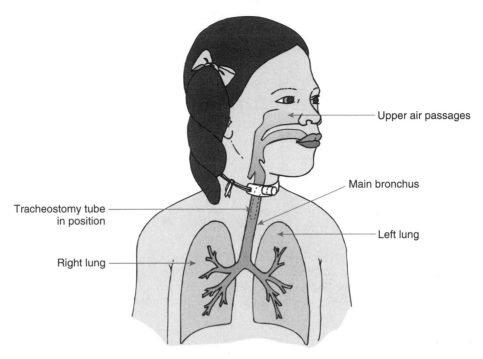

FIGURE 5-1 ▶ Respiratory system with artificial airway.

▶ Changing of the tracheostomy tube and trach strings
▶ Safe feeding techniques

ASSESSMENT DATA
Note signs of respiratory distress
Note ineffective ventilation
Note signs and symptoms of hypoxia
Assess color, consistency, and amount of mucus suctioned from tracheostomy
Note frequency that suctioning is needed
Evaluate caregiver's ability to change the trach tube without difficulty
Note signs of aspiration after feedings

RELATED NURSING DIAGNOSES
Impaired gas exchange
Ineffective airway clearance
Altered skin integrity
At risk for infection
Anxiety

SPECIAL CONSIDERATIONS
At no time should the caregiver attempt to change the tracheostomy tube alone. This is a two-person procedure and should be respected as such. In the child with a critical airway, if the care-

giver attempted to change the trach alone and was unable to reinsert the tube, a situation of grave consequences could occur.

Over time, granulation tissue grows around the inside of the tracheostomy site, which may cause reinsertion of the tube to become difficult. This situation should be reported to the physician immediately so that evaluation of the trach site can be made.

It is important to keep mucus in a liquified state to facilitate removal by suction or expectoration. For this reason humidifying devices must be placed over or near the trach, depending on design. Filtering devices can also be used over the trach site for the child who is ambulatory, permitting air purification during inspiration. As with any condition causing impaired gas exchange, the child should not be exposed to smoke, aerosols, dust, or any tracheal irritant that will promote increased mucus production.

The tracheostomy tube should be changed weekly, whenever an accumulation of secretions cannot be removed by suctioning, when there is a break in the flange, or in the event of a decannulation.

 THIS IS A 2 PERSON PROCEDURE. DO NOT ATTEMPT TO CHANGE THE TRACHEOSTOMY TUBE ALONE

TRANSCULTURAL CONSIDERATIONS
An interpreter will be needed for clients unable to speak English. Support and maintain the client's religious and cultural healthcare practices Acquire healthcare materials written in the client's native language, if available. Consider use of AT&T Language Line. See also the Culturological Assessment procedure in Unit 2 for general overview of cultural considerations.

▶ INTERVENTIONS
Tracheal Suctioning Technique

1. Wash hands.	*Prevents transmission of microbes*
	Prevents contamination
2. Select a suction catheter as ordered by the physician or one half the size of the diameter of the tracheal tube. One catheter should be used to suction the nose and mouth, and a separate catheter should be used to suction the tracheal tube. The suction catheter should have a suction port that can be manipulated by the thumb to control the force of suction.	
3. Measure the length of catheter insertion by placing the catheter near a spare tracheostomy tube of the same size currently in use. The end of the catheter should extend 0.5 cm beyond the end of the tracheostomy tube. Select a landmark on the catheter that will alert you to the length of insertion.	*Reduces chance of injury to the mucosal tissue below the tracheostomy tube*
4. Assure that the tracheostomy tube is secure and in place.	*Prevents inadvertent dislodging of the tube*
5. Open package containing the sterile catheter. Connect the distal end of catheter to tubing of the aspirator. Keep the sterile catheter in the package until ready to insert into tracheal tube.	*Sterile procedure prevents possibility of contamination*
6. Hyperventilate and oxygenate the child with a valved resuscitation bag, if ordered. Ventilate with 2–3 breaths.	*Offsets loss of oxygenation during suctioning*

7. Put on sterile gloves.

Prevents contamination

8. Insert sterile catheter into the tracheostomy tube until the premeasured length has been reached (see Figure 5-2). Do not apply suction.

Prevents trauma to the tracheal mucosa at end of trach tube

9. With a rotating twisting motion, apply intermittent suction while quickly withdrawing catheter from the trach tube (see Figure 5-3). Never suction for longer than 5–10 seconds at a time. Repeat this procedure until passage is clear.

Prolonged suctioning deprives the body of adequate oxygenation

10. If secretions are thick, instill 0.5 ml of sterile normal saline solution in the trachea before catheter insertion.

Liquifies secretions

11. Hand-ventilate and -oxygenate after suctioning, if ordered

Counteracts the hypoxia and atelectasis caused by suctioning

12. Rinse catheter with sterile water or normal saline solution after suctioning.

Clears catheter of secretions

13. Disconnect catheter from aspirator. Wrap catheter around gloved hand and pull glove off inside out, keeping soiled catheter inside the glove. Dispose of items in covered receptacle.

Keeps environment free of contaminated waste.

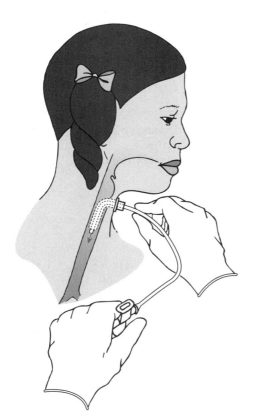

FIGURE 5-2 ▶ Proper technique for insertion of suction catheter with suction control open.

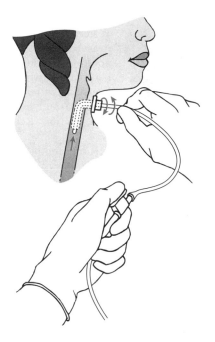

FIGURE 5-3 ▶ Proper technique for applying suction with thumb over suction control while removing catheter with twisting motion.

14. Ascultate lungs bilaterally.	*Ensures that all lung fields are ventilating adequately*
15. Empty aspirator bottle, discard waste, and rinse bottle.	*Maintains sanitary set-up*

Changing the Tracheostomy Tube

1. Wash hands.	*Retards transmission of microbes*
2. Attach twill tape or trach collar to flanges of tracheostomy tube, maintaining sterility of the tube.	*Prevents contamination*
3. Lubricate end of tracheostomy with sterile water.	*Enhances ease of insertion*
4. Position child with airway visible. Place a roll under shoulders.	*Maintains unobstructed view of airway*
5. If the child is old enough, elicit his/her participation by explaining the procedure and the need for cooperation.	*Allays anxiety*
6. Don gloves.	*Serves as protective barrier*
7. Administer supplemental oxygen and/or ventilate prior to changing the tube. This will assist the child to tolerate the procedure.	*Promotes optimum oxygenation during tube change*
8. Suction the trach prior to removal of the tube.	*Removes secretions to prevent blockage of airway*
9. The second person assists by holding the child, grasping the flanges, and on the count of three removes the tracheostomy tube (see Figure 5-4), while the caregiver quickly inserts the new tube in a downward motion guiding the tube along the airway.	*The two-person procedure minimizes the length of time needed for trach tube removal and reinsertion*

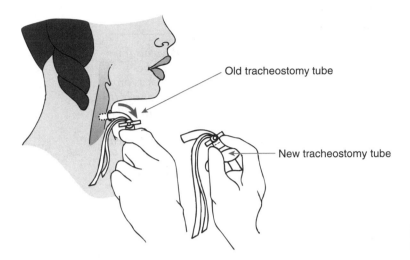

Old tracheostomy tube

New tracheostomy tube

FIGURE 5-4 ▶ Proper technique for changing of tracheostomy tube.

10. Assess breath sounds bilaterally with a stethoscope.

11. Fasten tape to flange and tie in place.

12. Insert dressing under flanges.

13. Assess security of tape and collar (one finger should be comfortably placed under the collar at the back or side of the neck)(see Figure 5-5).

Assures proper placement

Secures tube to prevent dislodging

Protects underlying skin surfaces

One-finger slack prevents trach ties from being too tight

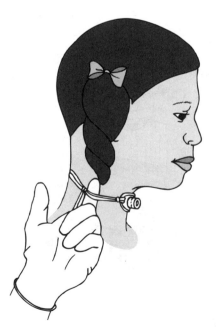

FIGURE 5-5 ▶ Checking for appropriate degree of tightness of tracheostomy ties.

Changing the Tracheostomy Tube Ties

1. Wash hands.

2. Don gloves.

3. If trach ties are used, instruct caregivers to check tracheostomy ties frequently, at least every 8 hours (see Figure 5-6). These ties should be securely attached to the flange of the trach tube and tied snugly in a double knot.

4. When applying new ties, place them along side the old ones, removing the old carefully after the new ties are in place. Never completely remove tracheostomy ties from the tracheostomy tube. This procedure requires two persons.

5. Always have a spare tracheostomy tube within reach in the event of accidental dislodgment or plugging.

6. Change tracheostomy tube weekly or as directed by physician.

7. Suction child after procedure if coughing is stimulated.

8. Ascultate lung fields.

9. Note color, consistency, amount, and odor of secretions.

Prevents transmission of microbes

Serves as protective barrier

Improperly fitting ties will cause dislodgment of the tracheostomy tube. A knot will prevent the ties from slipping.

Having a second person assures security in restraining the child from sudden moves

Allows for immediate replacement

Clean tracheostomy tubes prevent plugging and infection

Assures that the tube is patent

Ensures proper tube placement and evaluates adequacy of ventilation

Thick secretions result in plugging. A change in color and odor indicates infection.

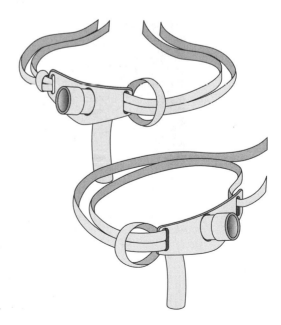

FIGURE 5-6 ▶ Techniques for tying tracheostomy ties.

Tracheostomy Skin Care

1. Instruct caregiver to cleanse tracheostomy site with half-strength hydrogen peroxide every 8–24 hours or as needed.

   Frequent cleansing decreases irritation on the skin from secretions.

2. Keep neck dry by removing secretions as needed.

   Moisture causes irritation leading to skin breakdown

3. Change tracheostomy ties as needed when they become soiled or wet from secretions.

   Wet ties irritate the skin and provide a warm, moist environment in which infection may develop

4. Change or clean suction cannister, nebulizer, or other respiratory equipment every 48 hours or as needed.

   Routine changing or cleaning of equipment decreases the risk of infection.

Oral Feeding the Child with a Tracheostomy

1. Position child in upright position during and after feedings.

   Sitting upright decreases the risk of aspiration

2. Do not suction child after meals.

   Suctioning stimulates the gag reflex that will cause vomiting.

DOCUMENTATION
The following should be noted in the nursing note:

Respiratory rate
Respiratory effort
Presence of cyanosis
Oxygen requirement
Stoma site-redness or skin breakdown around site
Frequency of need to suction
Characteristics of mucus-color, consistency, odor
Caregiver's ability to maintain tracheostomy and change trach tube
Feeding intolerance
Nutritional requirements
Family's ability to care for the child
Need for support services for the child and the family
All caregiver teaching
    Topics to include in the teaching plan:
        safe and correct handling of equipment/supplies
        emergency procedures
        underlying disease pathology
        appropriate community resources and contact persons

INTERDISCIPLINARY COLLABORATION
Any concerns and abnormal findings should be reported to the child's primary physician
Determine the need for additional supplies and order from DME company

Contact family social worker to aid in referral to community services that may be needed [1, 5, 8, 12–14, 32]

Cardiopulmonary Resuscitation

DESCRIPTION
Cardiopulmonary resuscitation (CPR) is an emergency procedure performed to restore respiratory and cardiac function to an individual who has suffered emergent hypoxemia and poor systemic perfusion

PURPOSE
To restore adequate gas exchange and circulation to the body

EQUIPMENT
Health assessment forms
CPR pocket mask or
Bag valve mask device
Suction apparatus if available

OUTCOMES
The child will maintain:

► Respirations sufficient to promote adequate gas exchange
► Pulses to promote circulation to vital organs
► Return to a conscious state
► Adequate urinary output
► A seizure-free status

ASSESSMENT DATA
Determine unresponsiveness
Look at chest movement for presence of respirations
Listen for presence of shallow respirations
Feel for pulses
Assess for evidence of airway obstruction

RELATED NURSING DIAGNOSES
Impaired gas exchange
Decreased cardiac output
Altered tissue perfusion
Ineffective airway clearance
Ineffective breathing patterns

SPECIAL CONSIDERATIONS
The care of a child who has been successfully resuscitated at home should include immediate notification of the physician regarding the incident, constant monitoring of vital signs, maintenance of body temperature with blankets, placement of the child in a side lying position to prevent aspiration from vomiting. The EMS team should have been notified at the start of the procedure to aid in the resuscitation and to transport the child to a healthcare facility.

TRANSCULTURAL CONSIDERATIONS

An interpreter will be needed for clients unable to speak English

Support and maintain the client's religious and cultural healthcare practices

Acquire healthcare materials written in the client's native language, if available

Consider use of the AT&T Language Line

See also the Culturological Assessment procedure in Unit 2 for general overview of cultural considerations.

▶ INTERVENTIONS
CPR of the Infant

1. Attempt to elicit a response and determine presence of breathing (see Figure 5-7)	*Determines client's unresponsiveness*
2. Call for help.	*One person cannot maintain CPR over a prolonged period of time*
3. Open airway—tilt head, lift chin (see Figure 5-8).	*Tongue is the most common cause of airway obstruction*
4. Do not hyperextend the neck.	*May collapse infant airway which is very supple*
5. Observe for chest movement. LOOK, LISTEN, FEEL.	*Indicates presence of spontaneous respirations*
6. Apply CPR mask and give two initial breaths.	*Mask forms airtight seal*
7. If lungs do not inflate, check for obstruction and remove by finger-sweeping the mouth or suctioning.	*Vomitus or foreign body my obstruct airway*

⚡ **DO NOT USE BLIND SWEEP IN INFANTS**

8. Determine a pulse—use brachial pulse (upper arm) (see Figure 5-9).	*Pulse rate and rhythm indicate adequacy of cardiac perfusion*

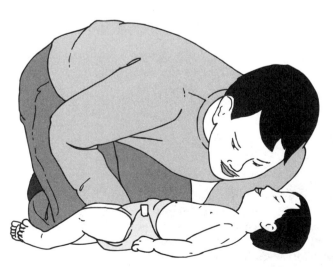

FIGURE 5-7 ▶ Determining presence of breathing in unresponsive infant.

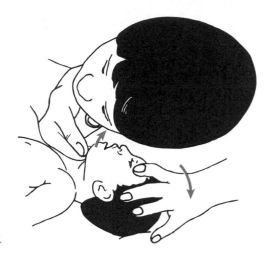

FIGURE 5-8 ▶ Opening the infant's airway.

a. If pulse is present—begin rescue breathing 1 breath every 3 seconds

b. If no pulse felt—start chest compressions. 5 compressions to 1 breath at a rate of 100/min. Place two fingers on lower third of sternum and compress at a depth of 1/2–1 inch (see Figure 5-10).

9. Check for a brachial pulse or spontaneous breathing after 1 minute.

10. Repeat cycle until emergency help arrives or spontaneous breathing and pulse return.

Assesses the return of respiration and perfusion

If breathing and circulation do not spontaneously return, the client will become anoxic if CPR is not continuously maintained

CPR of the Child 1–8 Years Old

1. Attempt to elicit a response.

2. Open airway—tilt head, lift chin—LOOK, LISTEN, FEEL.

Determines client's unresponsiveness

Tongue is the most common cause of airway obstruction.

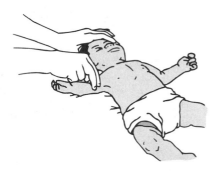

FIGURE 5-9 ▶ Assessing for presence of brachial pulse.

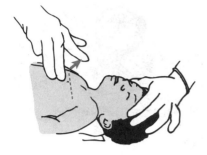

FIGURE 5-10 ▶ Locating position ot place fingers for chest compression in the infant.

3. Call for help.

One person cannot maintain CPR over a prolonged period of time.

4. Give two breaths.

Ventilates the airways and promotes chest expansion

5. Feel for pulse—use carotid site.
   a. If pulses are present—begin rescue breathing. One breath every 3 seconds until spontaneous breathing occurs
   b. If no pulses are felt—start chest compressions. Five compressions to 1 breath at a rate of 100/min. Place hands at lower third of sternum and compress at a depth of 1–1 1/2 inches (see Figure 5-11)

Correct positioning of the hands decreases chance of injury.

6. Check for pulses and spontaneous respirations after 1 minute. If still not present, repeat cycle.
7. Continue with compressions until emergency help arrives or spontaneous breathing and pulse return.

Assesses the return of respiration and perfusion

If breathing and circulation do not spontaneously return, the client will become anoxic if CPR is not continuously maintained

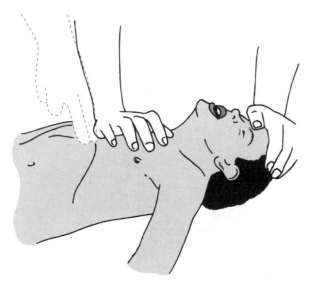

FIGURE 5-11 ▶ Correct placement of heel of heand for chest compression in the child.

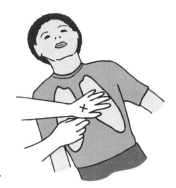

FIGURE 5-12 ▶ Chest compression in the child over 8 years of age.

CPR of the Child 8 Years and Older

1. Determine responsiveness.

Ensures that CPR is not performed on a conscious person

2. If unresponsive call for help.
3. Tilt head, lift chin, and hyperextend the neck (if a neck injury is not suspected).
4. LOOK, LISTEN, FEEL.

Mobilizes the EMS Team
Opens the airway

5. If no spontaneous respirations—give two slow breaths.
6. Feel for a carotid pulse.
    a. If present—give one breath every 5 seconds, 10–12 breaths/min.
    b. If no pulse present—start compressions. Give 15 compressions to every 2 breaths. Place both hands (heel of bottom hand) two fingers above child's ziphoid process and compress at a depth of 1 1/2–2 inches (see Figures 5-12, 5-13).
7. Repeat 15:2 cycle four times and check for a pulse and spontaneous respirations.

Determines the presence of spontaneous respirations
Restores ventilation
Detects the presence of a heartbeat

Simulates a heart rate of 80 to 100 beats per minute and provides ventilation

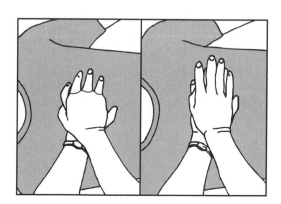

FIGURE 5-13 ▶ Hand placement for chest compression in child over 8 years of age.

8. Then, check for a pulse and respirations.

9. Continue with CPR until emergency help arrives or spontaneous breathing and pulse return.

Detects return of spontaneous breathing and circulation

If breathing and circulation do not spontaneously return, the client will become anoxic if CPR is not continuously maintained

DOCUMENTATION

The following should be noted in the nursing note:

General appearance of child prior to incident
Events leading up to incident
Child's response to interventions
Post resuscitation status
Vital signs pre and post resuscitation
All caregiver teaching:
    Topics to include in the teaching plan:
        safe and correct handling of equipment/supplies
        emergency procedures
        underlying disease pathology
        appropriate community resources and contact persons

INTERDISCIPLINARY COLLABORATION

Inform the physician of the events leading to the incident. The family may be able to participate in the resuscitation of the child until emergency help arrives. Notification of EMS at the start of the incident to administer care above what the nurse/caregiver is able to perform. [1, 5, 8, 12–14, 32]

PROCEDURE
Obstructed Airway Management, Pediatric

DESCRIPTION

Laryngeal obstruction is a life-threatening emergency. The larynx may be partially or fully obstructed by aspirated food or foreign objects, or may be obstructed secondary to edema due to inflammation, injury, or anaphylaxis. The most common manifestations of laryngeal obstruction include choking, coughing, gagging, dyspnea, use of accessory muscles of respiration and inspiratory stridor. See also Adult Respiratory System Procedure on Obstructed Airway Management, Adult.

PURPOSE

To remove the obstruction and restore adequate gas exchange

EQUIPMENT

Health Assessment Forms
CPR pocket mask or
Bag valve mask device
Suction apparatus if available

OUTCOMES

The child will maintain:

Respirations sufficient to promote adequate gas exchange

Return to a conscious state

A seizure-free status

ASSESSMENT DATA

Determine unresponsiveness

Look at chest movement for presence of respirations

Listen for presence of shallow respirations

Feel for pulses

Assess for evidence of airway obstruction

RELATED NURSING DIAGNOSES

Impaired gas exchange

Decreased cardiac output

Altered tissue perfusion

Ineffective airway clearance

Ineffective breathing patterns

SPECIAL CONSIDERATIONS

The care of a child who has been successfully resuscitated at home should include immediate notification of the physician regarding the incident, constant monitoring of vital signs, maintenance of body temperature with blankets, placement of child in side lying position to prevent aspiration from vomiting. The EMS team should have been notified at the start of the procedure to aid in the resuscitation and to transport the child to a healthcare facility.

TRANSCULTURAL CONSIDERATIONS

An interpreter will be needed for clients unable to speak English. Support and maintain the client's religious and cultural healthcare practices. Acquire healthcare materials written in the client's native language, if available. Consider use of AT&T Language Line. See also the Culturological Assessment procedure in Unit 2 for general overview of cultural considerations

> ▶ **I N T E R V E N T I O N S**
> *Infant: Obstructed Airway Emergency Management*

If the infant is conscious and choking:

1. Check for airway obstruction LOOK, LISTEN, FEEL.

Detects presence/absence of spontaneous respirations

2. Assess for blueness of lips.

Indicates presence of cyanosis

3. If obstructed:

Helps to dislodge obstruction

    give five back blows (head lower than trunk)
      (see Figure 5-14)
    give five chest thrusts (head lower than trunk)
      see Figure 5-15)

4. Repeat until airway is clear.

May be necessary to repeat the manuever several times to remove obstruction

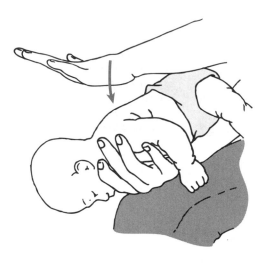

FIGURE 5-14 ▶ Correct position of infant for back blows.

If the infant becomes unconscious:

1. Call for help.

   Mobilizes EMS team

2. Open airway with tongue-jaw lift, remove foreign body **only if visible.**

   This manuever moves the tongue away from the back of the throat and opens the airway without moving the neck. Performing a blind sweep may inadvertently push the obstruction into the lower airways

3. Attempt to ventilate—if unsuccessful reposition head and attempt to ventilate again.

   Opens the airway

4. Give five back blows (head lower than trunk). Give five chest thrusts (head lower than trunk).

   Helps to dislodge the obstruction.

5. Open airway with tongue-jaw lift, remove foreign body **only if visible.**

   This manuever moves the tongue away from the back of the throat and opens the airway without moving the

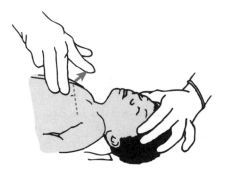

FIGURE 5-15 ▶ Position of fingers for chest thrusts in the infant.

	neck. Performing a blind sweep may inadvertently push the obstruction into the lower airways
6. Open airway with head-tilt, chin lift.	*Establishes full patency of the airway*
7. Attempt to ventilate.	*If the obstruction has been cleared, the rescuer will be able to restore ventilation*
8. Repeat sequence until effective.	*It may be necessary to repeat the manuever several times to dislodge the obstruction*

Child: Obstructed Airway Emergency Management

If the child is choking and conscious:

1. Follow steps above for the conscious-infant obstructed airway emergency management.
2. Instead of back blows, perform five Heimlich maneuvers (abdominal thrusts) until successful (see Figure 5-16).

    Creates an artificial cough that will dislodge an obstruction

   If the child becomes unconscious:

1. Call for help.
2. Open airway with tongue-jaw lift, remove foreign body **only if visible** (see Figure 5-17).

    Mobilizes the EMS Team

    This manuever moves the tongue away from the back of the throat and opens the airway without moving the neck. Performing a blind

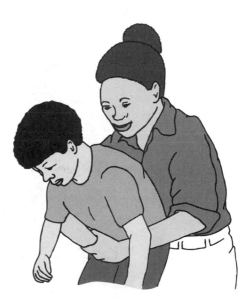

FIGURE 5-16 ▶ Position of abdominal thrusts.

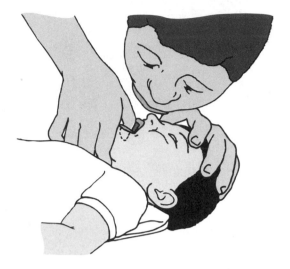

FIGURE 5-17 ▶ Performing the tongue-jaw lift to open airway.

3. Attempt to ventilate. If unsuccessful:
   Give five Heimlich maneuvers astride the child (see Figure 5-18).
   Open airway with tongue-jaw lift. Perform finger sweep to remove the foreign **only if visible** (see Figure 5-19).

sweep may inadvertently push the obstruction into the lower airways.
Creates an artificial cough that will dislodge an obstruction
This manuever moves the tongue away from the back of the throat and opens the airway without moving the neck. Performing a blind sweep may inadvertently

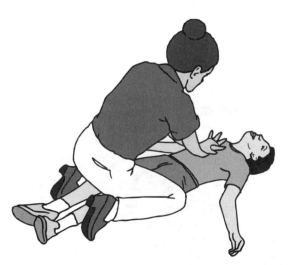

FIGURE 5-18 ▶ Performing abdominal thrusts in the child.

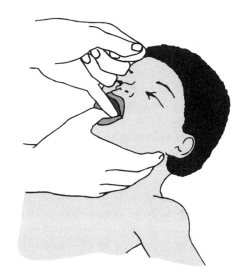

FIGURE 5-19 ▶ Performing the finger sweep in the child when the foreign object is visualized.

4. Open airway with head-tilt, chin lift, and attempt to ventilate.

push the obstruction into the lower airways
If the obstruction has been cleared, the rescuer will be able to restore ventilation

5. Repeat sequence until effective or emergency help arrives.

It may be necessary to repeat the manuever several times to dislodge the obstruction

DOCUMENTATION
The following should be noted in the nursing note:

General appearance of child prior to incident
Events leading up to incident
Child's response to interventions
Post-resuscitation status
Vital signs pre- and post-resuscitation
All caregiver teaching
    Topics to include in the teaching plan:
        safe and correct handling of equipment/supplies
        emergency procedures
        underlying disease pathology
        appropriate community resources and contact persons

INTERDISCIPLINARY COLLABORATION
Inform the physician of the events leading to the incident. The family may be able to participate in the resuscitation of the child until emergency help arrives. Notify the EMS team at the start of the incident to administer care above what the nurse/caregiver is able to perform. [4, 5, 12–14, 32]

PROCEDURE
Orophryngeal/Nasopharyngeal Suctioning

DESCRIPTION
Use of a nasal aspirator or bulb syringe is an easy way of clearing the nose and mouth of mucus. This is especially helpful in clearing the airway of an infant.

PURPOSE
To maintain a patent airway

EQUIPMENT
Health Assessment Forms
Bulb syringe or nasal aspirator
Stethoscope

OUTCOMES
The child will have:

▶ Adequate gas exchange
▶ Effective respirations
▶ Less anxiety
▶ Adequate nutrition due to ability to eat without difficulty

ASSESSMENT DATA
Note difficult respirations
Note discomfort
Note irritability
Note difficulty eating

RELATED NURSING DIAGNOSES
Impaired gas exchange
Ineffective breathing patterns
Anxiety
Altered nutrition, less than body requirements

SPECIAL CONSIDERATIONS
Saline nose drops are needed when mucus becomes dry and encrusted to povide liquification and to facilitate removal. To make a saline solution, mix 3/4 teaspoon of salt with 1 pint of tap water. Instill into nose with an eyedropper. This solution can be kept in a covered container but must be mixed fresh daily. Cleanse eyedropper after each time used.

Oropharyngeal/nasopharyngeal suctioning should be performed prior to initiating a feeding to improve the sucking reflex and to prevent gagging/choking during feedings.

TRANSCULTURAL CONSIDERATIONS
An interpreter will be needed for clients unable to speak English. Support and maintain the client's religious and cultural healthcare practices. Acquire healthcare materials written in the client's native language, if available. Consider use of the AT&T Language Line. See also the Culturological Assessment procedure in Unit 2 for general overview of cultural considerations.

▶ INTERVENTIONS

1. Squeeze rounded end of aspirator.	*Removes air from the aspirator*
2. Place the tip of the aspirator into nare.	*Positions syringe for effective removal of secretions*
3. Release bulb slowly.	*Creates a suction effect*
4. Remove from nare after bulb is inflated.	*Expanded bulb contains evacuated secretions*
5. Squeeze contents onto a tissue.	*Empties syringe of mucus waste*
6. Repeat steps 1 through 5 for the opposite nare.	
7. Repeat until nose and mouth are clear of excess mucus.	*Re-establishes a patent airway*
8. Cleanse the aspirator by filling with water, squeezing and removing water and mucus.	*Liquifies secretions for ease of removal*
9. Boil aspirator for 10 minutes, store in clean, dry container or plastic bag.	*Prevents the risk of infection*
10. Allow caregiver to perform the procedure.	*Documents client learning*

DOCUMENTATION
The following should be noted in the nursing note:

Child's tolerance of procedure
Color, consistency and amount of mucus removed
Respiratory status after intervention
Caregiver's ability to demonstrate procedure
All caregiver teaching:
    Topics to include in the teaching plan:
        safe and correct handling of equipment/supplies
        emergency procedures
        underlying disease pathology
        appropriate community resources and contact persons

INTERDISCIPLINARY COLLABORATION
Inform physician of inability to improve respiratory status
Obtain aspirating equipment from DME vendor or homecare agency [1, 4, 5, 12–14, 32]

PROCEDURE
Management of Home Mechanical Ventilation, Pediatric

DESCRIPTION
A wide variety of home mechanical ventilation devices are currently on the market to assist the infant/child to maintain adequate oxygenation. The choice of a ventilator to best meet the needs of an infant/child depends on several factors: underlying disease, mode of ventilation required, oxygenation and PEEP requirements, ventilator capability and functionality, and community experience. Prior to initiating home mechanical ventilation, the caregiver and family members must be assisted to become thoroughly trained in use of the equipment prior to hospital discharge, be provided with a

troubleshooting manual, have 24-hour servicing and access to a respiratory therapist, have back-up equipment, and be trained in the technique to perform manual ventilation in the event of equipment failure. See also Adult Respiratory System Procedure on home mechanical ventilation management.

PURPOSE
To maintain adequate ventilation

EQUIPMENT
Home ventilator equipment and supplies (tubing, circuitry, filters, pressure gauges, connectors/ adapters, humidifier, compressor, extra exhalation valve)
Oxygen equipment and related supplies (tubing, tank, concentrator, cylinder, nebulizer, mask/cannula)
Tracheostomy equipment and related supplies(ties, trach care kit, t-piece, gauze, extra trach tube)
Personal communication aid
Health assessment forms
Stethoscope
Resuscitation bag
Suction equipment (aspirator, tubing, collection container, suction catheter)
Distilled water for cascade
Sterile water and normal saline
Apnea monitor
Pulse oximeter
Alternate power source (generator or battery)
Back-up ventilator
Personal protective gear
Disinfectant cleaning equipment and storage supplies

OUTCOMES
The client/caregiver will:

▶ Maintain adequate ventilation
▶ Demonstrate ability to perform procedure
▶ Verbalize understanding of procedure to follow in the event of equipment malfunction

ASSESSMENT DATA
Note signs and symptoms of hypoxemia
Record type and amount of oxygen therapy
Document respiratory rate and character
Auscultate lung sounds and note adventitious sounds
Assess character of sputum
Review prescribed medication therapy
Assess growth and developmental parameters
Determine adequacy of nutritional status
Observe for evidence of fluid volume deficit/excess
Evaluate for evidence of cardiopulmonary compromise
Assess client/caregiver's knowledge base regarding the procedure

RELATED NURSING DIAGNOSES
Impaired gas exchange
Altered breathing patterns
Ineffective airway clearance
Anxiety

Powerlessness
At risk for altered parenting
At risk for ineffective family coping

SPECIAL CONSIDERATIONS

Prior to discharge to home, financial support for home ventilation should be thoroughly investigated. Third-party payors vary significantly in the amount of coverage that each can offer. Capitation for cost of medical equipment, supplies, prescriptions, homecare nursing services, and other services poses serious financial constraint. The medical social worker should be consulted to assist the family in determining eligibility for reimbursement and availability of community support programs. [1, 7, 8, 23, 27]

To ensure a more successful transition to the home setting, the discharge planner should discuss with the family options for having 24-hour homecare nursing service for the first few weeks, tapering to 8 hours of nursing service per day as the medical needs of the infant/child dictate. Additionally, because of the time commitment required to meet the needs of the ventilator-dependent infant/child, the family must be assisted to consider respite care to relieve caregivers periodically. [1, 7, 8, 23, 27]

Types of ventilators used for infants and children fall into two main categories: invasive/non-invasive positive-pressure ventilators, and noninvasive negative-pressure devices. Positive-pressure ventilation supports the child's respiratory system by pushing air into the lungs and holding pressure for a predetermined amount of time per physician order and then permitting pressure levels to return to baseline. Positive-pressure ventilation can be delivered via a tracheostomy tube, or face/nose mask, and can be provided by volume-controlled, pressure-controlled, or bilevel positive airway pressure (BiPAP).

> **Volume Ventilator**—Various models of the Bear, Aequitron, and Lifecare volume ventilators are commonly used in the home. The ventilator is regulated at a preset tidal volume, depending on the needs of the infant/child, with controlled pressure limits to deliver the necessary volume.

> **Pressure Ventilator**—Pressure ventilation is used primarily in the acute care setting and only occasionally in homecare. With this device air is moved into the lungs at a preset pressure limit, depending on the needs of the child, while the tidal volume that the lung receives varies. These devices require a continuous air source that may be difficult to maintain in the home.

> **BiPAP**—The bilevel positive pressure airway pressure is a low-pressure ventilatory support system that delivers pressurized air to the infant through a face/nose mask. On inspiration, the device is set to deliver a breath at a prescribed level. On expiration, the pressure level is lowered to permit an exhaled breath. BiPAP can be set in several modes to permit the infant/child's specific needs including continuous positive airway pressure (CPAP) [1, 7, 8]

Negative-pressure ventilation moves air into and out of the lungs by applying subatmospheric pressure around the chest. Inhalation occurs when the chest cavity expands as a result of a decrease in atmospheric pressure, and exhalation occurs by passive relaxation of chest wall and lungs. There are two negative-pressure ventilation systems in use in homecare: invasive and noninvasive negative-pressure ventilators.

▶ *Invasive Negative Pressure Ventilator*—Several ventilator models (Emerson, Lifecare, Thompson Maxivent) are positive pressure ventilators with a negative pressure capability.
▶ *Noninvasive Negative Pressure Ventilator*—Body devices that can wrap around the chest (Pulmo-Wrap, Nu-Mo, Poncho) are used to create negative pressure and are powered by a respirator

Prior to discharge, the caregivers will need to be instructed in use care and management of the infant/child and equipment. A manual containing a set of written instructions should be available at all times listing troubleshooting procedure, emergency telephone numbers, and guidelines for emergency intervention. The caregivers should understand the underlying pathology causing the client's compromised respiratory state. The teaching plan should include:

▶ *Ventilator:* operational controls and prescribed settings, procedure and schedule for cleaning circuitry, alarms, troubleshooting, use of manual ventilation, alternative power source, cleaning/disinfecting equipment
▶ *Respiratory equipment:* apnea monitor, pulse oximetry, tracheostomy management, oxygen therapies
▶ *Emergency care:* access to EMS, nearest hospital facility, electrical and telephone suppliers and back-up system during power failure, signs and symptoms of respiratory distress, criteria for initiating CPR and for calling DME vendor, rescue squad, physician, homecare agency
▶ *Daily maintenance:* supply inventory, medication administration, nutrition needs, physician follow-up, developmental program (occupational/physical/speech therapy), and plans for travel, transportation, and schooling [1, 7, 8, 23]

Once the child has been discharged to home, the family will also need to consider and plan for transportation of the child to physician visits or other outings. Arrangements must be made for ventilation during transportation. Depending on ventilator used, external battery power or portable ventilators may be an option. Age-appropriate car seats or wheelchairs that can be anchored in the van or specially designed car will be needed. There must always be two adults in the car, one to attend to the child, the other to drive the vehicle. Families should be given information on how to obtain handicapped parking permits/license to facilitate parking. When no other option is available, families may use ambulance services or special para-transit services provided by public transportation in some communities. [1, 7, 8]

The caregiver will also need to be informed of the risks associated with long-term mechanical ventilation and to know the signs and symptoms of fluid imbalance, decreased cardiac output, cardiorespiratory compromise, respiratory infections, and pneumothorax/pneumomediastinum. To prevent atelectasis the caregiver should be instructed to reposition the infant/child frequently, to perform postural drainage and percussion as ordered, to suction as needed, and to periodically hyperinflate/hyperoxygenate the child as ordered. To prevent tampering with settings, the family should childproof ventilator controls using plastic panels, which can be purchased from the DME vendor or ventilator manufacturer. To troubleshoot the alarm system, the caregivers must know how to assess the infant/child first before determining the nature of the cause for the alarm. The infant should be removed from the ventilator and manually ventilated if the cause requires more than a simple reconnection of circuitry. The caregiver should be instructed to observe for air leak around the tracheostomy tube, need for suctioning or nebulizer treatment, an empty oxygen tank, etc. [1, 7, 8, 23]

The family must also be aware of the need to exercise caution when handling oxygen equipment in the home.

▶ Place "no smoking" signs throughout the home where oxygen is stored or in use
▶ Do not store oxygen tank near stove or source of heat
▶ Keep source of oxygen at least 5 feet from electrical outlets and appliances
▶ Do not use heating pad/blanket or other electrical appliance near source of oxygen
▶ Use cotton linens/clothing to prevent buildup of static electricity
▶ Do not use oil or alcohol near oxygen source
▶ Keep oxygen container in upright position and securely anchored
▶ Regularly check oxygen levels
▶ Keep fire extinguisher in same room with source of oxygen

► Do not adjust level of oxygen without medical order
► With an oxygen compressor, keep a 3-day supply of oxygen in the home
► With an oxygen concentrator, do not use an extension cord, clean filter two times/week; during power failure use back-up source of oxygen
► For liquid oxygen, do not touch metal parts with bare hands, may cause frostbite [1, 7, 8, 23]

TRANSCULTURAL CONSIDERATIONS

An interpreter will be needed for the client/caregiver unable to speak or understand the English language. Obtain educational materials in the client/caregiver's native language, if available. Consider use of AT&T Language Line. See also Culturological Assessment procedure in Unit 2 for general discussion of cultural considerations.

▶ INTERVENTIONS

1. Verify physician order.	*Reduces risk of error*
2. Wash hands.	*Prevents transmission of microbes*
3. Perform physical assessment.	*Establishes baseline information of physiological data findings*
4. Explain procedure.	*Allays anxiety*

5. Perform safety check of equipment:
  Inspect for evidence of excessive wear
  Check connections for tightness
  Perform routine cleaning per manufacturer's recommendations
  Inspect battery level and operational hours
  Drain water from all tubing
	Assures proper functioning of equipment

6. Set up/maintain oxygen source.	*Maintains adequate oxygenation*
7. Set up the ventilator circuits and attach to ventilator.	*Maintains integrity of system*
8. Set up the suction equipment.	*Makes available for immediate use*
9. Set up manual resuscitator bag.	*Allows ventilation to be maintained while client is off mechanical ventilator*
10. Put on personal protective gear (gloves, mask, gown as needed).	*Serves as barrier*
11. Turn on/maintain ventilator and ensure attachment to client's airway.	*Establishes/maintains power source*
12. Suction airway as needed.	*Establishes airway clearance*
13. Give in-line aerosol treatments if prescribed.	*Liquifies secretions/dilates bronchioles*
14. If child is old enough, demonstrate use of communication board/aid.	*Maintains dialogue with client*
15. Instruct client/caregiver in home mechanical ventilation procedure and permit return demonstration.	*Documents client/caregiver's ability to implement ordered procedure*
16. Notify local emergency medical system and power supply company for priority service.	*Establishes emergency preparedness protocol*

For Positive-Pressure Devices

Invasive Positive-Pressure Ventilation

MECHANICAL VENTILATOR

1. Assess mode setting.	*Determines number of assisted/nonassisted breaths/minute*
Set rates per physician order for: a. Control volume; or b. Rate or assist control rate; or c. Intermittent mandatory ventilation rate, or d. Synchronized intermittent mandatory ventilation rate.	
2. Assess respiratory rate setting and compare with client's actual respiratory rate.	*Counts the number of breaths per minute*
3. Assess tidal volume setting and compare with client's actual expired volume.	*Documents amount of gas client receives with each breath*
4. Assess the sigh volume, if ordered.	*Stimulates production of surfactant by maintaining expansion of the alveolar bed*
5. Assess low-pressure and high-pressure alarm settings and compare with client's breath efforts.	*Alerts client/caregiver of abnormal situation*
6. Assess the fraction of inspired oxygen.	*Registers the percentage of oxygen concentration.*
7. Assess the peak flow or inspiratory time	*Determines how fast the prescribed tidal volume is to be delivered*
8. Assess positive end-expiratory pressure, if ordered.	*Prevents alveolar collapse*
9. Assess expiration time.	*Determines length of exhaled breath*
10. Evaluate heat temperature settings.	*Allows for warming of air prior to inspiring*

Noninvasive Positive-Pressure Ventilation

Full-Mask Mechanical Ventilation (FMMV)—Avoids tracheostomy tube placement by using a tight-fitting mask which forms an airtight seal to deliver forced air into the upper airways

1. Ensure that mask fits tightly over face.	*Maintains tight airseal*

Nasal Intermittent Positive-Pressure Ventilation (NIPPV)—Avoids tracheostomy tube placement by using a tight-fitting mask over the nose to deliver forced air into the upper airways. Because of the potential for air leakage out of the mouth, NIPPV is not as effective as FMMV.

1. Ensure that mask fits tightly over nose.	*Maintains tight air seal*

BiPAP—This is a bilevel respiratory system that maintains a constant level of positive airway pressure. The inspiratory pressure levels provide the client with a pressure boost, while the expiratory pressure level maintains positive end-expiratory pressure to keep alveoli open and facilitate gas exchange.

1. Ensure that mask fits tightly over nose or mouth as ordered.	*Maintains tight airseal*

Continuous Positive-Airway Pressure (CPAP)—This device uses a nasal mask to maintain continuous positive pressure to prevent the collapse of soft upper airway tissue in the treatment of sleep apnea (See Figure 5-20).

1. Ensure that mask fits tightly over the nose.	*Maintains tight airseal*

For Noninvasive Negative Pressure Devices

NU MO Suit—Can be a chest shell or an upper-body or full-body garment that forms a tight seal around the external chest surface to permit the intermittent generation of negative pressure. During the negative-pressure cycle, the air from the higher pressured external atmosphere enters the air passages of the body. When the negative pressure stops, passive exhalation begins. The suit is powered by a negative-pressure respirator, which is connected to the garment.

1. Ensure a tight seal around all connectors	*Maintains tight airseal*

DOCUMENTATION

The following should be noted in the nursing note:

Client response to the procedure
Untoward responses reported to the physician
Interventions as a result of deviations from the norm
Respiratory physical assessment findings (character of sputum, lung sounds, vital signs, trach site, oxygen saturation)
Safety of home setting
Ventilator settings
Family dynamics/interactions and coping ability
Growth and developmental findings
Consultations with physical/occupational/therapist, and speech-language pathologist
Consultations with nutritionist, respiratory therapist, DME vendor
All caregiver teaching:
Topics to include in the teaching plan:
safe and correct handling of equipment/supplies

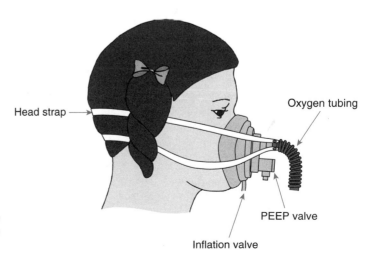

FIGURE 5-20 ▶ Administering oxygen by face mask with continuous positive airway pressure (CPAP).

emergency procedures
underlying disease pathology
appropriate community resources and contact persons

INTERDISCIPLINARY COLLABORATION

Inform physician of presence of adventitious lung sounds, and compare with previous findings

Document interventions employed to treat untoward responses. Collaborate with respiratory therapist or equipment maintenance.

Determine adequacy of supplies/equipment and need to initiate reorder from DME vendor

Consult with social worker to determine client's eligibility for financial assistance/reimbursement for supplies and equipment, and to identify community resources [1, 5, 7, 8, 12, 23, 27]

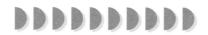

Pediatric Cardiovascular System Procedures

PROCEDURE

Management of Heart Disease

DESCRIPTION
Heart disease is classified as either congenital or acquired. Congenital heart disease is defined as abnormal anatomy or function of the heart that is present at birth. Acquired heart disease develops after birth in a normal heart as the result of infection, autoimmune responses, drug toxicities, metabolic deficiencies, or familial patterns.

PURPOSE
To instruct caregiver in the implementation of ordered interventions to maintain adequate cardiac function

EQUIPMENT
Weight scale
Stethoscope
Sphygmomanometer
Thermometer
Health Assessment forms
Oxygen supplies and equipment, as ordered
Pulse oximeter for oxygen monitoring, as applicable

OUTCOMES
The child will be:

- ▶ Adequately oxygenated
- ▶ Able to tolerate a level of activity
- ▶ Free from pain and discomfort
- ▶ Able to meet nutritional requirements
- ▶ Free from signs and symptoms of heart failure
- ▶ Able to maintain growth and development status

ASSESSMENT DATA
Note color of lips, nailbeds, skin, and oral cavity, and evidence of circumoral cyanosis
Evaluate capillary refill
Auscultate lungs for presence of wheezing or crackles, also note rate and pattern of respirations
Note dyspnea at rest or on exertion, presence of sternal retraction
Auscultate heart sounds for rate, rhythm, murmur, gallop, or missed beats

Note irritability and/or lethargy

Assess skin for color, temperature, dry, clammy, or mottled-like appearance

Note ability to eat without distress and adequacy of nutritional intake

Evaluate intake and output, assess for edema of eyelids and face

Obtain vital signs and pulse oximetry reading, as ordered

Evaluate growth and development; chart growth on growth curve to evaluate nutritional status

Assess dietary intake: types of foods, amount, frequency of feedings, use of food supplements

Document history of sickling crisis and family history of sickle cell disease

Review laboratory results for evidence of infection and chronic anemia

Review caregiver knowledge of medication regimen and client compliance

RELATED NURSING DIAGNOSES

Altered cardiac output

Altered tissue perfusion

Impaired gas exchange

Altered nutrition, less than body requirements

Altered growth and development

Activity intolerance

At risk for infection

SPECIAL CONSIDERATIONS

Children with cyanotic heart disease have a lower oxygen saturation even after surgical correction, which may result in a slightly bluish appearance to lips and nailbeds. In addition to signs of potential respiratory compromise, the nurse should also observe for symptoms of congestive heart failure (CHF), see Display 5-1.

DISPLAY 5-1 *Clinical Symptoms of CHF*

Cardiovascular

Tachycardia

Precordial impulse

Gallop rhythm

Nasal flaring

Periorbital edema

Rapid weight gain

Peripheral cyanosis

Distended neck veins (rare)

Respiratory

Tachypnea

Dyspnea, orthopnea

Retractions

Enlarged liver

Grunting respirations

Fine rales

Decreased pulse oxygen saturation level

Related

Feeding difficulties, anorexia

Diaphoresis

Oliguria

Irritability

Fatigability

Note: Some of these signs in isolation may resemble characteristics of the underlying respiratory problem; therefore, it is important to perform an overall assessment of the infant.

Reprinted/adapted with permission from: Ahmann, E. *Home care for the high-risk infant: A family centered approach.* Gaithersburg, MD: An Aspen Publication. 1996, p. 181.

TRANSCULTURAL CONSIDERATIONS

In children with dark skin pigmentation, it may be difficult to assess cyanosis, the oral cavity and gums may be the best and most reliable area of assessment. An interpreter will be needed for clients unable to speak English. Support and maintain the client's religious and cultural healthcare practices. Acquire healthcare materials written in the client's native language, if available. Consider use of AT&T Language Line. See also the Culturological Assessment procedure in Unit 2 for general overview of cultural considerations.

▶ INTERVENTIONS

1. Wash hands.	*Prevents transmission of microbes*
2. Don gloves.	*Serves as protective barrier*
3. Perform physical assessment.	*Establishes baseline information of physiological data findings*
4. Verify medical orders.	*Reduces risk of error*
5. Instruct caregiver in the signs and symptoms of heart failure.	*Early recognition can prevent distress*
6. Instruct caregiver in use of oxygen if needed.	*Oxygen saturation may be low*
7. Instruct caregiver on importance of medications, side effects, and administration.	*Evaluates effectiveness of medication*
8. Encourage diet high in calories or maintain tube feedings, as ordered.	*Meets body's needs for greater energy expenditure*
9. Provide age-appropriate stimulation and activities, as tolerated.	*Promotes growth and development*
10. Monitor intake and output.	*Assesses fluid retention*
11. Weigh twice weekly, as ordered, and maintain weight log.	*Evaluates presence of fluid volume excess/deficit*
12. Evaluate caregiver knowledge of CPR and instruct as needed.	*Reinforces learning*

DOCUMENTATION

The following should be noted in the nursing note:

Vital signs and weight
Color of skin, lips, and nailbeds
Capillary refill
Presence of edema
Need for oxygen, amount being administered, how administered
Heart and lung sounds
Diet, route of feeding, tolerance of feedings
Activity level and tolerance
Presence of pain or discomfort
Urinary output
Stooling pattern
Oxygen saturation
Family's understanding of disease, medications, and signs and symptoms of complications, ability to cope and care for child

All caregiver teaching:
    Topics to include in the teaching plan:
        safe and correct handling of equipment/supplies
        emergency procedures
        underlying disease pathology
        appropriate community resources and contact persons

INTERDISCIPLINARY COLLABORATION

Inform the primary care physician and cardiologist of changes in condition or abnormal clinical findings: increased oxygen requirements or decreased oxygen saturation, decreased urinary output, decreased appetite, and decreased activity level. Any complaints of pain or discomfort should be reported.

Support groups can be helpful in providing coping skills for families. [1, 4, 5, 7, 12–14, 32]

PROCEDURE
Management of Sickle Cell Disease

DESCRIPTION

Sickle cell anemia is a hereditary disorder in which an erythrocyte containing hemoglobin S becomes sickle in shape because of a decrease in oxygen. This sickled-shaped cell either hemolyzes or causes sluggish blood flow. External stressors such as vigorous exercise, illness, and exposure to high altitudes cause a decrease in oxygen. In the absence of these external stressors, clients may be asymptomatic. However, in the event of severe crisis, sickle cell anemia may be a life-threatening condition.

PURPOSE

To assess for signs and symptoms of sickle cell crisis

EQUIPMENT

Related healthcare instructional materials
Health Assessment forms
Oxygen supplies, if ordered
Intravenous supplies, if ordered
Thermometer

OUTCOMES

The child will:

▶ Avoid situations that reduce oxygen saturation
▶ Be adequately hydrated
▶ Be free from infection
▶ Be free from pain

ASSESSMENT DATA

Assess for signs and symptoms, including:

Pain in joints, back or abdomen
Pain and swelling in hands and feet (hand-foot syndrome)
Enlarged spleen and liver
Respiratory distress/pneumonia-like symptoms
Hematuria

Pale mucous membranes
Poor wound healing

RELATED NURSING DIAGNOSES

Impaired gas exchange
At risk for injury
At risk for fluid volume deficit
Pain
Ineffective coping skills
Altered urinary elimination
Altered tissue perfusion

SPECIAL CONSIDERATIONS

Because sickle cell disease is an abnormality of the blood, major organs are affected. The nurse should perform a general assessment of client noting symptoms of sickle cell disease:

- ▶ Overall: developmental delay, chronic anemia, delayed sexual maturation, and potential for infection
- ▶ Crisis: pain and evidence of ischemia in areas of involvement, such as
    extremities: swelling of hands, feet and joints
    abdomen: severe pain
    cerebrum: stroke, visual disturbance
    lungs: pulmonary disease
    liver: obstructive jaundice
    kidney: hematuria
- ▶ Potential long-term effects on:
    heart: cardiomegaly, systolic murmurs
    lungs: decreased pulmonary function, pulmonary insufficiency
    kidneys: enuresis, inability to concentrate urine, renal failure,
    genital: priapism
    liver: cirrhosis, intrahepatic cholestasis, liver enlargement
    spleen: reduction in splenic activity, splenomegaly, increased risk of infection
    eyes: visual disturbances, retinal detachment, blindness
    extremities: chronic leg ulcers, at risk for salmonella osteomyelitis, skeletal deformity (lordosis, kyphosis)
    central nervous system: seizures, hemiparesis

Surgical treatment of this condition may include removing of the spleen to decrease the production of RBCs.

TRANSCULTURAL CONSIDERATIONS

This disorder is usually found in the black population, although individuals from the Arabian Peninsula, Greece, Turkey, and India are also susceptible. Consider use of AT&T Language Line. See also the Culturological Assessment procedure in Unit 2 for general overview of cultural considerations.

▶ INTERVENTIONS

1. Wash hands.	*Prevents transmission of microbes*
2. Perform physical assessment.	*Establishes baseline information of physiological data findings*

3. Verify medical orders.

4. Minimize situations of excessive physical exertion and emotional stress.

5. Encourage child to drink enough liquids to maintain fluid intake as ordered.

6. Instruct caregiver to closely monitor urinary output for amount, color, and consistency.

7. Report signs and symptoms of infection immediately to physician.

8. Administer pain medication to relieve discomfort as ordered.

9. Assess the need for genetic counseling/referral, if newly diagnosed.

Reduces risk of error

Conserves oxygen supply to blood cells

Prevents dehydration

Assesses renal function and fluid status

Early treatment prevents stress on the body

Prevents emotional stress

Assists the family to make informed reproductive decisions

DOCUMENTATION
The following should be noted in the nursing note:

Vital signs
Presence of any signs of respiratory distress
Quality of breath sounds in all lobes
Swelling or pain in joints of hands and feet
Pain or discomfort in abdomen or lower back
Frequency and use of analgesics
Change in mental status
Child/caregiver's knowledge of disease and treatment plan
Altered urinary output
All caregiver teaching:
    Topics to include in the teaching plan:
        safe and correct handling of equipment/supplies
        emergency procedures
        underlying disease pathology
        appropriate community resources and contact persons

INTERDISCIPLINARY COLLABORATION
All treatment is collaborated between the primary care physician and the hematologist. Any abnormal findings should be reported to one or both of these physicians.

Families benefit greatly from support groups who offer suggestions in coping with a chronic illness. The child should be encouraged to participate in group activities with children who also suffer from sickle cell anemia. [1, 4, 5, 12–14, 32]

PROCEDURE
Management of Hemophilia

DESCRIPTION
A bleeding disorder caused by a deficiency in one of the normal clotting factors VIII, IX, X. Factor VIII is the most common deficiency. The disorder is caused by a recessive gene passed on maternally to male children almost exclusively. Bleeding may occur either spontaneously or after an injury that may sometimes be very minor.

PURPOSE

Instruct the caregiver on signs and symptoms of internal bleeding, treatment during bleeding episode, and prevention of complications

EQUIPMENT

Health Assessment forms
Stethoscope
Sphygmomanometer
Thermometer
Educational materials

OUTCOMES

The child will be:

Free from injury
Free from pain
Physically mobile

ASSESSMENT DATA

Assess signs and symptoms including:
Frequent bruising or bleeding which is difficult to stop
Hemarthrosis
Epistaxis
Abdominal pain indicative of internal bleeding
Joint pain or stiffness
Hematuria
Intense unexplained pain
Any precipitating factors leading to frequent bruising or bleeding, since this disorder is often
    brought on by stressors

RELATED NURSING DIAGNOSES

Altered mobility
Altered growth and development
Altered comfort level
Ineffective coping skills
Impaired skin integrity

SPECIAL CONSIDERATIONS

Most cases are diagnosed within 12 to 18 months of age after an episode of prolonged bleeding following a minor injury.

Genetic testing is highly recommended for the parents of children with this disease.

TRANSCULTURAL CONSIDERATIONS

An interpreter will be needed for clients unable to speak English. Support and maintain the client's religious and cultural healthcare practices. Acquire healthcare materials written in the client's native language, if available. Consider use of AT&T Language Line. See also the Culturological Assessment procedure in Unit 2 for general overview of cultural considerations.

▶ INTERVENTIONS

1. Wash hands.

Prevents transmission of microbes

2. Perform physical assessment.	*Establishes baseline information of physiological data findings*
3. Verify medical orders.	*Reduces risk of error*
4. Treat swollen painful joints with ice packs and immobilize as ordered.	*Relieves pain*
5. If child placed on bedrest, begin active range of motion exercises after acute phase.	*Maintains limb mobility*
6. Instruct caregiver to avoid use of aspirin or aspirin-like analgesics.	*Inhibits platelet formation*
7. Instruct caregiver on maintaining safe environment.	*Prevent injury*
8. Encourage parent/child to: Pad infant cribs, use helmets, maintain a clutter-free play area, use *no* throw rugs on floor, discourage contact sports in older children. Use soft toothbrush for dental hygiene. Use knee and elbow pads.	*Reduces potential for injury*
9. Maintain adequate nutrition and prevent excessive weight gain.	*Decreases strain on joints*
10. Provide emotional support to child and caregiver through open communication and support groups.	*Strengthens coping skills*
11. Instruct or reinforce with caretaker the administration of Factor VIII during bleeding episodes, as ordered.	*Early administration of clotting factor prevents complications*
12. Review signs and symptoms of disease complications.	*Reinforces client learning*
13. Assess the need for genetic counseling/referral, if newly diagnosed.	*Assists the family to make informed reproductive decisions*

DOCUMENTATION
The following should be noted in the nursing note:

Vital signs
Growth and development
Signs of any overt or covert bleeding
Frequency, severity, and duration of bleeding
Presence of pain or discomfort
Any treatments administered (i.e., ice packs, Factor VIII, etc.)
Instructions given to caretaker/child and their comprehension of treatment
Coping skills of child/family
All caregiver teaching:
    Topics to include in the teaching plan:
        safe and correct handling of equipment/supplies
        emergency procedures
        underlying disease pathology
        appropriate community resources and contact persons

INTERDISCIPLINARY COLLABORATION
Anyone who interacts with these children should be informed about their condition: daycare workers, school nurses, teachers, coaches. Other healthcare providers such as dentists and physical therapists should be included in this group. Any and all abnormal signs should be reported to the

physician immediately. Consider the need to consult with the medical social worker to determine the family's eligibility for financial assistance/reimbursement for medication and supplies. [1, 4, 5, 32]

PROCEDURE
Administration of Antihemophilic Factor (Factor VIII)

DESCRIPTION
Administering Factor VIII replaces the missing clotting factors in clients with hemophilia A. The drug corrects or prevents bleeding episodes by assisting in the conversion of prothrombin to thrombin

PURPOSE
To restore blood clotting function

EQUIPMENT
Intravenous supplies
Ordered medication
Health Assessment forms
Gloves
Protective equipment (goggles, apron, face shield, etc), as needed

OUTCOMES
The client will:

▶ Demonstrate no symptoms of bleeding
▶ Report decrease in discomfort
▶ Demonstrate improved ambulation and joint movement

ASSESSMENT DATA
Observe for evidence of ecchymosis, petechiae, hematuria, hemetemesis, hemoptysis, tarry stool
Assess for allergic reaction
Watch for excessive bleeding from minor cuts
Check for excessive gingival bleeding
Monitor changes in clotting times, CBC, urinalysis
Observe changes in vital signs: hypotension, tachycardia, tachypnea
Question client regarding increase in menses
Observe joints for swelling

RELATED NURSING DIAGNOSES
Altered comfort level
At risk for altered cardiac output
Impaired mobility

SPECIAL CONSIDERATIONS
Drug must be stored in refrigerator but not allowed to freeze. After reconstituting, the solution should appear clear, colorless, or yellow. The reconstituted drug will be stable for 24 hours but must be used within 1–3 hours. Do not refrigerate reconstituted drug.

When monitoring blood pressure do not overinflate cuff to avoid risk of bruising. Remove adhesive tape from any pressure dressing carefully to avoid injury to skin.

TRANSCULTURAL CONSIDERATION

Some religious groups will not permit the administration of blood products to replace loss during
episodes of hemorrhage

Consider use of AT&T Language Line

See also Culturological Assessment procedure in Unit 2 for general overview of cultural considerations
tions

▶ INTERVENTIONS

1. Verify physician order.	*Reduces risk of error*
2. Wash hands.	*Prevents transmission of microbes*
3. Obtain vital signs prior to initiating infusion.	*Establishes baseline data*
4. Remove concentrate and diluent from refrigerator and allow to reach room temperature.	*Concentrate dissolves easier at warmer environmental temperature*
5. Reconstitute drug per manufacturer's recommendations.	*Ensures accuracy of protocol*
6. Don gloves and other protective gear as needed.	*Serves as protective barrier*
7. Perform venipuncture.	*Establishes intravenous site*
8. Determine patency of intravenous site.	*Prevents infiltration*
9. Follow physician order and homecare agency protocol for intravenous administration by injection or infusion.	*Reduces risk of error*
10. Check pulse and blood pressure during infusion.	*May indicate evidence of hemorrhaging*

⚡ **IF HYPOTENSION DEVELOPS STOP ADMINISTERING THE DRUG.**

11. After administering, apply prolonged pressure to venipuncture site and monitor site every 5–15 minutes for 2 hours after administration.	*Monitors evidence of bleeding*
12. Obtain specimens for laboratory analyses of urine, clotting factors, and CBC as ordered.	*Indicates trends in response to interventional strategies*

DOCUMENTATION

The following should be noted in the nursing note:

Client's tolerance of the procedure
Pertinent laboratory results
Vital signs pre-, during, and post- procedure
Untoward reactions
All caregiver teaching:
    Topics to include in the teaching plan:
        safe and correct handling of equipment/supplies
        emergency procedures
        underlying disease pathology
        appropriate community resources and contact persons

INTERDISCIPLINARY COLLABORATION
Report all untoward reactions to physician
Consult social worker to evaluate client's eligibility for financial assistance
Follow up all laboratory results with homecare agency's contracted laboratory service
Collaborate with pharmacy to have drug delivered to home
Place order for all necessary supplies with DME company [5, 6, 11, 23, 32]

PROCEDURE
Home Total Parenteral Nutrition Therapy, Pediatric

DESCRIPTION
Home total parenteral nutrition (TPN) refers to a process of delivering nutrients intravenously via a central or peripheral line. Peripheral parenteral nutrition is used to deliver intravenous nutrients containing concentrations of glucose below 12.5%. The more concentrated dextrose solutions must be administered via a central line, and they typically combine in varying concentrations water, carbohydrates, protein, lipids, seven major electrolytes, minerals, and thirteen trace elements. See also Adult Cardiovascular System Procedure on Home Total Parenteral Nutrition Therapy, Adult.

PURPOSE
To improve, maintain, or restore the client's nutritional status

EQUIPMENT
Ordered TPN solution
Intravenous tubing with inline filter
0.22 micron filter or 1.2 micron filter if solution contains lipids or albumin
Dressing supplies
Antiseptic ointment
Gauze
Vials of normal saline solution for parenteral use
Gloves and mask
Sterile saline solution for irrigation
Alcohol pads
Plastic trash bag
Tape
Label and pen
22 G to 25 G needles (if used) or needleless connectors
Agency-approved flush solution
Infusion pump or controller
Replacement caps for catheter ends
5-cc and 10-cc syringes
Intravenous pole
Glucometer
Urine test strips
Refrigerator
Emergency care
    Thrombolytics as ordered
    Hemostats with covered ends
    Repair kit for catheter (correct type, size, lumen)

OUTCOMES

The caregiver will:

► Administer prescribed nutritional therapies to achieve adequate nutritional status
► Administer prescribed hydrational requirements
► Use aseptic technique to insure that client will be free of infection
► Demonstrate competency in the administration and management of TPN therapy

ASSESSMENT DATA

Monitor intake and output; observe for evidence of fluid volume excess/deficit

Monitor stool output (< 20 cc/kg/day)

Record results of related laboratory data, and report findings outside of clinical parameters [culture and sensitivity, CBC, electrolytes, iron, albumin, transferrin, glucose, blood urea nitrogen, creatinine, liver function studies, ammonia, bicarbonate, triglycerides, calcium, phosphorus, magnesium, alkaline phosphatase, transferase, zinc, copper, cholesterol, bilirubin, and vitamins A and D]

Assess vital signs, height weight, head circumference, and plot on growth chart

Assess vulnerability to infection, evaluate immune and nutritional status

Observe skin surfaces around central venous line, enteral tube insertion sites, ostomy sites, perianal area

Monitor parenteral infusion to ensure intake of prescribed therapy

Assess achievement of developmental milestones

Consult with occupational/physical therapist and speech-language pathologist as needed

Document caregiver's ability to correctly perform all procedures

Assess family's plan for emergencies

Determine caregiver's ability to troubleshoot equipment

Ensure that safety measures are known by all caregivers

Record daily urine glucose and specific gravity

RELATED NURSING DIAGNOSES

At risk for infection

Fluid volume excess/deficit

Altered skin integrity

Altered nutrition less than body requirements

At risk for altered parenting

At risk for ineffective family coping

SPECIAL CONSIDERATIONS

Infants and children are typically discharged to home with "all-in-one" or "three-in-one" total parenteral nutrition solutions. Such solutions combine glucose, amino acids, and lipids into one bag. This combination of nutrients has been found to be easier and more convenient to administer. In the pediatric client, the concentration of calcium and phosphorus in the TPN solution will be higher than that required for the adult. Unfortunately, the higher the concentration of calcium and phosphorus the greater the chance for the development of precipitates and drug incompatibility. Therefore, the amount of calcium and phosphorus added to the TPN must be carefully assessed. Routinely, the nurse will draw blood for laboratory analysis and report all findings to the physician and pharmacist for regulation of TPN components. Because frequent blood draws can lead to anemia in the child, the nurse will need to exercise care in obtaining the smallest amount of blood necessary for accurate laboratory analyses. [1, 8, 23, 31]

The components of TPN therapy include fluid, calories, carbohydrates, protein, fats, and metabolites. Fluid calculation will be based on the child's fluid requirements or 1 1/2 times maintenance. Children with high stool output (>20 cc/kg/day) will have greater fluid requirements, as will the child with an ileostomy or fever. The nurse will carefully monitor weight, intake and output, hydrational status, and temperature in the management of the child's fluids. Based on those assessments, the physician may order an increase in oral intake, if possible, depending on underlying condition, or an increase in intravenous fluids. [1, 8, 23, 31]

Calories administered parenterally are usually 5 to 15% less than the calorie intake required for enteral feeds. The caloric distribution should generally be divided so that carbohydrates constitute the main source of energy at 30–50%; proteins are maintained at 15% of total calorie count; and fats represent less than 60% of the total calories. The child's weight is an important measurement of the adequacy and tolerance of the nutritional intake, and weight should be obtained weekly. [1, 8, 23, 31]

Glucose is the main source of carbohydrate used in the TPN solution and is monitored by blood and urinary sugar levels. A pediatric preparation of amino acids will be used in the TPN solution to meet the child's protein needs. The child will need to be closely monitored for protein losses as occurs with increase in metabolic demands associated with fluid losses from wounds, inflammatory response, or sepsis. BUN, bicarbonate, ammonia, and albumin levels will be routinely monitored to control for protein losses. [1, 8, 23, 31]

Fats will be administered in the form of Intralipids 20% and will be monitored by triglyceride levels. The quantity and type of electrolytes and minerals will vary with each child. Dosages will be regulated according to serum levels. [1, 8, 23, 31]

During hospitalization, a central catheter will placed in a subclavian, internal, or external jugular vein and advanced into the superior vena cava. A tunneled catheter will be surgically inserted for use in homecare and is pulled through the subcutaneous tissue to exit on the chest (Figure 5-21). The catheter is equipped with a cuff, which is implanted under the skin to serve as a barrier to infection by sealing off the skin tunnel. The catheter can be single- or double-lumen and varies in size from 4 to 9 French. Care must be taken not to puncture the catheter. A needleless system or small bore, short needle is used to access the catheter. A clamp comes already attached to the catheter and should be the only clamp used. If necessary, a padded hemostat can be substituted for clamping the catheter. On occasion, the catheter may become damaged or torn. An emergency repair kit should be available in the home at all times. [1, 8, 23]

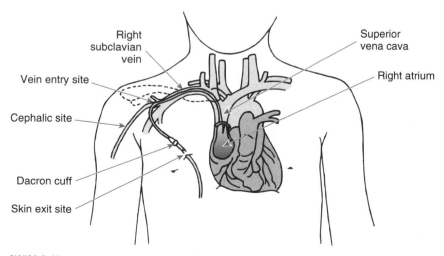

FIGURE 5-21 ▶ Insertion of central venous catheter.

The primary caregiver and a backup person should be thoroughly trained in safely administering TPN therapies and must be knowledgeable in the strategies to promote infant and child development. Additionally, they should be well informed with regard to the potential risks and benefits of home TPN therapy, and they should be informed of all necessary responsibility. Caregivers should know that the access site will need to be evaluated for evidence of infection; the infusion device will need to be monitored for rate of flow and evidence of malfunction; and the home will need to be assessed for its ability to support all aspects of care. The family and caregivers will need to realize that 24 hours of care will be required for the child, and that an emergency preparedness plan of action must be in place. The home and environment will be assessed for adequacy of refrigeration for TPN solutions, storage space for supplies, electrical safety, cleanliness of the home, emergency medical system access, functioning telephone line, and backup power supply in event of power outage. Caregivers should be instructed to go to nearest emergency room for accidental removal of catheter, catheter fracture, too rapid infusion of TPN solution or rapid deterioration in clinical status. All caregivers should be trained to perform CPR [1, 8, 23]

There are several complications of central line placement for which the caregiver must be trained to monitor and report:

Infections: Use of aseptic technique is crucial in reducing the risk of infection. Hand washing, gloving, masking, and use of other protective equipment as needed will prevent the transmission of microbes. Change the TPN solution and tubing every 24 hours. Care should be planned so that the number of times the catheter must be accessed is minimized. If the catheter becomes contaminated, it will need to be surgically removed if the infection does not respond to antibiotic therapy. Routine care of catheter-induced infections should include obtaining blood cultures for all temperature elevations. Cultures should be obtained from all lumens of the catheter and blood cultures should be drawn from the child. If possible, the antibiotic of choice should be compatible with the TPN solution so that the solution will not need to be stopped during the antibiotic infusion. If the antibiotic is not compatible with TPN, the nurse will need to collaborate with the physician and pharmacist in selecting the concentration of dextrose to be used to infuse the antibiotic. Sudden reduction in the rate of the TPN solution may place the child at risk for a hypoglycemic reaction. [1, 8, 23]

Occlusions: Drugs and admixtures may form precipitates with the TPN solution, a thrombus may form in the catheter itself, and blood allowed to return into the catheter may clot off. These and other factors place the catheter at risk for occlusion. With a physician order and according to agency policy, the nurse may be instructed to administer various kinds of thrombolytic agents to dissolve the occluding substance. [1, 8, 23]

Catheter Dislodgment/Breakage: The catheter must be looped and secured with tape and a dressing to prevent its accidental displacement. The nurse will need to be creative in helping the family devise strategies to keep the catheter out of the child's reach. A catheter repair kit should be in the home at all times. The nurse will follow and instruct the caregiver in the agency protocol to follow to repair the catheter and prevent formation of air emboli. [1, 8, 23]

Irritation: The caregiver will be instructed by the nurse in aseptic dressing changes as per agency protocol and physician order. The site will need to be observed for evidence of redness, tenderness, warmth, rash, exudate, or other signs of infection. [1, 8, 23]

Air Emboli/Extravasation of fluid: The nurse will instruct the caregiver to observe for evidence of cardiopulmonary compromise in the event of the formation of air emboli. The caregiver will be instructed to initiate the emergency medical system and to initiate CPR if indicated. In the event of leakage of fluid around the catheter site or edema of the chest, face, or extremity on the side of the insertion site, the caregiver will be instructed to stop the infusion and prepare for emergency transport to the nearest hospital. [1, 8, 23]

Pump malfunction, rupture of the TPN bag or lack of delivery of the TPN solution from pharmacy or the DME company: Caregivers will need to have a backup plan. An intravenous bag of the same concentration of glucose as the ordered TPN solution should be in the home at all times. Caregivers should be trained to routinely perform an inventory of supplies and equipment, to notify the DME company or agency when routine troubleshooting does not correct the malfunctioning equipment, and to know how long the child can be without the TPN solution before hypoglycemia becomes evident. [1, 8, 23]

TRANSCULTURAL CONSIDERATIONS

A translator may be needed to assist with instruction and training for the family that is not fluent in English. The nurse will need to determine the availability of health-related materials in the primary language of the caregivers. Consider use of AT&T Language Line. See Culturological Assessment procedure in Unit 2 for general overview of cultural considerations.

▶ INTERVENTIONS

1. Verify physician order.	*Reduces risk of error*
2. Explain procedure.	*Allays anxiety*
3. Wash hands.	*Prevents transmission of microbes*
4. Perform physical assessment.	*Establishes baseline clinical data*
5. Identify a clean work area and gather all supplies.	*Promotes efficiency*
6. Have the caregiver remove TPN solution from the refrigerator 2 to 4 hours prior to instillation, per agency protocol.	*Avoids hypothermia and venous spasm and constriction which may result from infusing a chilled solution*
7. Check the solution label against medical order, noting components, expiration date, and client name.	*Reduces risk of error*
8. Check the TPN container and assess for leaks, assess the solution for evidence of precipitation or evidence that lipid emulsion has separated out of solution (forms brown layer); question any unusual finding and return solution to pharmacy, obtain new TPN solution bag and perform same checks.	*Assesses for evidence of poor quality solution*
9. Don gloves.	*Serves as protective barrier*
10. Wipe off tops of normal saline vials with alcohol pad.	*Prevents contamination*
11. Fill three 10-cc syringes with normal saline or use agency-approved flush solutions (Figure 5-22).	*Prepares syringes to flush the line*
12. Using sterile technique, spike TPN bag, squeeze, and release drip chamber.	*Initiates flow of solution*
13. Prime the line, invert the filter at the distal end of the tubing, open the roller clamp.	*Removes air from tubing*
14. Tap the line to dislodge air bubbles trapped in Y-ports.	*Removes air from tubing*
15. Connect intravenous line to infusion device per manufacturer's recommendations.	*Reduces risk of error*

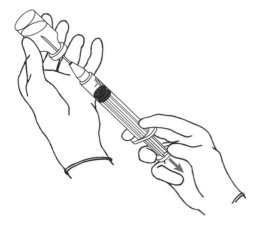

FIGURE 5-22 ▶ Technique for holding syringe and removing solution from a vial.

16. Have caregiver perform the procedure.	*Assesses caregiver's ability to correctly perform the procedure*

For Continuous Infusion [note: always follow specific physician orders and agency guidelines]

1. Wash hands.	*Prevents transmission of microbes*
2. Explain procedure.	*Allays anxiety*
3. Don gloves.	*Serves as protective barrier*
4a. If connecting to capped lumen:	*Establishes patency and ensures compatibility*
▸ Wipe cap with alcohol pad and allow to air dry, use saline-filled 10-cc syringe to flush the lumen per agency protocol (Figure 5-23).	
▸ After flushing the catheter, keep thumb on plunger while withdrawing the syringe and clamp catheter.	*Prevents blood back up into catheter*
4b. If connecting directly to uncapped catheter:	
▸ Use saline-filled 10-cc syringe to flush the lumen per agency protocol;	*Establishes patency and ensures compatibility*
▸ Then, clamp the catheter with in-line clamp.	*Prevents air emboli*
5. Remove cap and attach distal end of intravenous line to catheter then tape ends in place	*Secures connection*
6. Unclamp tubing and turn on infusion device	*Initiates infusion*
7. Set rate of infusion and program the device, physician may order the solution to be tapered up at the start of the infusion and tapered off at the completion of the infusion	*Allows pancreas to slowly adjust to increase/decrease in glucose levels*
8. If ordered, cycle the TPN rate to infuse over 12 to 18 hours	*Gives body a period of fasting to help lower circulating insulin levels during rest periods*
9. Discard sharps and waste appropriately	*Reduces risk of needle stick and spread of contamination*

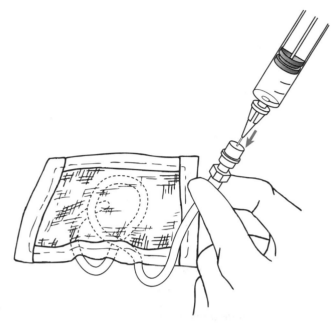

FIGURE 5-23 ▶ Flushing the central venous catheter

10. Remove gloves and wash hands	*Prevents transmission of microbes*
11. Review procedure with caregiver and permit return demonstration	*Assesses caregiver's ability to implement the procedure*

For Changing the Solution

1. Prepare solution per physician order.	*Reduces risk of error*
2. Spike the intravenous bag, prime the intravenous line, and close clamp.	*Prevents formation of air emboli*
3. Hang the new TPN bag next to the old bag.	*Minimizes time required to change to new solution*
4. Turn off the infusion device, disconnect old intravenous tubing (clamp central catheter first), and attach new tubing per manufacturer's recommendation.	*Reduces risk of error*
5. Attach distal end of intravenous tubing to capped or uncapped lumen of central line flushing the line with saline solution as above.	*Establishes patency and ensures compatibility*
6. Open clamp, turn on infusion device, and set rate as ordered.	*Initiates infusion*
7. Discard sharps and waste appropriately.	*Reduces risk of needle stick and spread of contamination*
8. Remove gloves and wash hands.	*Prevents transmission of microbes*
9. Review procedure with caregiver and permit return demonstration.	*Assesses caregiver's ability to implement the procedure*

For Changing Central Line Dressing

1. Wash hands.

2. Explain procedure.
3. Don gloves and mask.
4. Remove old dressing and discard appropriately.

5. Remove gloves, don sterile gloves.
6. Cleanse skin per agency-approved protocol, using circular motion and ordered cleansing agent start at insertion site, repeat cleansing action three times (Figure 5-24).
7. Allow area to dry then cover with gauze or transparent dressing, label and date (Figure 5-25).
8. Discard sharps and waste appropriately.

9. Remove gloves and wash hands.

10. Repeat procedure routinely per agency protocol and/or when dressing becomes soiled or wet.

11. Review procedure with caregiver and permit return demonstration.

Prevents transmission of microbes
Allays anxiety
Serves as protective barrier
Prevents spread of contamination
Use strict aseptic technique
Disinfects the skin

Documents time of dressing change
Reduces risk of needle stick and spread of contamination
Prevents transmission of microbes
Permits direct observation of site for evidence of infection, irritation, dislodging, leaks, catheter breakage
Assesses caregiver's ability to implement the procedure

To Discontinue the Infusion

1. Wash hands.

2. Explain procedure.
3. Don gloves.
4. Fill flush syringes per agency protocol.

5. Open package containing connector caps.

Prevents transmission of microbes
Allays anxiety
Serves as protective barrier
Prepares solution to flush intravenous line and capsi
Promotes efficiency

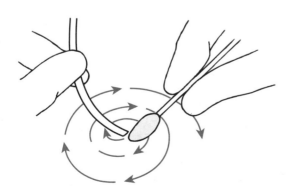

FIGURE 5-24 ▶ Using a circular motion to cleanse central catheter insertion site.

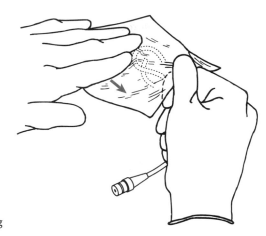

FIGURE 5-25 ▶ Placement of trasparent dressing

6. Wipe caps with alcohol swab and ordered antiseptic solution.	*Disinfects caps*
7. Flush caps with ordered flush solution.	*Prevents formation of air emboli*
8. Stop the infusion and clamp intravenous line.	*Prevents inadvertent infusion of remaining TPN solution*
9. Clamp catheter line with in-line clamp.	*Prevents formation of air embolus*
10. Disconnect intravenous line from central line catheter.	*Separates central line from continuous infusion*
11. Remove old cap and replace with new cap quickly.	*Minimizes exposure to environment*
11. Review procedure with caregiver and permit return demonstration.	*Assesses caregiver's ability to implement the procedure*

DOCUMENTATION
The following should be included in the nursing note:

All untoward clinical findings and interventions implemented to correct
Record all intake and output, vital signs, height/weight/head circumference measurements
Insertion site evaluation
Type of TPN solution rate of infusion and client tolerance
All laboratory results
Growth and developmental status
Nutritional status
Family interaction/dynamics
Safety measures implemented
Emergency plan
Home/environmental assessment
Caregiver instruction and ability to implement procedures
All caregiver teaching
    Topics to include in the teaching plan:

safe and correct handling of equipment/supplies
emergency procedures
underlying disease pathology
appropriate community resources and contact persons

INTERDISCIPLINARY COLLABORATION

Inform the physician of all untoward clinical findings and actions taken to correct

Discuss with the physician the need to obtain referrals for nutritionist, speech and/or occupational and/or physical therapist, or other health professional depending on need

Consult with pharmacist for all TPN solutions and concentrations

Consult with laboratory technologist to obtain all laboratory results

Review with homecare agency protocol to follow for obtaining/transporting lab specimens

Consult with social worker to determine family's eligibility for reimbursement for cost of supplies/equipment, and to access community support groups

Consult with DME vendor for ordering of equipment/supplies [1, 4, 5, 8, 10–14, 21–23, 24, 26, 31, 32]

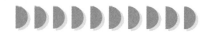

Pediatric Gastrointestinal System Procedures

3

Colostomy Care and Management

DESCRIPTION
A colostomy is a surgical opening made into the colon for diversion of fecal contents. A portion of the colon is brought through an abdominal incision and sutured to the abdominal wall to form a stoma. The procedure may be performed as a temporary measure to promote healing status post a bowel resection, or the procedure may be permanent following removal of the distal colon.

PURPOSE
Maintain skin integrity around stoma
Prevent skin irritation and break down

EQUIPMENT
Health Assessment forms
Gloves
Wash cloth
Pouch/appliance
Rinse bottle
Stoma paste
Skin barrier
Wafer

OUTCOMES
The client/caregiver will:

- ▶ Keep the area around the stoma clean, dry, and free from stool
- ▶ Be able to change the pouch and reapply a skin barrier
- ▶ Maintain cleanliness of the intact pouch
- ▶ Verbalize knowledge of signs/symptoms of complications

ASSESSMENT DATA
Note color and consistency of stool
Note change in bowel pattern
Assess color of stoma, change in size
Note bleeding from stoma other than during cleaning
Note bleeding from skin around stoma
Note elevation in temperature
Evaluate child/caregiver's ability to perform procedure

Evaluate coping skills of child/caregiver
Assess nutritional status and dietary intake

RELATED NURSING DIAGNOSES
At risk for impaired skin integrity
Altered body image
Noncompliance
Ineffective coping
Altered bowel elimination

SPECIAL CONSIDERATIONS
Children are almost always discharged to home with a functioning colostomy. While not always possible, the ideal plan includes instruction of the family and child on all aspects of care. However, the often overwhelming care and change in lifestyle assumed by some families necessitate intensive followup homecare nursing. It is important to note the child and family's response to the colostomy. In the older child, problems of altered body image and low self-esteem may be evident. Family support must be present to help the child display positive behaviors. The homecare nurse must help the family understand that proper care of the colostomy can lead to a life filled with educational, social, and athletic activities.

TRANSCULTURAL CONSIDERATIONS
Some cultures may regard the colostomy as a sign of disgrace because it does alter body image and it deals with excreta in an abnormal manner. An interpreter will be needed for clients unable to speak English.

Support and maintain the client's religious and cultural healthcare practices. Acquire healthcare materials written in the client's native language, if available. Consider use of AT&T Language Line. See also the Culturological Assessment procedure in Unit 2 for general overview of cultural considerations.

▶ INTERVENTIONS

Intervention	Rationale
1. Verify physician order.	*Reduces risk of error*
2. Wash hands.	*Reduces the transfer of microorganisms*
3. Organize equipment, prepare colostomy apparatus, use a template to cut/trim wafer to size	*Promotes efficiency*
4. Explain procedure.	*Decreases anxiety and eliminates fear*
5. Perform physical assessment.	*Establishes baseline clinical data findings*
6. Don gloves.	*Serves as protective barrier*
7. Remove old pouch and wafer.	*Permits direct observation of the stoma site*
8. Assess skin around stoma and under wafer. Review signs and symptoms of skin breakdown with caregiver.	*A proactive skin care regime decreases potential complications*
9. Discuss appropriate skin care protocol, per physician order, with caregiver. Apply skin barriers as ordered, and allow area to dry.	*Permits feedback and facilitates communication to ensure that orders are followed* *Protects skin from irritation*

10. Cut wafer to size following standard colostomy-measuring technique.	*Appliance devices must be precisely measured to fit to decrease risk of leakage of stool*
11. Place new wafer with adhesive side to skin around stoma.	*Keeps stool away from the skin*
12. Attach colostomy pouch to wafer by placing over stoma pressing firmly to seal	*Accurate and tight seal is needed to prevent leaking*
13. Take the open lower part of the pouch and roll three to four times and fasten with a self-clamp or rubber band.	*Prevents the pouch from leaking*
14. Empty pouch when it is about one-third full by opening the lower end.	*Prevents leakage*
15. Cleanse pouch with warm soapy water and rinse using rinse bottle.	*Eliminates odors and keeps stoma clean*
16. Remove gloves and wash hands following procedure.	*Prevents cross-contamination*
17. Have caregiver/client demonstrate their ability to provide colostomy care as ordered.	*Documents caregiver/client's understanding of the treatment protocol*
18. Have caregiver/client verbalize understanding of complications requiring physician notification: ribbon-like stools, excessive diarrhea, bleeding, prolapse, constipation, or absence of flatus.	*Verifies caregiver/client knowledge of appropriate actions to take when complications occur*

DOCUMENTATION

The following should be noted in the nursing note:

Vital signs, weight, and age
Developmental milestones
Location and condition of stoma
Evidence of structure, bleeding, prolapse, retraction, or infection
Characteristics of stools
Stooling pattern
Compliance with ostomy care
All teaching that includes diet, nutrition, medications, and any referrals to support agencies
All caregiver teaching:
    Topics to include in the teaching plan:
        safe and correct handling of equipment/supplies
        emergency procedures
        underlying disease pathology
        appropriate community resources and contact persons

INTERDISCIPLINARY COLLABORATION

Inform the physician of any abnormal findings or noncompliance issues
Inform school nurse, teacher, or day care workers about child's condition and instruct in ostomy care
Consult with WOC nurse to provide a support person whom the family can contact to assess the stoma and recommend skin care protocol
Maintain inventory of colostomy supplies and have caregiver notify DME company for reorders
    [4, 5, 13, 14, 23, 32]

Cleft Lip and Cleft Palate Care and Management

DESCRIPTION
Cleft lip and cleft palate are developmental malformations of the oral cavity which occur in utero. This incomplete fusion at the lip's upper border and or palate is a common facial abnormality evident at birth.

PURPOSE
To provide adequate nutrition and safety for the child with cleft lip and or cleft palate

EQUIPMENT
Health Assessment Forms
Feeding bottle
Cross-cut, soft nipple
Feeding formula

OUTCOMES
The child will:

► Demonstrate appropriate weight gain and growth
► Be free from risk of aspiration
► Be free from infection

ASSESSMENT DATA
Take vital signs and weigh daily
Evaluate infant's ability to suck and swallow
Evaluate mother's ability to breastfeed
Evaluate respiratory status during feeds
Assess suture line on the upper lip
Evaluate family's coping skills in caring for the child

RELATED NURSING DIAGNOSES
Altered nutrition, less than body requirements
At risk for aspiration
At risk for infection (respiratory, otitis media)
At risk for injury

SPECIAL CONSIDERATIONS
Surgical management of this defect is a series of staged surgical corrections for the infant. Within 1–2 months of age, surgical fusion of the cleft in the lip is performed. Surgical closure of the cleft palate begins from 4–18 months. This may also be a staged procedure depending on the severity of the cleft.

It is important that the family receives adequate support from support groups and appropriate agencies to cope with the many years of medical management that is needed.

TRANSCULTURAL CONSIDERATIONS
An interpreter will be needed for clients unable to speak English Support and maintain the client's religious and cultural healthcare practices Acquire healthcare materials written in the client's native

language, if available. Consider use of AT&T Language Line. See also the Culturological Assessment procedure in Unit 2 for general overview of cultural considerations.

▶ INTERVENTIONS

1. Wash hands.	*Prevents transmission of microbes*
2. Verify physician order for formula-fed infant.	*Reduces risk of error*
3. Elevate head during and after feedings.	*Prevents aspiration*

Prior to surgical repair

4. For the formula-fed infant, use a special feeding appliance:

    ▶ Soft nipple with a cross-cut (premie nipple works well).

    ▶ Position the nipple between the infant's tongue and existing palate.

       ▶ When using devices without nipples (asepto syringe, Breck feeder), place formula on back of tongue and control flow of formula in accordance with infant's ability to swallow.

5. Assess infant's ability to suck and maintain an adequate intake in breast-fed infant.

6. Offer 1–2 ounces of water after feeding.

7. Burp infant after every ounce.

Compensates for infant's feeding difficulty

Allows the infant to suck without difficulty

Facilitates compression of the nipple

Prevents aspiration

Breastfeeding should be discontinued if unable to maintain nutrition

Cleanses the mouth to prevent a source of infection

Infant will have tendency to swallow excessive air when feeding

Post-surgical repair

1. Cleanse suture line of lip as per physician direction.	*Keeps area free from infection*
2. Maintain lip protective device.	*Protects the suture line*
3. Use nontraumatic feeding technique.	*Reduce risk of injury*
4. Avoid placing objects in mouth (straw, pacifier, spoon, tongue depressor).	*Avoids trauma to incision line*
5. Weigh weekly and compare with growth and development scale.	*Evaluates growth and developmental status*
6. Observe caregiver's ability to perform procedure and re instruct as needed.	*Documents caregiver's ability to implement plan of care*

DOCUMENTATION
The following should be noted in the nursing note:

Weight and vital signs
Condition of lip repair
Feeding techniques and positioning

Difficulty in sucking and swallowing
Signs of respiratory distress during feeds
Level of discomfort or irritability
Family dynamics and bonding with infant
All caregiver teaching
    Topics to include in the teaching plan:
        Safe and correct handling of equipment/supplies
        Emergency procedures
        Underlying disease pathology
        Appropriate community resources and contact persons

INTERDISCIPLINARY COLLABORATION

The members of the healthcare team needed to manage the child's care include the: pediatrician, plastic surgeon, speech language pathologist, and audiologist nutritionist, dentist and orhodontist. [5, 32] Parent support groups have a very important role in providing families with the coping skills needed to care for their child.

PROCEDURE
Gastroesophageal Reflux (GER) Care and Management

DESCRIPTION

Gastroesophageal reflux is a condition in which gastric contents return to the esophagus and pharynx because of the incompetence of the sphincter located between the lower esophagus and the stomach. The condition may become a chronic problem if not treated with medication or surgery.

PURPOSE

To provide adequate nutrition to support normal growth and development

EQUIPMENT

Health Assessment forms
Feeding bottle
Choice of appropriate nipple for bottle feeding, as ordered
Feeding formula
Enteral feeding tube and feeding bag, if applicable
Oxygen supplies, if ordered

OUTCOMES

The child/caregiver will:

▶ Be free from feeding intolerance
▶ Maintain adequate caloric intake to support weight gain for age
▶ Be free from upper respiratory infections
▶ Maintain a patent airway

ASSESSMENT DATA

Monitor weight gain
Assess respiratory status for apnea, dyspnea, choking, chronic upper respiratory infection
Note vomiting associated with feedings
Note hematemesis or melena caused by irritation from gastric contents

RELATED NURSING DIAGNOSES

At risk for ineffective airway clearance
Altered nutrition, less than body requirements
At risk for ineffective family coping
Altered bowel elimination
At risk for ineffective airway clearance

SPECIAL CONSIDERATIONS

The medical management of this disorder is initially treated with medication such as antacids and muscle-toning agents. Enteral feeds may be started to rest the GI tract and provide nutrition. When these therapies prove to be ineffective surgical correction may be considered.

TRANSCULTURAL CONSIDERATIONS

An interpreter will be needed for clients unable to speak English. Support and maintain the client's religious and cultural healthcare practices. Acquire healthcare materials written in the client's native language, if available. Consider use of AT&T Language Line. See also the Culturological Assessment procedure in Unit 2 for general overview of cultural considerations.

▶ INTERVENTIONS

1. Wash hands.

   Prevents transmission of microbes

2. Perform physical assessment.

   Establishes baseline information of physiological data findings

3. Instruct caregiver on positioning the child upright in an infant seat before, during, and after feedings.

   Prevents aspiration

4. Thicken feedings with cereal if ordered. Enlarge holes in the nipple, if appropriate for infant's sucking ability and thickness of feeding, for bottle feedings.

   Provides consistency to feeds

5. Instruct in need for oxygen.

   Relieves respiratory distress

6. Instruct in medication administration and effectiveness of medication.

   Reinforces plan of care

7. Provide high-caloric formulas for feedings.

   Provides a higher caloric intake to meet energy expenditure requirements

8. Observe caregiver's ability to use and maintain feeding tube, if applicable.

   Evaluates knowledge deficit

DOCUMENTATION

The following should be noted in the nursing note:

Child's general appearance
Respiratory status, especially signs of respiratory effort
Instructions given on positioning, medications, and nutrition
Administration of oxygen
Caregiver's ability to care for child
All caregiver teaching
   Topics to include in the teaching plan:
      safe and correct handling of equipment/supplies

emergency procedures
underlying disease pathology
appropriate community resources and contact persons

INTERDISCIPLINARY COLLABORATION

Inform primary care physician of any signs of respiratory effort especially dyspnea, apnea, and the need for oxygen. Consistent weight loss can also be of concern.

Enlisting the help of a nutritionist will aid the family in providing adequate nutrition essential for normal growth and development.

Support groups assist the family in developing coping skills especially if the child requires feeding tubes to maintain nutrition. [4, 5, 10, 1, 25, 32]

PROCEDURE
Gastrostomy Tube (GT) Care and Management

DESCRIPTION

Gastrostomy tubes are used for children with poor oral-motor function as the result of CNS dysfunction, head injury or multiple trauma with long-term recovery, oral and esophageal burns, and recovery from GI surgery.

This method of feeding requires the creation of a surgical opening into the child's stomach, and the placement of a catheter through which feedings are instilled. The procedure is performed under general anesthesia. Gastrostomy tubes come in a variety of types. See Special Considerations in section below.

PURPOSE

To provide adequate nutrition to support normal growth and development

EQUIPMENT

Health assessment forms
Foley catheter with a 5-cc balloon
10-cc syringe
Water
Nipple
Scissors
Tweezers
Clamp
Toomey syringe 30 or 60 cc

OUTCOMES

The caregiver will be able to:

▶ Replace a gastrostomy tube using the foley catheter tube
▶ Maintain skin integrity around the site
▶ Instill feedings.

ASSESSMENT DATA

Note redness or swelling around gastrostomy tube site
Note presence of drainage or gastric contents from site
Assess pain or discomfort expressed by child
Note abdominal distention

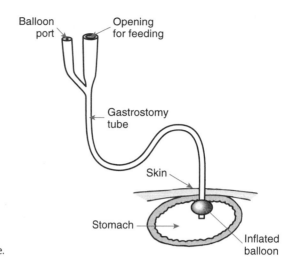

FIGURE 5-26 ▶ Placement of gastrostomy tube.

RELATED NURSING DIAGNOSES
Altered growth and development
At risk for infection
Impaired skin integrity
Altered nutrition; less than body requirements

SPECIAL CONSIDERATIONS
When selecting the appropriate feeding method to be used for the child, several factors must be considered. Client history should include any documentation of disorders causing rapid gastric emptying, vomiting secondary to limited gastric volume, and diarrhea due to dumping syndrome. Tube feedings are administered by any one of three methods: bolus, gravity, and continuous feeds. The bolus method is selected for children who fatigue easily during regular oral feeding, and those who must be placed on long-term tube feeding. For the bolus method, the feeding is administered through a 60-cc straight-tip syringe into a nasogastric tube or through a 60-cc catheter tip syringe through a gastrostomy tube. The feeding is instilled over approximately 20 minutes, and the rate of flow is regulated by elevating or lowering the syringe. The bolus method most closely resembles natural feeding. The gravity feeding method is accomplished by instilling the feeding into a feeding bag attached to an infusion tubing set with clamp. The feeding bag is hung on a pole or hanger. The rate of flow is regulated with a clamp, which is set to deliver the feeding over a 45-minute period. The gravity method is used for the client who develops diarrhea or vomiting with the bolus feeding. The most expensive of the methods is the continuous feeding method, which is used when the child must receive a slow accurate feeding, as in the child with failure to thrive or GER. The feeding is instilled into an enteral feeding bag designed to connect to a feeding pump. The pump is set to infuse electronically to prevent overfilling of the stomach and to reduce the risk of vomiting. There are several brands of feeding pumps. Typically, the brand is selected by the infusion company. Selection is based on the following criteria: size, portability, weight, complexity of use, power source, reliability, and technical support. [1, 8, 24, 31, 32]

In the last decade, several advances have been made in the design of gastrostomy tubes to correct some of the problems associated with long-term tube insertion: skin irritation at the stoma site, tube migration and blockage of the pyloric valve, and issues related to altered body image (Table 5-1). Currently two new types of tubes are in use: the foley catheter with an antimigration

TABLE 5-1 Types of Enteral Feeding Tubes

Type	Insertion	Maintainence
Foley	Inserted by nurse or trained caregiver after the site has healed	Change monthly or as ordered Replace immediately if accidentally removed Clean site daily with soap and water No dressing needed at site
G-Tube	Inserted by nurse after site has healed	Change every 3 months or as ordered Clean site daily with soap and water No dressing needed at site
Gastrostomy Buttons	Mic-Key Button inserted by nurse or trained caregiver Corpak or Bard Button inserted by surgeon	Change only when malfunction occurs Clean site daily with soap and water No dressing needed at site
NGT	Inserted by nurse or trained caregiver	Change weekly alternating nares Verify placement prior to initiating all feedings
PEG Tube	Inserted by surgeon	Changed by surgeon Hold all feedings for 24 hours post insertion Change dressings daily until site heals, then Clean site daily with soap and water No dressing needed at healed site

Adapted from *Coram Healthcare Corporation Nursing Orientation Program Manual.* Denver CO: The Corporation, 1995. Used with permission.

device and skin surface devices (gastrostomy buttons). Gastrostomy feeding buttons are available in two types: Malecot-type button (which requires an obturator for placement) and the balloon-type button. While gastrostomy buttons are preferred by caregivers, there are several disadvantages, which must be considered with their use. Feeding, administering medications, and venting of the button requires attaching a feeding extension set or decompression tube to open the button's one-way valve, which is a step not required with traditional foley catheter tubes. Additionally, the small diameter of the venting or decompression tube reduces the amount of gas or emesis that can be expelled. Consequently, care must be taken in choosing to use these tubes in the child who requires frequent venting after feeding. When the buttons can be used, they are ideal because they are stationery, do not require tape for securing, and rarely occlude. See reinsertion of the gastrostomy button under Adult Gastrointestinal System. [1, 8, 23, 24, 32]

The following are guidelines for the caregiver to become familiar with when caring for the child with a traditional gastrostomy tube (GT):

▶ A nipple with air vents is used to keep the foley snug against the abdominal wall. These air vents allow the skin around the site to breathe.
▶ The GT site should be cleansed one to three times daily, as ordered.
▶ Some bleeding may occur at the stoma if the tube is accidentally pulled out and reinsertion may cause a degree of discomfort.

▶ Gastrostomy tubes are changed when they become soft, are blocked with medication/food, when the balloon deflates, and as ordered. The gastrostomy tube may be changed preventatively every 6 to 12 months

▶ Always change the tube **Prior** to feeding

⚡ **ALWAYS CHECK PLACEMENT OF THE TUBE BEFORE FEEDING**

TRANSCULTURAL CONSIDERATIONS

An interpreter will be needed for clients unable to speak English. Support and maintain the client's religious and cultural healthcare practices. Acquire healthcare materials written in the client's native language, if available. Consider use of AT&T Language Line. See also the Culturological Assessment procedure in Unit 2 for general overview of cultural considerations.

▶ INTERVENTIONS

Caring for the Initial Surgically Inserted GT

1. Wash hands.	*Prevents transmission of microbes*
2. Don gloves.	*Serves as protective barrier*
3. Cleanse the site daily with soap and rinse with water or as ordered, once the site has healed.	*Cleanliness decreases chance of infection*
4. Dry area surrounding the insertion with site with clean gauze.	*Moist areas tend to harbor infection and cause skin breakdown*
5. Check the site every 4–8 hours for signs of leakage, redness or infection.	*Early detection of leakage helps to prevent development of complications*
6. Apply gauze around GT site, as ordered, if drainage is consistent.	*Gauze helps to remove moisture*
7. Clothe child in loose-fitting garments.	*Loose clothing will not press the GT against the skin*

Changing the Gastrostomy Tube

1. Wash hands.	*Prevents transmission of microbes*
2. Don gloves.	*Serves as protective barrier*
3. Test the balloon of the Foley catheter by instilling 5 cc of water; test for 2 minutes then remove water.	*Detects any leaks in the balloon*
4. Cross-cut the tip of a nipple and slide the nipple over the tip of the foley catheter about 4 inches.	*Stabilizes tube at base of insertion site*
5. Attach Toomey syringe to end of new catheter.	*Prevents leakage of stomach contents during insertion*
6. Attach 10-cc syringe filled with 5 cc of water to balloon port of the new catheter.	*Water is used to inflate the balloon to secure its position at the insertion site*
7. Lubricate tip of catheter.	*Facilitates easier insertion*

8. Withdraw water from balloon of old catheter.

   Assures that current balloon is fully deflated allowing for easier removal

9. Gently pull the old GT out.

   Decreases trauma to stoma site

10. Insert new Foley immediately about 2–3 inches into stomach depending on age and size of the child clamp closed.

   Prevents closure of site

11. Instill 5 cc of water into balloon and gently pull back on catheter until resistance is met.

   Balloon keeps catheter in place

12. Unclamp lower end of catheter with Toomey and allow stomach contents to drain by gravity.

   Checks placement of catheter

13. Cleanse skin with soap and water. Dry well.

   Prevents skin breakdown

14. Pin GT to inside of child's clothing [note: the gastrostomy button will not require securing].

   Prevents dislodgment

15. Clothing should be loose- not tight-fitting.

   Loose fitting clothing will not press the GT against the skin

16. If leakage occurs, instruct caregiver to attach a 10-cc syringe to the balloon port and withdraw water from the balloon, then re-add 5cc of water as ordered.

   Refills balloon to desired level

17. If leak persists, tube will need to be changed.

   Balloon has a slow leak

18. Remove gloves and wash hands following procedure.

   Prevents cross contamination

Feeding the Child with a Gastrostomy Tube

1. Wash hands.

   Prevents transmission of microbes

2. Schedule feedings along with family meals or as ordered.

   Includes child in family activities

3. Infants should be held and offered a pacifier during feedings (Figure 5-27). Toddlers should sit at the table with the family; offer finger foods if allowed.

   Promotes growth and development

4. Prior to initiating the feeding, check for gastric residual and follow medical orders for holding the feeding.

   Evaluates adequacy of peristaltic activity or detects presence of intestinal obstruction

5. Feeds may be instilled by bolus, gravity, or through a feeding pump, as ordered.

   Selection of method of feeding depends on underlying condition and client's feeding tolerance

6. Keep feedings at room temperature or warm slightly.

   Prevents stomach cramps

7. Infants require the feeding to be interrupted for burping.

   Prevents distention

8. In the child with a Nissen Fundoplication, leave tube unclamped for 30 minutes, or as ordered, after feed and then clamp until next feeding.

   Allows air to escape

9. Unclamp tube if the child begins to vomit or have abdominal distention.

   Decompresses the stomach

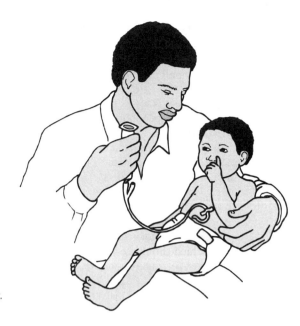

FIGURE 5-27 ▶ Positioning the child for gastrostomy feeding.
Tip of syringe should be at level of child's shoulder.

10. Have caregiver demonstrate ability to provide gastrostomy care as ordered.

Documents caregiver's understanding of the treatment protocol

11. Have caregiver verbalize understanding of complications requiring physician notification: abdominal distension, gastric residual, vomiting, abdominal pain, diarrhea, constipation.

Verifies caregiver's knowledge of appropriate actions to take when complications occur

DOCUMENTATION
The following should be noted in the nursing note:

Child's tolerance of procedure
Skin integrity around stoma
Drainage from stoma site
Tolerance of feedings
Any vomiting or distention
Growth and developmental status
Caregiver's ability to care for child
All instruction given on care
Date and time of tube change and description of type of tube inserted
All caregiver teaching
    Topics to include in the teaching plan:
        safe and correct handling of equipment/supplies
        emergency procedures
        underlying disease pathology
        appropriate community resources and contact persons

INTERDISCIPLINARY CONSIDERATIONS:
Any problems or concerns should be reported to the child's physician
Consider need to consult nutritionist for feeding intolerance
Consult with WOC nurse for management of ostomy. [1, 8, 12–14, 21, 23, 24, 29, 32]

PROCEDURE
Duodenal/Gastric Tube Care and Management

DESCRIPTION
Enteral feedings provide nourishment through the instillation of a special feeding formula via a tube inserted orally or nasally into the stomach, duodenum, or jejunum. These feedings may be intermittent or by continuous drip, and the catheter may be left in place or inserted and removed with each feeding. Conditions requiring the implementation of this feeding procedure include the following: anomalies of the throat, esophagus, or bowel; severe debilitation from a neurological or cardiac event; respiratory distress; and, coma. The type of feeding selected is determined by age, underlying pathology, tolerance, and site of insertion of the enteral tube. [1, 8, 23, 32]

EQUIPMENT
Health Assessment forms
Feeding tube appropriate for age of the child or infant.
5–20-cc syringe
30–50-cc syringe
Feeding pump bag
1/2–inch waterproof tape
Tincture of benzoin
Water soluble lubricant
Bottle brush
Feeding formula
Stethoscope
Feeding pump, if ordered

PURPOSE
To insert, maintain or remove enteral feeding catheters, to correctly administer enteral feedings, and to insure adequate caloric intake for the child or infant unable to nipple feed or coordinate sucking

OUTCOMES
The client/caregiver will:

▶ Maintain adequate nutritional status to promote growth and development
▶ Demonstrate ability to correctly insert feeding tube
▶ Check placement of tube before feedings
▶ Administer feedings as ordered
▶ Verbalize knowledge of tolerance parameters for enteral feedings including: gastrointestinal tolerance, stool frequency, and body weight

ASSESSMENT DATA
Correlate child's age with appropriate growth measurement scales and determine adequacy of nutritional status
Assess child's tolerance of feeding formula

Document bowel and bladder function
Obtain diet history to include: current dietary intake, feeding history, allergies, food likes/dislikes

RELATED NURSING DIAGNOSES
Knowledge deficit
Altered nutrition; less than body requirements
Altered growth and development
At risk for impaired skin integrity

SPECIAL CONSIDERATIONS
Caregivers are usually sent home from the hospital with a small amount of supplies to make it through the first few days. It is important to determine on initial contact with the family the type of equipment that will be used in the home. If a pump is required, an electrical safety assessment must be performed. Checking with the insurance company for coverage of DME supplies prior to the visit would be very helpful. Having the right supplies ordered for the family decreases anxiety. Tube feedings may be a short-term intervention or a lifetime endeavor. Helping the caregiver incorporate these feedings into the daily schedule is an important part of the homecare teaching plan. When it is not made part of the daily routine from the start, the family's mounting anxiety could cause the feedings to be missed. If feedings are continuous throughout the night, professional nursing care may be initially ordered around-the-clock. Evaluation of the family's ability to administer feedings safely due to the risk for aspiration is vital. Arranging the home visit during a scheduled feed is the optimal time to evaluate the family's ability to follow the medical regimen. Report to the homecare agency and/or third-party payor the need to authorize the scheduling of more nursing visits, if warranted, to ensure the caregiver's comprehension of and ability to safely perform all related feeding procedures. Additionally, consider the need to periodically evaluate the level of caregiver fatigue and need for respite care. [1, 8, 23, 32]

Silastic tubes are typically used for long-term feedings. Typically, indwelling catheters, other than silastic catheters, are replaced every 3 days, alternating nares at the point of insertion. Indwelling catheters tend to coil and knot, and may perforate the stomach or cause gastric ulceration. Secure indwelling catheters to the face with transparent bandage and replace as needed. Prior to initiating the feeding, check for tube placement. During and after the feeding, place the child in a sitting position or elevate the head (Figure 5-28). [1, 8, 23, 32]

TRANSCULTURAL CONSIDERATIONS
Some families follow a community approach to taking care of sick family members. If the caregiver is uncomfortable with inserting a nasogastric tube, another family member will need to be taught the procedure. Members of some cultures believe that breastfeeding is the only way to incorporate the baby into the family and may have some reluctance with use of enteral tube feedings. Encouraging the mother to put the baby to the breast while the tube feeding is running may be an acceptable approach. Encourage the mother to pump and use the breastmilk for the feeding if special formula for extra calories has not been ordered. Remember to check with the physician prior to suggesting this alternative.

An interpreter will be needed for clients unable to speak English. Support and maintain the client's religious and cultural healthcare practices. Acquire healthcare materials written in the client's native language, if available. Consider use of AT&T Language Line. See also the Culturological Assessment procedure in Unit 2 for general overview of cultural considerations.

❱ INTERVENTIONS

1. Wash hands.   *Prevents transmission of microbes*

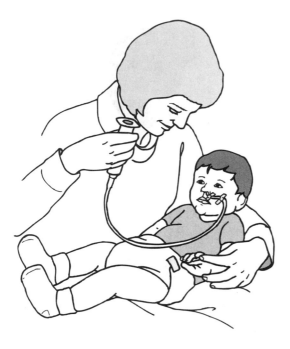

FIGURE 5-28 ▶ Positioning the infant for nasogastric feeding. Tip of syringe should be at level of child's shoulder.

2. Explain procedure to older child and caregiver.	*Reduces anxiety*
3. Organize equipment.	*Promotes efficiency*
4. Don gloves.	*Serves as protective barrier*
5. Premeasure the feeding catheter.	*Ensures accuracy of tube placement*
a. To measure for insertion of a *nasogastric* tube, measure from the nose to the earlobe and then to a point midway between the xiphoid process and the umbilicus (Figure 5-29).	
b. to measure for insertion of an *orogastric* tube, measure from the mouth and proceed in the same manner as above for nasogastric tube measurement.	
6. Have caregiver securely hold the toddler or older child	*Ensures that child is adequately restrained*
7. Lubricate the premeasured catheter with water or water soluble lubricant	*Allows for easier insertion*
8. Insert catheter	*The initial direction will allow the tube to pass easily*
a. For *nasogastric tube placement*, insert catheter into nares, direct toward the occiput and follow down the passage of the pharynx until the premeasured mark on the catheter has been reached	
b. For *orogastric tube placement*, insert catheter into the mouth and direct the catheter toward the direction of the throat passing the catheter until the premeasured mark has been reached	
9. Tape catheter to nose and face (Figure 5-30).	*Secures position*
10. Check for proper placement by instilling 3 ml of air into the end of catheter. Place stethoscope over stomach and	*Feedings cannot be started if tube is not in correct posi-*

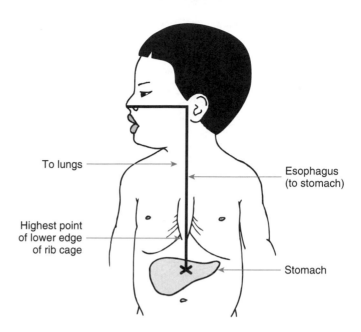

To lungs

Esophagus
(to stomach)

Highest point
of lower edge
of rib cage

Stomach

FIGURE 5-29 ▷ Measuring for placement of nasogastric tube.

listen for a "pop." Aspirate stomach contents and test with PH paper for acidity and note gastric residual.

tion or if there is evidence of excessive gastric residual

11. REMOVE THE CATHETER IMMEDIATELY IF THE CHILD BEGINS TO COUGH, BECOME SHORT OF BREATH, OR LOOKS CYANOTIC.

Tube has passed into the bronchus

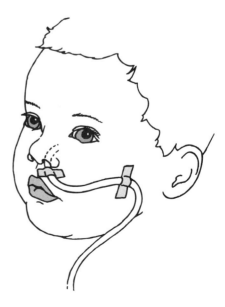

FIGURE 5-30 ▷ Securing the nasogastric tube

12. Check the medical order for accuracy of type of feeding, amount and rate of infusion.

Ensures that medical orders are being appropriately followed

13. If by gravity feed, teach caregiver to attach end of catheter to end of 50-cc syringe or feeding bag and elevate to level of the infant's/child's shoulder.

Feeding should be instilled slowly to prevent discomfort

14. If by low-volume pump, teach caregiver to use feeding pump safely, connecting syringe or feeding to pump as designed.

Enhances comfort level of caregiver with the enteral feeding process

15. When feeding is completed, remove the catheter and feeding bag. Rinse the feeding bag with water. Wash the catheter with soap and water and store in a clean covered container.

Reduces incidence of bacterial growth

16. If the tube is to remain indwelling, clamp and secure to clothing after flushing with water.

Prevents reflux of feeding

Reduces amount of tension on the tube and potential inadvertent displacement between feedings

17. Review signs of feeding intolerance with caregiver: vomiting, diarrhea, abdominal distension, gastric residual prior to feeding, choking, or difficulty breathing.

Reinforces caregiver learning

18. Encourage caregiver to allow infant or toddler to engage in nonnutritive sucking during the tube feeding.

Helps infant/toddler associate sucking with satiety

19. Obtain anthropometric measurements and compare with normal growth and development scale.

Monitors infant or child's nutritional status

20. Obtain serum specimens for laboratory studies as ordered: electrolytes, glucose, creatinine, BUN, albumin, liver function tests.

Provides physiological data to analyze nutritional status

DOCUMENTATION

The following should be noted in the nursing note:

Caregiver's ability to perform procedure
Child's tolerance of procedure
Signs of vomiting or distention, discomfort
Child's tolerance of feed
Any instruction given to caretaker about treatment plan
All caregiver teaching
    Topics to include in the teaching plan:
        safe and correct handling of equipment/supplies
        emergency procedures
        underlying disease pathology
        appropriate community resources and contact persons

INTERDISCIPLINARY COLLABORATION

Inform the physician and dietician of poor weight gain status, food intolerance, or untoward clinical findings

Coordinate ordering of supplies with DME company and/or homecare agency. Consult with WOC nurse for management of ostomy.

Consult social worker to assist family in finding appropriate support groups in the community [1, 2, 5, 6, 8–10, 12–14, 19–21, 23, 24, 26, 29, 31, 32]

PROCEDURE
Management of Failure To Thrive

DESCRIPTION
Failure to thrive (FTT) is a chronic condition characterized by a failure to maintain weight and sometimes height above the fifth percentile on age-appropriate growth charts. Most children are diagnosed before the age of 2 years. This condition has the potential of becoming life-threatening if ignored. The etiology of FTT is associated with underlying physical, emotional, or psychological problems. Some of the organic causes of the disease are associated with physical anomalies or conditions affecting major organ systems. Some of the nonorganic causes are associated with poor caregiver-infant interactions.

PURPOSE
To instruct the caregiver on feeding and parenting skills that encourage the child to maintain adequate nutrition for growth and development

EQUIPMENT
Health Assessment forms
Sphygmomanometer
Stethoscope
Thermometer
Weight scale
Educational materials

OUTCOMES
The child/caregiver will:

► Demonstrate knowledge of meal planning that provides adequate caloric intake required for growth
► Demonstrate effective feeding techniques
► Maintain steady weight gain over a period of time
► Demonstrate a healthy caregiver-child relationship

ASSESSMENT DATA
Note child's general appearance and medical history
Assess development status, plot development on growth chart
Obtain prenatal/neonatal history
Obtain nutritional history (see Unit 2 Evaluation of Nutritional Status)
Obtain developmental history (see Unit 2 Developmental Assessment)
Evaluate family/social history and dynamics
Evaluate caregiver-child interaction
Review medication profile with caregiver and determine level of understanding

RELATED NURSING DIAGNOSES
Altered growth and development
Knowledge deficit
Altered nutrition, less than body requirements

Ineffective family coping
Altered parenting

SPECIAL CONSIDERATIONS

If FTT is organic in nature, the focus of care will be oriented toward procedures dealing with the anomaly or condition. If FTT is found to have a nonorganic component, work with the caregiver and infant to improve feeding interactions. Providing for family support and advocating for other services will be part of the evaluation. Referrals for home speech-language pathology evaluation, which for infants is a feeding issue, can be obtained if not already in place. Many states have programs for early intervention. If the infant was not enrolled in any program prior to discharge from the hospital, discuss a social work evaluation with the insurance company to connect the family to available services in their area

Be aware of the need to reinforce caregiver education regarding FTT. Set-up the nursing visit to take place during feeding. Avoid authoritative intervention, suggestions, or criticism. Use positive reinforcement when the caregiver demonstrates nurturing behaviors.

Note recommended caloric intake and weight per age, and compare normal anthropometric measurements with client findings.

TRANSCULTURAL CONSIDERATIONS

Interpreting bonding between infant and caregiver can be very subjective, and cultural differences must be considered prior to judging if positive bonding is occurring. Lack of confidence on the part of mothers, especially teenage mothers, can be misread. Evaluating how the family unit functions is a vital component of the nursing visit. Encourage participation in parent support groups, such as teen mother groups, and parents of children with special needs support groups. An interpreter will be needed for clients unable to speak English. Support and maintain the client's religious and cultural healthcare practices.

Acquire healthcare materials written in the client's native language, if available. Consider use of AT&T Language Line. See also the Culturological Assessment procedure in Unit 2 for general overview of cultural considerations.

▶ INTERVENTIONS

1. Perform physical assessment.

   Establishes baseline information of physiological data findings

2. Weigh and measure child. Measure head circumference.

   Provides a baseline assessment

3. Instruct caregiver to weigh weekly.

   Tracks weight gain/loss

4. Assess developmental and growth status using age-appropriate charts (see Appendices 2-5 and 2-6).

   Evaluates findings with same age children

5. Observe interaction between caregiver and child. Assess bonding behaviors and child's response to caregiver.

   Evaluates emotional attachment

6. Observe caregiver and child during a feeding.

   Assess feeding techniques

7. Encourage caregiver to keep a food diary for 1 week of all food eaten.

   Provides data for MD and assists in meal planning

8. Instruct in meal planning using Food Guide Pyramid.

   Assures intake of balanced nutrients

9. Instruct in parenting skills by demonstrating proper holding, stroking, feeding techniques. For older children, instruct in communication skills through age appropriate words and gestures.

   Eliminates knowledge deficit

10. Provide age-appropriate stimulation for child and encourage appropriate activities.

Encourages growth and development

DOCUMENTATION
The following should be noted in the nursing note:

Child's height, weight, head circumference, general appearance, developmental status
Any feeding intolerances—vomiting, diarrhea, abdominal distention
Caregiver/child interactions, parenting skills
Family and environmental dynamics
Instructions given on diet, developmental stimulation, parenting skills, and coping strategies
Referral to community agencies
All caregiver teaching:
    Topics to include in the teaching plan:
        safe and correct handling of equipment/supplies
        emergency procedures
        underlying disease pathology
        appropriate community resources and contact persons

INTERDISCIPLINARY COLLABORATIONS
All findings from the homecare nurse should be reported to the primary physician. Collaboration with a nutritionalist can provide the caregiver with information on meal planning and calorie requirements specific to age. Referral to community services serve as a source of education in parenting and coping skills, and may aid in providing social, emotional, and financial support. [1, 5, 14, 22, 31, 32]

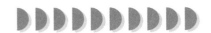

4

Pediatric Renal System Procedures

Intermittent Bladder Self-Catherization

DESCRIPTION
Intermittent bladder self-catherization is a clean procedure performed by the child or the caregiver to relieve the bladder of urine. This procedure becomes necessary following the development of a neurogenic bladder. Whenever there is an interruption or injury to the reflexes necessary for bladder control, and the bladder is unable to empty itself or does not empty completely, catherization becomes necessary. Conditions leading to a neurogenic bladder are spinal bifida or spinal cord injury.

PURPOSE
Removal of urine from the bladder which may be stagnant, thereby decreasing the risk of infection and urinary reflux

EQUIPMENT
Health Assessment forms
Catheter and storage container (size appropriate for age)
Gloves (unsterile and disposable)
Water soluble lubricant
Iodine solution surgical scrub
Cotton balls
Soap/water/washcloth
Collection receptacle
Storage container
Clean tissue or paper towel

OUTCOMES
The child/caregiver will:

▶ Be free from the risk of infection
▶ Not experience discomfort from distention
▶ Be knowledgeable in performing the procedure

ASSESSMENT DATA
Note concentration of urine (clear or cloudy)
Note color of urine (clear or pale yellow)
Note presence of strong odor
Hematuria

RELATED NURSING DIAGNOSES
Altered urinary elimination
Urinary retention
Reflex incontinence
Knowledge deficit

SPECIAL CONSIDERATIONS
An older child who has experienced a spinal cord injury may have difficulty accepting this condition. There may be a loss of self-esteem and some degree of noncompliance resulting from altered body image. When approaching the child in the home it is essential to provide privacy in performing this procedure to maintain modesty.

TRANSCULTURAL CONSIDERATIONS
An interpreter will be needed for clients unable to speak English. Support and maintain the client's religious and cultural healthcare practices Acquire healthcare materials written in the client's native language, if available. Consider use of AT&T Language Line. See also the Culturological Assessment procedure in Unit 2 for general overview of cultural considerations.

▶ INTERVENTIONS

1. Verify medical orders.	*Reduces risk of error*
2. Wash hands.	*Prevents transmission of microbes*
3. Prepare a clean work area; place tissue or paper towel on flat surface.	*Preparation and organization will hasten the procedure*
4. Gather supplies and equipment; keep catheter in container until ready to use.	*Keeps catheter clean*
5. Explain procedure to the child, and position the child either sitting or supine.	*Relieves anxiety*
6. Don clean gloves.	*Serves as protective barrier*
7. Remove clean catheter from container, lubricate with water soluble lubricant, place on clean surface.	*Eases insertion of catheter*
8. Cleanse perineal area with soap and water.	*Provides a clean area and prevents contamination*
9. Remove gloves and discard, wash hands.	*Prevents contamination*
10. Don clean gloves.	*Serves as protective barrier*

11. Cleanse area around urinary meatus with iodine solution on a cotton ball if ordered.
    For boys: hold the penis in an upright position, pull back foreskin in uncircumcised child and wipe tip of penis
    For girls: separate the labia, wipe from front to back using cotton ball once and discarding. Repeat two times.
	Disinfects area around catheter insertion

12. Identify urinary meatus (for the girl child who is learning to perform the procedure, use a mirror to permit visualization of site).	*Ensures accuracy of insertion*
13. Insert catheter into opening until urine begins to flow (Figures 5-31, 5-32). Place open end of catheter into collection container.	*Permits measurement of urine volume*

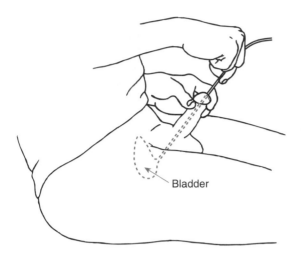

Bladder

FIGURE 5-31 ▶ Technique for male self-catheterization.

14. Instruct the child to take slow deep breaths and to bear down.

Relaxes the child and helps to empty the bladder

15. When urine begins to slow or stop, gently pull back on catheter until there is no further flow and catheter is removed.

Remove catheter slowly to prevent muscle spasms

16. Wash catheter in soap and water, dry thoroughly, and place back in container or dispose of catheter if taught to use new catheter each time.

Catheter can be used again when cleaned properly

17. Remove gloves, discard, and wash hands.

Prevents contamination

18. Praise the child for helping.

Encourages participation

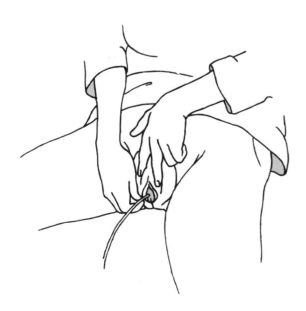

FIGURE 5-32 ▶ Technique for female self-catheterization.

19. Allow the older child and caregiver to perform the procedure.

Documents client/caregiver's ability to implement the plan of care

DOCUMENTATION
The following should be noted in the nursing note:

Vital signs, especially any elevation in temperature
Presence of abdominal distention
Complaints of pain or discomfort
Characteristics of urine (color, consistency, odor)
Trouble with insertion of catheter
Amount of urine removed
Frequency of catheterization
Child/caregiver's knowledge of procedure and ability to demonstrate
Onstructions on fluid and dietary intake to keep urine neutralized
All caregiver teaching
   Topics to include in the teaching plan:
      safe and correct handling of equipment/supplies
      emergency procedures
      underlying disease pathology
      appropriate community resources and contact persons

INTERDISCIPLINARY COLLABORATION
For the child that attends school, the school nurse should be instructed on the catherization procedure. The nurse may be required to assist the child who is unable to self catheterize. All signs and symptoms of complications, any concerns, or abnormal findings should be reported to the physician immediately. Anticipate the need to reorder supplies from the DME vendor. Consult with the medical social worker to determine the family's eligibility for financial assistance/reimbursement for supplies, and to locate support groups.

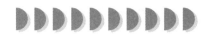

Pediatric Endocrine System Procedures

5

Management of Diabetes Mellitus, Pediatric

DESCRIPTION

Diabetes mellitus is an endocrine disorder resulting in insufficient insulin production by the pancreas. This insufficiency may be the result of a genetic predisposition, autoimmune defect, illness, and stress.

Diabetes mellitus is a disease, which if not controlled can be fatal for the child. Neurological complications, vascular changes, poor wound healing, retinal and kidney damage are some of the potential complications that may occur. It is important to stress the importance of followup medical care throughout the child's lifetime to prevent these complications from rapidly occurring.

PURPOSE

To assess caregiver's knowledge of the disease process and dietary management, to evaluate caregiver's ability to administer medications, to monitor caregiver's ability to perform glucose testing, to instruct the caregiver in signs and symptoms of complications and implementation of treatment modalities

EQUIPMENT

Health Assessment Forms
Glucometer
Finger lancets
Insulin syringes, consider use of U-30 syringes with microfine needle
Alcohol pads
Chemstrips specifically to test urine ketones
Educational materials
Daily log

OUTCOMES

The child/caregiver will:

► Be knowledgeable about the disease process and the treatment required
► Demonstrate use of glucometer to test blood sugar
► Know how to draw up prescribed insulin in a syringe and administer injection
► Be knowledgeable about diet and how to regulate intake during tiles of illness and stress
► Be free from complications of the disease process, know signs and symptoms of hyper- and hypoglycemia
► Verbalize the importance of exercise as a daily activity, routine foot care, and eye examinations

ASSESSMENT DATA
Assess home environment for learning, cleanliness, storage of supplies, and public utilities
Observe use of glucometer and chemstrips
Observe insulin preparation and administration
Evaluate knowledge of dietary regimen
Evaluate personal hygiene
Evaluate exercise program
Evaluate compliance to treatment

RELATED NURSING DIAGNOSES
At risk for infection
Altered growth and development
Knowledge deficit
Noncompliance
Self-esteem disturbance

SPECIAL CONSIDERATIONS:
Developmental

Infant/Toddler: Select a home glucose monitor that requires the smallest amount of blood for testing. There are also pediatric lancets that will decrease the pain of testing. As children grow older, the nurse can include them in the process by asking them to identify the finger to be tested or the site for the insulin injection.

School aged: Education of the child's teachers and classmate can reduce problems at school. Teachers should understand and be equipped to handle episodes of hypo- and hyperglycemia. Changes may be needed in the school schedule to permit midmorning and late afternoon snacks. During the summer children can be encouraged to attend summer camps to participate in normal camp fun while learning to control diabetes.

Adolescent: Peer pressure and the desire to fit in are the challenges associated with this age group. Social situations require advanced planning and wise choices. Adolescents should be encouraged to participate fully in their own care but be carefully supervised until proven to be responsible. Eating disorders pose a serious problem for any adolescent but are vastly complicated by diabetes. Professional help may be required to assist the adolescent with this problem.

TRANSCULTURAL CONSIDERATIONS
For clients with predominant ethnic food choices, appropriate list of foods with guidelines on how to incorporate into the diabetic diet should be provided. An interpreter will be needed for clients unable to speak English. Support and maintain the client's religious and cultural healthcare practices. Acquire healthcare materials written in the client's native language, if available. Consider use of AT&T Language Line. See also the Culturological Assessment procedure in Unit 2 for general overview of cultural considerations.

▶ **INTERVENTIONS**

1. Allow child/caregiver to verbalize understanding of disease process and treatment (see Table 5-2).	*Assesses knowledge*
2. Observe child/caregiver's use of glucometer blood testing of glucose, and use of chemstips for urine testing of ketones.	*Reinforces knowledge and corrects misinformation*

TABLE 5-2   Diabetic Client Education

Topical Areas	Educational Content
Medication	Insulin administration
	Site selection rotation
	Types of insulin
	Insulin storage
	Measuring/mixing of insulin
	Oral hypoglycemic combination therapy
Diet	Age appropriate diet
	Nutritional consultation
Exercise	Types of exercise
	Timing of exercise
	When to avoid exercise
Home Glucose Monitoring	Performing finger puncture
	Testing procedure
	Quality control testing
	Supply requisition
Sick Day Management	Testing for ketones
	Maintaining fluids
	When to call physician
	When to test blood glucose
Hypoglycemia/Hyperglycemia	Signs and symptoms
	Treatment
	Prevention
Skin/Dental/Foot Eye Care	Areas of concern
	Skin/dental/foot eye care
Complications	Neuropathy
	Nephropathy
	Retinopathy
	Cardiovascular

3. Observe child/caregiver with insulin administration. Instruct/reinforce child/caregiver's knowledge of action of insulin in the body, times of administration, rotation of injection sites, and adjustments of dose per MD orders.

Evaluates client's knowledge base

4. Instruct on accurate and consistent record keeping of glucose levels, activity, and insulin dose.

Documents trends in blood glucose control

5. Instruct meal preparation following diet plan from nutritionist (see Table 5-3). Stress importance of snacks.

Dietary planning is the basis for individualized meal plan and calorie/carbohydrate control

6. Instruct on importance of daily bathing and assessment for any breaks in the skin (cuts, scratches), periodic dental and eye exams.

Diabetic children are more prone to infection

7. Explain importance of exercise, how glucose levels are effected, and the need for food before and after exercise.

Exercise promotes interaction with peers and good self esteem

8. Instruct on vigilant monitoring of blood glucose levels and the presence of urine ketones during times of illness and stress.

Alert child/caregiver to signs and symptoms of diabetic acidosis or ketoacidosis

TABLE 5-3 Diabetic Meal Planning Approaches

Meal Planning Tool	Description
Healthy Food Choices	A simple meal planning tool used to teach clients how to use the food exchange system
	Appropriate for clients/caregivers with a sixth to seventh grade reading level
Exchanges Lists for Meal Planning	A tool used to promote consistency in meal content to achieve blood glucose control using the food exchange system
	The tool is designed to be personalized for the client by the dietitian
	Increases variety and flexibility in meal planning
	Designed for clients needing a fixed daily caloric intake, or those with limited food composition knowledge
Carbohydrate Counting	A tool consisting of three pamphlets:
	−*Getting Started, Level I* encourages consistency of carbohydrate intake
	−*Moving on, Level II* teaches clients how to adjust medication/food/activity based on "pattern reading"
	−*Intensive Diabetes Management Using Carbohydrate/−Insulin Ratios, Level III* instructs clients on how to change insulin requirements based on food intake
	Simplifies diabetic meal planning
	Uses a more precise method of estimating carbohydrate intake
	Focuses on the amount of carbohydrate eaten per meal
Total Available Glucose (TAG)	A tool which defines food based on the amount of glucose obtained from proteins, fats, and carbohydrate.
	The insulin requirement is adjusted according to the glucose content consumed
	This approach requires that the food be weighed for calculate intake
	To be used most effectively, the client/caregiver must be very motivated with above average cognitive ability.
Single Topic Diabetes Resources	An educational packet containing reproducible client handouts covering 21 diabetes nutrition-related topics
Faciliating Lifestyle Change: A Resource Manual	A tool containing monitoring forms for nutrition assessment, goal setting and lifestyle changes
The First Steps in Diabetes Meal Planning	A tool which uses a diabetic food guide pyramid poster to provide basic nutrition information for newly diagnosed diabetics

© 1998. The American Dietetic Association. *Pediatric Manual of Clinical Dietetics.* Modified with permission.

9. Instruct the child to wear or carry identification describing condition.

Source of immediate information for all healthcare providers

DOCUMENTATION

The following should be noted in the nursing note:

General physical condition
Environmental assessment
Observations, demonstrations by child/caregiver in treatment plan
All instructions given while in the home
Compliance of child/caregiver to treatment

Coping skills
All caregiver teaching:
    Topics to include in the teaching plan:
        safe and correct handling of equipment/supplies
        emergency procedures
        underlying disease pathology
        appropriate community resources and contact persons

INTERDISCIPLINARY COLLABORATION

Inform physician of all concerns that will affect the health of the child. All healthcare providers who provide treatment to the child need to be aware of the child's condition (i.e., dentist, opthalmologist). In the school-aged child, teachers and school nurses should be advised of the specific plan and should know the child's prescribed insulin doses.

Support groups are often necessary for both the child and family to accept and deal with the chronic illness of diabetes.

A nutrition consult may need to be ordered for special dietary concerns [5, 12–14, 24, 25, 26, 31, 32]

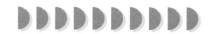

 # Pediatric Immune System Procedures

6

Organ Transplant Care and Management, Pediatric

DESCRIPTION
The general treatment of children who have received organ transplants is essentially similar regardless of the organ that has been transplanted. Long term immunosuppression therapy and organ rejection are the two areas of concern that direct the management of the patient. See also section on Adult Immune System Procedures. Organ Transplant Care and Management, Adult.

PURPOSE
To instruct the child/caregiver on recognition of signs and symptoms that could indicate organ rejection.

EQUIPMENT
Health assessment forms
Stethoscope
Sphygomomanometer
Thermometer
Infusion equipment/supplies, as ordered
Venipuncture supplies
Weight scale

OUTCOMES
The child/caretaker will:

▶ Be knowledgeable in medication administration
▶ Recognize signs and symptoms of rejection
▶ Demonstrate a positive self-image
▶ Demonstrate age appropriate growth and development
▶ Be familiar with adequate support systems needed to enhance coping

ASSESSMENT DATA
Assess caregiver's knowledge of treatment plan and medication protocol
Note caregiver's ability to care for the child
Note child's psychological status in regard to treatment plan
Evaluate caregiver's knowledge of signs and symptoms of rejection
Assess child's dietary intake
Assess for signs of infection

Note the need for supportive services
Review medication profile with caregiver and determine level of understanding

RELATED NURSING DIAGNOSES
Anxiety
Fear
Body image disturbance
At risk for injury
At risk for infection
Ineffective coping skills

SPECIAL CONSIDERATIONS
A child who returns home after an organ transplant will create a strain on the family structure. Whether the child has suffered from a chronic illness resulting in transplantation or the reason for transplantation resulted from an acute infection, the family now copes with the life-threatening situation of organ rejection. Since this reaction can occur rapidly with subtle symptoms, there is always some degree of stress and fear lurking within the family unit.

TRANSCULTURAL CONSIDERATIONS
An interpreter will be needed for clients unable to speak English
Support and maintain the client's religious and cultural healthcare practices
Acquire healthcare materials written in the client's native language, if available
Also see Cultural Assessment procedure in Unit 2 for general overview of cultural considerations.

▶ INTERVENTIONS

1. Instruct child/caregiver on purpose and use of each ordered medication and their adverse reactions such as:
   Increased risk for infection
   Delayed growth and development
   Weight gain
   Cushingoid appearance
   GI irritation
   Hyperglycemia
   Hypertension
   Increased hair growth
   Bone marrow suppression
   Personality changes

   Assures accurate medication administration and alerts family to seek prompt medical attention when needed

2. Instruct on the signs and symptoms of organ rejection:
   Elevated temperature
   Pain or discomfort
   Swelling or tenderness at graft site
   Loss of appetite
   Fatigue
   General malaise
   Abnormal drug levels
   Abnormal lab values

   Alerts caregiver to prompt medical attention

3. Explain importance of frequent assessment for signs and symptoms of infection (respiratory, urinary, mouth, and skin).

   Immunosupression medication decreases the body's ability to fight infection

4. Instruct on universal precautions and meticulous hand washing. Avoid infected individuals with URIs and communicable diseases. Daily oral hygiene with frequent dental care.	*Reduces risk of infection*
5. Encourage rest periods with return to normal activity level. Encourage age appropriate activities and peer interaction for the older child.	*Promotes age appropriate development and fosters self esteem and positive body image*
6. Encourage maintenance of nutritionally adequate diet.	*Supports general health*
7. Instruct child to wear or carry identifying medical information.	*Alerts healthcare providers to administer proper treatment in an emergency*
8. Explain the importance of keeping scheduled MD and lab appointments for followup care.	*Ongoing medical attention and care is required throughout therapy*
9. Initiate referrals to social services and support groups both for the child and the family.	*Assists in the development of effective coping skills*

DOCUMENTATION

The following should be included in the nursing note:

Vital signs
General appearance
Diet and any feeding intolerance
Activity level
Growth and development status
Compliance with medical treatment
Instructions given to caregivers on medical treatment
Complications and signs and symptoms to report to physicians as well as any child/family concerns
Referrals to social services and support groups
All caregiver teaching
        Topics to include in the teaching plan:
            safe and correct handling of equipment/supplies
            emergency procedures
            underlying disease pathology
            appropriate community resources and contact persons

INTERDISCIPLINARY COLLABORATION

The child who has received an organ transplant relies on a network of health professionals to manage the medical treatment required. The transplant team maintains a close relationship with the child and family. This includes, not only the physician in charge, but the transplant nurse, physical therapists, social workers, pharmacists, and the primary care physician. It is also important that the school nurse of a school-aged child be instructed in medications and signs and symptoms that may be of concern. [5, 6, 15, 32]

DDDDDDDDD

7 Pediatric Integumentary System Procedures

PROCEDURE

Burn Wound Management

DESCRIPTION

A burn is an injury to any layer of the skin caused by the sun, heat, electricity, chemicals, scalding fluids, or gases. The deeper the burn the greater the tissue damage (see Table 5-4).

PURPOSE

To assess wound healing and prevent the complications of infection

EQUIPMENT

Health Assessment Forms
Sterile dressing supplies as prescribed by the physician
Antibiotic cream prescribed by the physician

OUTCOMES

The child will:

► Exhibit signs of complete wound healing
► Be free from infection/complications
► Be pain free
► Have full function and mobility of burned areas
► Have a positive body image
► Maintain adequate nutritional intake
► Maintain fluid balance

ASSESSMENT DATA

Assess vital signs, especially any elevation of temperature
Note any redness or blistering of burn
Note any wound drainage-color consistency, amount, or foul odor
Evaluate frequency in need to change dressings
Observe level of discomfort/pain, frequency and need for analgesics
Evaluate caregivers ability to perform dressing change

RELATED NURSING DIAGNOSES

Impaired skin integrity
Fluid volume deficit
At risk for infection

TABLE 5-4   Burn Types, Causative Agents and Treatment Measures

Type	Causative Agent	Priority Treatment
Thermal	Open flame	Extinguish flame
	Steam	Flush with cool water
	Hot liquids	Consult fire department
	[water, grease, tar, metal]	
Chemical	Acid	Neutralize or dilute chemical
	Strong alkalis	Remove clothing
		Consult Poison Control Center
Electrical	Direct current	Disconnect power source and move to area of safety
	Alternating current	Initiate CPR as indicated
	Lightning	Consult electrical experts
Radiation	Solar [ultraviolet]	Shield the skin appropriately
	Xrays	Limit time of exposure
	Radioactive materials	Move client away from source of radiation
		Consult radiation expert

McNeal, GJ. (1996). Nursing Care of Clients with Burns. In: P.LeMone and K. Burke: *Medical-Surgical Nursing: Critical Thinking in Client Care.* Menlo Park, California: Addison Wesley Publishers.

Impaired mobility
Altered nutrition, less than body requirements
Pain
Ineffective coping
Altered body image

SPECIAL CONSIDERATIONS

It is very important to allow older children to participate in the dressing change. This allows them to become part of the care they need, and it also alleviates some of the stress they feel when the dressings are changed. Teaching the caregivers the proper procedure for wound care and the signs and symptoms of complications provides an opportunity for them to take an active role in the child's treatment plan.

TRANSCULTURAL CONSIDERATION

Children with dark pigmented skin have a greater tendency for scar formation and development of keloids when the burns are the result of extensive tissue damage.
Consider use of AT&T Language Line.
See also the Culturological Assessment procedure in Unit 2 for general overview of cultural considerations

▶ INTERVENTIONS

Pain Management

1. Assess the client's level of pain.

Pain tolerance is the duration and intensity of pain that the client can endure

1 Premedicate the child 30 minutes before procedure.

Reduces pain associated with the procedure

2. Explain procedure to child.

Relieves stress and anxiety

3. Allow the child to verbalize the experience.

Clients experience and express pain in their own manner, using various sociocultural adaptation techniques

Powerlessness

1. Allow an older child to choose which part of the procedure he or she wants to do.

Relieves stress and fear

2. Allow the child to express feelings.

The nurse assists the client to cope by therapeutically listening, displaying a caring presence, and by providing positive feedback

3. Set short-term, realistic goals.

Small incremental gains are easier to achieve and allow for frequent positive feedback

At Risk for Infection

1. Wash hands.

Prevents transmission of microbes

2. Monitor and record body temperature.

Elevated temperature indicates the presence of infection

3. Observe for signs and symptoms of infection.

Continuous assessment enables the nurse to evaluate interventional strategies

4. Culture all wounds and body secretions as ordered.

Culture and sensitivity reports identify the presence of infectious microbes and indicate appropriate antimicrobial therapies

5. Maintain aseptic technique.

Prevents contamination

6. Don gloves.

Serve as a protective barrier

7. Follow orders for using the open or closed wound dressing procedure.

Prevents infection

If Closed Method Is Used

a. Remove old dressing. May need to be soaked in warm water prior to removal

Alleviates discomfort

b. Wash hands and don sterile gloves

Prevents contamination

c. Cleanse wound with normal saline or solution prescribed by the physician and pat dry if ordered

Friction from the cleansing improves blood supply to the area

d. Cover the wound with antibiotic cream if ordered (see Display 5-2)

Prevents infection

e. Cover with sterile pads or vaseline gauze as ordered. Keep dressing intact with surgical tape or gauze roll

DISPLAY 5-2 *Topical Antimicrobial Burn Medications*

Mafenide Acetate (Sulfamylon)

Action:

Bacteriostatic agent effective against gram positive and negative organisms

Nursing Responsibilities:

Use with caution in clients with renal or pulmonary disease

Observe for the development of hypersensitivity and metabolic acidosis

Assess for evidence of superinfection within the burn wound

Client Education:

Explain that a burning sensation will follow drug application. Premedicate to control for discomfort

Apply the drug to clean burn wounds once or twice daily as ordered

Discontinue use if an allergic response occurs

Report any sudden or prolonged increase in respiratory rate

Silver Nitrate

Action

Bacteriostatic agent that inhibits growth of wide variety of gram negative and positive organisms

Nursing Responsibilities

The drug has limited penetrating ability and should not be used more than 72 hours following burn injury

The drug interacts with chloride ions to form a black percipitate that discolors the burn wound and hampers visual inspection

High concentrations of the drug results in cellular toxicity to surrounding tissue

Observe for hyponatremia and hypochloremic alkalosis

Client Education

Report any signs of hypotonicity: swelling, weight gain, difficulty breathing

Because the black percipitate which forms with use of this drug obscures direct observation of the wound site, clients must be told to watch for systemic signs and symptoms of infection: fever, malaise, rapid pulse, listlessness

The wound should be saturated with a 0.5% aqueous solution of the drug with bid dressing change as ordered

Silver Sulfadiazine (Silvadene)

Action

Bacteriocidal agent that is effective against a variety of gram negative and positive organisms

Nursing Responsibilities

The drug may cause a marked leukopenia during initial therapy which tends to subside over course of therapy

Observe for evidence of hypersensitivity and report findings

If sulfa crystals form in the urine keep the client well hydrated

Client Education

Apply thin coating of the drug daily to clean burn wound as ordered

Continue the drug until healing is apparent

Discontinue drug if allergy develops

Watch for evidence of concentrated urine and report to physician

If not contraindicate, drink plenty of fluids to prevent formation of sulfa crystals in the urine

1) apply dressings circumferentially in a distal to proximal manner

Retards the formation of dependent edema

2) All fingers and toes are wrapped separately

Prevents friction and breakdown of skin surfaces

f. For wet to dry dressings, a thick gauze is applied to maintain moisture and is soaked frequently with the ordered solution

Assures that antiseptic dressing is kept moist to saturate wound

If Open Method Is Used

a. Maintain strict adherence to protective isolation

Reduces presence of environmental contaminants

b. Cleanse wound with normal saline or solution prescribed by the physician

Friction from the cleansing improves blood supply to the area

c. Apply antimicrobial agent as ordered, leave open to air, reapply as needed

Because of tendency to rub off on clothing, the topical agent will need to be applied frequently

8. Stress the importance to caregiver of keeping wound or dressing clean

Prevents infection

Impaired Mobility

1. Instruct client and caregiver to perform active and passive ROM exercises to joints as ordered (see Table 5-5).

Prevents contractures

2. Apply splints as ordered.

Retards formation of contractures

3. Maintain limbs in functional alignment.

Preserves joint mobility

TABLE 5-5   Positioning the Client with Burn Wounds

Area Burned	Positioning
Head and Neck	to achieve hyperextension, place a rolled towel under the neck or shoulder to achieve extension, use no pillow
Shoulder/axilla	to achieve abduction/external rotation of the anterior shoulder, abduct the arm 90 degrees from the side of the trunk, to achieve flexion/internal rotation of the posterior shoulder, position the arm slightly behind the midline of the body
Elbow	to achieve extension/supination, maintain the joint in the extended position, palm upward
Wrist	to achieve extension, use a splint to maintain 30- to 45-degree extension
Fingers	to achieve flexion/extension, use splints
Legs	to maintain slight abduction, place a pillow between the legs, use a trochanter roll to prevent external rotation
Knee	to achieve extension, position the client in a supine position with the knees extended and in the supine position with the feet hanging over the lower end of the mattress, knee splints may also be used, while the client sits in a chair, legs should be elevated and extended
Ankle	to achieve a neutral position, use a padded footboard and ankle splints to avoid inversion or eversion

McNeal, GJ. (1996). Nursing Care of Clients with Burns. In: P.LeMone and K. Burke: *Medical-Surgical Nursing: Critical Thinking in Client Care.* Menlo Park, California: Addison Wesley Publishers.

Altered Nutrition, Less than Body Requirements

1. Encourage daily intake of nutritious foods from each of the four food groups.

   Adequate nutritional intake facilitates wound healing

2. Weigh the client weekly, and assess growth and development.

   Anthropometric measurements indicate the adequacy of nutritional support therapies

3. Obtain blood specimens for protein, iron, CBC, glucose, and albumin as ordered.

   Decreased serum values indicate inadequate nutritional intake

4. Encourage frequent intake of oral fluids as ordered.

   Prevents fluid volume deficit

Prevention of Hypertrophic Scarring

1. Apply tubular support bandages or custom-made elastic garment to affected area as ordered

   Pressure garments reduce risk of scar tissue formation

DOCUMENTATION

The following should be noted in the nursing notes:

Vital signs especially any elevation in temp
Size and appearance of wound
Presence of any drainage-color, amount, or foul odor
If skin graft present appearance of graft site-color of skin, tissue perfusion. Also assess the donor
    site
Functional mobility of affected area
Child/caregivers compliance to treatment plan
Presence of altered body image or low self-esteem in the child
Knowledge of medication administration
Instructions on home safety and accident prevention
All caregiver teaching
    Topics to include in the teaching plan:
        safe and correct handling of equipment/supplies
        emergency procedures
        underlying disease pathology
        appropriate community resources and contact persons

INTERDISCIPLINARY COLLABORATION

The severity of the burn will dictate if other services may need to be involved (nutrition, plastic surgery, occupational therapy, psychology and others). Extensive burns to the limbs will require physical therapy to regain normal function. The homecare nurse plays a very important role in providing instruction and support to the family. Frequent visits to assess the wound keep the physician informed of the child's recovery. [5, 11, 18, 28, 30, 32]

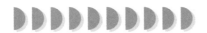

8 *Pediatric Musculoskeletal System Procedures*

Cast Care and Management

DESCRIPTION

A cast is utilized to immobilize an extremity and to promote proper bone alignment.

The most common categories of casts include those that are used on upper and lower extremities, hip and knee (Spica casts), and spinal and cervical casts. The cast may be made from plaster or a synthetic material such as fiberglass.

EQUIPMENT

Health Assessment Forms
Pillows
Adhesive tape or moleskin
Plastic wrap or a plastic bag

PURPOSE

To maintain the integrity of the cast and the surrounding skin until proper bone healing has occurred

OUTCOMES

The child will:

▶ Maintain skin integrity
▶ Have good tissue perfusion
▶ Maintain mobility and sensation
▶ Be free from pain
▶ Not experience physical injury
▶ Maintain normal bowel and bladder functioning

ASSESSMENT DATA

Monitor cardiovascular status—assess peripheral pulses, capillary refill distal to the fractured extremity
Check cast for tightness—you should be able to insert two fingers inside the cast
Assess for pain, swelling, coldness, cyanosis, or pallor of the extremity
Assess ability to move fingers or toes on command
Note sensation of tingling or numbness
Check condition of the cast for integrity, hot spots, areas of drainage or bleeding
Assess skin around the cast for irritation and/or breakdown or pressure areas

Assess vital signs for signs of infection
Assess respiratory status—signs of respiratory effort or compromise especially with a spica cast
Assess the need for pain medication
Assess for altered bowel elimination/constipation especially with spica cast

RELATED NURSING DIAGNOSES
Altered tissue perfusion
Altered skin integrity
Pain
Altered physical mobility
At risk for injury

SPECIAL CONSIDERATION:
A child with a fractured femur is susceptible to frequent muscle spasms, which may require pain management to relieve discomfort over a period of several days.

Any complaints of chest pain or difficulty breathing should be reported immediately to the physician to rule out the possibility of a pulmonary or fat embolism.

TRANSCULTURAL CONSIDERATION:
In those children who have been diagnosed with hematological disorders such as sickle cell anemia, an injury or fracture may cause such physical stress on the body that, for example, a sickle cell crisis may occur. Consider use of AT&T Language Line. See also the Culturological Assessment procedure in Unit 2 for general overview of cultural considerations.

▶ INTERVENTIONS
Care of the Wet Cast

1. Inform the caregiver that the cast made of plaster will be wet for many hours.
    While the cast is drying handle as little as possible
    Touch the cast only with the palms of the hands, never with the fingers (Figure 5-33)
    Turn the child in a spica cast every 2 hours to facilitate drying
    Do not use a heated fan or dryer to dry the cast

Caregivers may be unaware of the length of time needed for complete drying of the plaster cast

Skin care

1. Keep skin between fingers and toes clean and dry. Area above and below the cast should also be washed with soap and water and well dried.

Prevents irritation and skin breakdown

2. Once the cast is dry, cover rough edges on cast by "petalling." Cut several strips of adhesive bandage or moleskin 3 inches by 1–2 inches wide. Tape one end of the strip inside the cast and the other end on the outside. Do this all around the edge of the cast (Figure 5-34).

Prevents skin irritation from the cast rubbing on the skin. Also relieves pressure areas

3. Keep the cast dry especially if it is made from plaster. Fiberglass casts may be wiped off with a wet cloth. To keep a body cast clean and dry, place plastic around the

When plaster becomes wet it will become soft and has the ability to indent if pres-

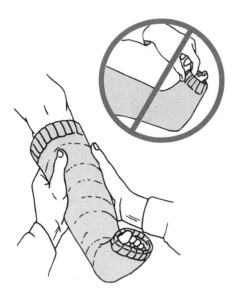

FIGURE 5-33 ▶ Handling the wet cast with the palms of the hands.

opening in the genital area. Remind caregiver to not place diapers over the cast
4. Tub baths are not advised, although an arm cast may be covered with plastic if tub bathing is necessary.
5. Instruct the child to never put anything inside the cast to relieve an itch on the skin.

sure is applied causing pressure on the skin.

Increases risk of wetting the cast

Objects may become lodged inside the cast

Positioning

1. Keep extremities elevated on a pillow to keep proper alignment of the body and redistribute the weight from the cast (Figure 5-35).

Prevents dependent edema

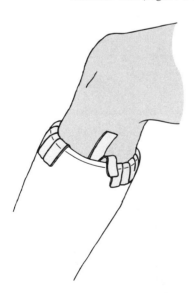

FIGURE 5-34 ▶ Covering the rough edges of the cast.

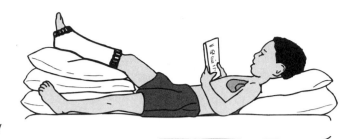

FIGURE 5-35 ▶ Positioning the casted extremity above the level of the heart to prevent edema.

2. Turn the child in a spica cast every 2–4 hours or as ordered.

Reduces pressure from prolonged immobility

Transfer Technique

1. Lift cast with two hands under the cast. *Never* try to use only one hand. A cast is heavier than you think.

Misjudgment can lead to inadvertant dropping of the affected limb resulting in pain and injury

2. Always have two people lift or move a child in a body cast (spica cast). Never use the bar between the legs to lift or move.

Prevents injury

Safety Considerations

1. Instruct in proper crutch walking.
2. Instruct family to keep pathways clutter free, floors should be void of loose rugs, and rough play should be discouraged.

Prevents injury
Prevents injury

DOCUMENTATION
The following should be noted in the nursing note:

Vital signs
Condition of the skin around the cast
Condition of the cast
Need for pain medication
Neurovascular, cardiovascular assessment
Family/child education
Function and mobility status
All caregiver teaching
    Topics to include in the teaching plan:
        safe and correct handling of equipment/supplies
        emergency procedures
        underlying disease pathology
        appropriate community resources and contact persons

INTERDISCIPLINARY COLLABORATION

With any immobilization of a body part, physical therapy is needed to restore proper function and mobility

The family is instructed in ROM exercises by the therapists to continue in strengthening the effected extremity

Community resources may be contacted to provide transportation to and from therapies [5, 12–14, 21, 23, 29, 32]

PROCEDURE
Management of Traction Devices

DESCRIPTION
The most frequently used types of traction are:

Manual traction: traction applied to the body part by the clinician's hand positioned distal to the fracture site for the purpose of establishing proper bone alignment during casting.

Skin traction: traction applied directly to the skin surface and indirectly to the skeletal structures.

Cervical traction: traction used to manage cervical spine injuries

Skeletal traction: traction applied directly to the skeletal structure by a pin, wire, or tongs inserted distal to the fracture site by an orthopedic surgeon.

EQUIPMENT
Depending on the type of traction used:
Weights
Pulleys
Ropes
Spreader block

> *For Buck's Extension Traction*
> elastic bandage
> heel protector

> *For Skeletal Traction*
> See Pin Site Care Equipment

> *For Halo-Vest Device*
> Metal frame
> removable vest
> See also Pin Site Care Equipment

PURPOSE
Traction is used to immobilize a body part and promote bone realignment

OUTCOMES
▶ Skin integrity will be maintained
▶ Function and mobility will be restored
▶ Family will maintain traction and report untoward clinical findings

ASSESSMENT DATA

Note the line of pull exerted by the traction; it should be upward, abducted, or adducted
Check the condition of ropes, pulleys, weights, frame, bandages, or splints
Check the alignment of child in relation to the traction
Assess the child's behavior in relation to the presence of pain as caused by the traction
Observe and report evidence of infection
Assess nutritional status
Determine psychosocial adjustment

RELATED NURSING DIAGNOSES

Altered mobility
Altered urinary/bowel elimination
Pain
Altered growth and development
Diversional activity deficit
Altered skin integrity
At risk for infection
At risk for altered tissue perfusion
At risk for impaired gas exchange
Altered body image

TRANSCULTURAL CONSIDERATIONS

An interpreter will be needed for clients unable to speak English. Support and maintain the client's religious and cultural healthcare practices. Acquire healthcare materials written in the client's native language, if available. Consider use of AT&T Language Line. See also the Culturological Assessment procedure in Unit 2 for general overview of cultural considerations

▶ INTERVENTIONS

1. Wash hands.

Prevents transmission of microbes

2. Verify physician order.
3. Apply appropriate type of traction.

Reduces risk of error

For Skin Traction or Buck's Extension Traction

a. Replace any elastic bandage or nonadhesive straps when needed by applying new straps/bandages to medial and lateral aspect of lower affected extremity. A second person should help maintain the traction

Interruption of traction may cause injury when reapplied. Bandages should be kept clean.

b. Assess that bandages are reapplied not too tight or too loose in order to assure proper traction

Improperly placed bandages can cause malalignment

c. Attach a spreader block to the distal end of the tape

Spreader block prevents pressure along the side of the foot

d. Attach a rope to the spreader block and pass the rope over a pulley, which has been secured to the end of the bed

Faciliates suspension of the extremity

e. Apply weights as ordered and allow to hang freely (see Figure 5-36)

Traction cannot be maintained when weights are permitted

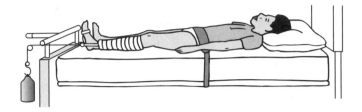

FIGURE 5-36 ▶ Child in Buck's extension traction with freely hanging weights.

	to touch the floor or the bed
f. Apply heel protector	Reduces risk of heel ulcer formation

For Skeletal Traction

a. Perform pin care as often as ordered	Prevents infection
b. Assess site of insertion for evidence of drainage, redness, swelling, excessive pain	Detects presence of infectious process

For Halo-Vest Device

a. Connect metal frame of halo ring to removable vest per manufacturer guidelines	Secures attachment
b. Assess skin under the vest daily by unbuckling one side of the vest at a time to maintain traction	Detects evidence of skin irritation
c. Encourage frequent position changes	Prevents skin breakdown
d. Wash and dry skin of chest and back through side openings	Maintains cervical traction while bathing torso
e. Turn the client and vest as a unit	Log rolling maintains proper head neck and body alignment
f. Keep vest wrench taped to front of vest or follow manufacturer's recommendations for emergency vest removal	Procedure to remove vest varies with type of vest device used
g. Perform pin care as ordered	Prevents infection
h. Note stability of pin sites, stabilize the head and inform physician of evidence of pin detachment	Cervical pin detachment constitutes a medical emergency
4. Check the pull of the traction to assure proper balance.	Prevents injury
5. Change position frequently relieving pressure on hips, buttocks, coccyx, shoulders, and back of head.	Prevents pressure areas and skin breakdown
6. Always maintain alignment after moving child.	Prevent injury and pain
7. Check pulses on affected limb and compare to unaffected side.	Assesses circulatory status
8. Assess neurovascular status of affected limb, as apropriate.	Determines nerve involvement
9. Perform ROM exercises to unaffected limbs, as appropriate.	Promotes joint mobility Prevents contractures
10. Encourage fluids.	Promotes kidney function
11. Provide a diet high in fiber.	Prevents constipation

12. Provide age-appropriate activities for the child.	*Encourage normal growth and development*
13. Encourage deep breathing exercises hourly.	*Facilitates lung expansion and movement of respiratory secretions*
14. Provide emotional support.	*Helps client adjust to altered body image*
15. Instruct caregiver in safe management and care of traction devices and permit return demonstration.	*Prevents risk of injury and evaluates caregiver learning*

DOCUMENTATION
The following should be noted in the nursing note:

Vital signs
Skin integrity of entire body—redness, swelling, edema, drainage
Traction set up noting amount of weight used
Circulatory, neurovascular status
Degree of discomfort or pain, frequency of pain medication
Bowel habits
Urinary output
Coping skills of child and family
Education provided to the child/caregiver
All caregiver teaching
    Topics to include in the teaching plan:
        safe and correct handling of equipment/supplies
        emergency procedures
        underlying disease pathology
        appropriate community resources and contact persons

INTERDISCIPLINARY COLLABORATION
Inform physician of all abnormal findings, increased pain, or poor coping skills.
Collaborate with physical therapist to provide instructions on exercises to promote joint mobility.
    The instructions should be given to both the caregiver and child.
Collaborate with occupational therapist who can instruct family on age-appropriate activities.
Encourage home-study programs for school aged children during their recovery phase. [5, 13, 20, 23, 32]

PROCEDURE
Pin Site Care

DESCRIPTION
Surgical placement of pins or wires restore alignment and give support to an extremity or affected bone

EQUIPMENT
Health Assessment forms
Saline solution
Sterile gauze pads
Cotton swab

Hydrogen peroxide
Iodine or antibiotic ointment

PURPOSE
To keep pin sites clean, free from infection, discomfort and pain

OUTCOMES
▸ Pin sites will be infection free
▸ Caregivers will demonstrate knowledge of pin care
▸ Pain and discomfort will be controlled by analgesics

ASSESSMENT DATA
Note signs and symptoms on infection
Record drainage color, amount, odor
Assess pin site location
Monitor level of pain
Review medication profile with caregiver and determine level of understanding

RELATED NURSING DIAGNOSES
Altered mobility
Impaired skin integrity
Pain
At risk for infection
Knowledge deficit

SPECIAL CONSIDERATIONS
It is important to always note the placement of the pins on the skin so that any signs of the pins becoming dislodged can be noted and reported immediately to the physician.

TRANSCULTURAL CONSIDERATIONS
An interpreter will be needed for clients unable to speak English. Support and maintain the client's religious and cultural healthcare practices. Acquire healthcare materials written in the client's native language, if available. Consider use of AT&T Language Line. See also the Culturological Assessment procedure in Unit 2 for general overview of cultural considerations.

▶ INTERVENTIONS

1. Verify medical orders.	*Reduces risk of error*
2. Wash hands.	*Prevents transmission of microbes*
3. Don gloves.	*Serves as protective barrier*
4. Pour hydrogen peroxide, as ordered, onto the sterile gauze pad and cotton-tipped applicator clean around each pin site. Use a clean gauze pad and cotton swab for each pin.	*Removes old drainage and skin bacteria.*
5. Rinse site with saline solution as ordered.	*Removes peroxide residue*
6. Place antibiotic cream or iodine solution, as ordered, on cotton swab and apply to pin site.	*Prevents the growth of bacteria*
7. Leave site open to air or cover sterile gauze pad as ordered.	*Permits direct visualization of site*
8. Remove gloves wash hands.	*Prevents transmission of microbes*

DOCUMENTATION

The following should be noted in the nursing note:

Vital signs
Condition of skin around pin sites
Presence of drainage, redness, or swelling
Level of pain and discomfort
Family knowledge of skin care
Family/child education on physical therapy
All caregiver teaching
   Topics to include in the teaching plan:
      safe and correct handling of equipment/supplies
      emergency procedures
      underlying disease pathology
      appropriate community resources and contact persons

INTERDISCIPLINARY COLLABORATIONS:

Inform physician of the presence of any signs of infection, family compliance to treatment plan, and/or any safety issues in the home.

Physical therapy has a large role in the treatment to restore normal function and mobility [5, 13, 21, 23, 32]

Pediatric Neurological System Procedures

PROCEDURE
Ventriculoperitoneal/Ventriculoatrial Shunt Management

DESCRIPTION

A ventriculoperitoneal (VP) or ventriculoatrial (VA) shunt is a surgical procedure that permits the placement of a drainage system in the ventricle of the brain to remove excess cerebral spinal fluid (CSF), or to relieve an obstruction that impedes ventricular circulation. Shunt systems typically consist of a ventricular catheter, flush pump, a one-way valve, and a distal catheter to transport excess CSF to either the peritoneal cavity or the right atrium of the heart. Hydrocephalus is the most common defect that requires this type of intervention. The ventricular-gallbladder or ventricular-pleural shunt procedure may be performed when the VP or VA shunt procedure cannot be implemented.

EQUIPMENT

Sterile dressing supplies for wound care
Health Assessment Forms

PURPOSE

Assessment of child's neurological status to detect signs and symptoms of increased intercranial pressure and or shunt obstruction

OUTCOMES

The child will:

▶ Be free from infection due to surgical intervention
▶ Maintain appropriate growth and development behaviors

The caregiver and/or child will:

Be knowledgeable about shunt function and signs and symptoms of increased ICP

ASSESSMENT DATA

Note signs and symptoms of depressed neurological status (hypertension, bradycardia, slowing respirations)
Measure head circumference especially in infants and note any increase in size
Note changes in feeding patterns, loss of appetite or vomiting
Note level of conscious, irritability, high pitched cry
Assess signs and symptoms of infection
Evaluate growth and development status

Assess knowledge and coping skills of caregivers in the treatment plan
Review medication profile with caregiver and determine level of understanding

RELATED NURSING DIAGNOSES
At risk for infection
Adaptive capacity intracranial: altered
Anxiety
Altered growth and development

SPECIAL CONSIDERATIONS
The onset of increased ICP may be abrupt or gradual. It is therefore critical that the caregiver know how to assess for neurological changes and know when to report such changes to the physician. The major shunt complications include infection and malfunction. A malfunctioning shunt occurs secondary to kinking, plugging, or migration of the catheter. When such malfunctions occur, the child is at risk for increased ICP. Shunt infections are serious complications which must be treated with intravenous antibiotic therapy. Wound infection, meningitis, ventriculitis, septicemia, and bacterial endocarditis are possible types of shunt infections.

TRANSCULTURAL CONSIDERATIONS
An interpreter will be needed for clients unable to speak English. Support and maintain the client's religious and cultural healthcare practices. Acquire healthcare materials written in the client's native language, if available. Consider use of AT&T Language Line. See also the Culturological Assessment procedure in Unti 2 for general overview of cultural considerations.

▶ INTERVENTIONS

1. Verify medical orders.	*Reduces risk of error*
2. Wash hands.	*Prevents transmission of microbes*
3. Perform physical assessment.	*Establishes baseline information of physiological data findings*
4. Demonstrate wound care to the caregiver if the child has recently had a shunt placed and has been discharged with instructions for dressing changes.	*Reinforces aseptic technique taught in the hospital*
5. Instruct the caregiver on signs and symptoms of ICP, shunt infection, shunt malfunction, and seizure activity.	*The caregiver is the primary source of information on any changes in the child's condition*
6. Instruct in diet and importance of fluids.	*Proper nutrition promotes growth*

DOCUMENTATION
The following should be noted in the nursing note:

Vital signs, especially elevation of temperature
Change in neurological status, bulging or tight fontanel lethargy, decreased responsiveness, irritability, confusion, eyes that appear deviating downward and sunken, ataxia, headache, seizure activity

Redness or swelling along shunt tract or operative site
Change in feeding patterns, loss of appetite, vomiting
Instructions given to family on signs, symptoms, and complications
Child's developmental status
Coping skills of the family and knowledge deficit
All caregiver teaching
   Topics to include in the teaching plan:
      safe and correct handling of equipment/supplies
      emergency procedures
      underlying disease pathology
      appropriate community resources and contact persons

INTERDISCIPLINARY COLLABORATION
It is important to provide support for these families through parent groups, social services, and community agencies. Such support will assist in the development of coping skills and will help to reduce the fears associated wth caring for the child with a neurological disorder [1, 5, 21, 32].

PROCEDURE
Seizure Management

DESCRIPTION
Seizures are transient alterations of the brain's electrical system. These alterations are characterized by a change in level of consciousness, motor, sensory, or autonomic functioning. Seizures can be classified as:

1) petit mal: a loss of consciousness without motor movement
2) grand mal: generalized tonic, colonic muscle movements
3) febrile: tonic, colonic movements due to extreme elevation in body temperature
4) status epilepticus: repetitive tonic, colonic seizures without regaining consciousness.

PURPOSE
To enforce seizure precautions with the family/caregiver

EQUIPMENT
Health Assessment forms
Educational materials
Seizure activity log

OUTCOMES
The child/caregiver will:

▶ Be free from injury
▶ Maintain good dental hygiene
▶ Be knowledgeable about seizure disorder

ASSESSMENT DATA
Note type of seizure observed
Record date, time of onset, and duration of seizure
Note activity of child at time of onset
Note postictal status of the child
Review medication profile with caregiver and determine level of understanding

RELATED NURSING DIAGNOSES
At risk for injury
Knowledge deficit
Anxiety
Fear

SPECIAL CONSIDERATIONS
The most important consideration is that the family/caregiver be knowledgeable and comfortable in caring for the child. The caregiver must remain calm and in control when the child is experiencing a seizure to be of any assistance.

TRANSCULTURAL CONSIDERATIONS
An interpreter will be needed for clients unable to speak English. Support and maintain the client's religious and cultural healthcare practices. Acquire healthcare materials written in the client's native language, if available. Consider use of AT& T Language Line. See also the Culturological Assessment procedure in Unit 2 for general overview of cultural considerations.

▶ INTERVENTIONS

1. Wash hands.

Prevents transmission of microbes

2. Perform physical assessment.

Establishes baseline information of physiological data findings

3. Reinforce seizure precautions with family by providing a safe environment for the child having a seizure.
    Move child to floor
    Remove any article in the vicinity that may cause harm
    Loosen all restrictive clothing
    Never restrain a child having a seizure
    Position child on his or her side or stomach to prevent aspiration in vomiting
    Position head midline not hyperextended to maintain airway
    Do not place anything in child's mouth
    Stay with child until seizure is over and support child

Prevents injury

4. Instruct caregiver to keep a log of all seizure activity

Provides essential data for physician

5. Encourage child safety in daily living by:
    Promoting safe age-appropriate activities
    Avoiding dangerous play activities (i.e., tree climbing)
    Using helmet during bike riding
    Supervising bathing and water sports

Eliminates risk of injury

6. Instruct caregiver on importance of complying with medication administration. Stress the importance of periodic drug levels to assure therapeutic dose is maintained.

Increases caregiver's knowledge base

7. Encourage regular dental check-ups and good dental hygiene.

Some anticonvulsants may cause tooth and gum disorder

8. Child should wear medical ID tag.

Source of immediate information for healthcare providers

DOCUMENTATION

The following should be noted in the nursing note:

Any observed seizure activity
Instruction given to child or caregiver
Concerns or fears of child/caregiver
Developmental and emotional status of the child
Compliance and coping skills of family/child
All caregiver teaching
    Topics to include in the teaching plan:
        safe and correct handling of equipment/supplies
        emergency procedures
        underlying disease pathology
        appropriate community resources and contact persons

INTERDISCIPLINARY COLLABORATION

Consider refering the caregiver to community and parent support groups to aid in the development of coping skills.

All professionals that care for the child with seizures should be instructed in seizure precautions. This includes day care workers, teachers, and camp counselors.

The physician should coordinate the medical management of the child and all those involved. [1, 5, 12, 21, 32]

PROCEDURE

Impaired Motor Function and Muscle Tone Management

DESCRIPTION

Children diagnosed with impaired motor function and muscle tone are classified as chronically ill. Characteristics of these disease processes result in multisystem dysfunction, a developmental delay in both physical and mental status, and immobilization. Often these children are bedridden and wheel chairbound.

PURPOSE

To instruct the family in the care of a chronically ill child

EQUIPMENT

Health Assessment forms
Assistive devices for mobilization
Splints
Educational materials

OUTCOMES

The child/caregiver will:

▶ Maintain skin integrity
▶ Be free from infection
▶ Receive adequate nutritional intake

▶ Evaluate bowel and bladder function
▶ Provide ROM exercises to extremities
▶ Demonstrate ability to provide care for the child
▶ Provide age specific developmental activities

ASSESSMENT DATA

Perform general physical assessment
Note presence of respiratory compromise
Note skin redness caused by pressure on an area
Evaluate nutritional status
Evaluate feeding pattern; diet, frequency, and route
Evaluate tolerance to feedings
Observe motor function status, presence of contractures, spasticity of extremities
Note developmental milestones
Evaluate family's understanding of disease process and ability to provide care
Review medication profile with caregiver and determine level of understanding

RELATED NURSING DIAGNOSES

Impaired gas exchange
Altered skin integrity
Altered nutrition less than body requirements
At risk for infection
Altered growth and development
Altered mobility
Ineffective family coping skills

SPECIAL CONSIDERATIONS

The coping skills of families who have a chronically ill child are tested over and over. Stress becomes overwhelming at times for the caregiver in the family. Because the sick child requires so much attention, the entire family structure is reorganized to meet those needs. A great deal of support is necessary to guide the family to provide as near a normal environment as possible.

TRANSCULTURAL CONSIDERATIONS

An interpreter will be needed for clients unable to speak English. Support and maintain the client's religious and cultural healthcare practices. Acquire healthcare materials written in the client's native language, if available. Consider use of AT&T Language Line. See also the Culturological Assessment procedure in Unit 2 for general overview of cultural considerations.

▶ INTERVENTIONS

1. Wash hands.	*Prevents transmission of microbes*
2. Perform physical assessment.	*Establishes baseline information of physiological data findings*
3. Instruct family on how to care for the child.	*Eliminates knowledge deficit*
4. Instruct caregiver in performance of ADLs and permit return demonstration.	*Documents caregiver's ability to maintain child's basic needs*
5. Maintain proper body positioning: Keep head midline Use pillows, rolls, cushions to position and stabilize child	*Supports skeletal alignment*

Keep a neutral body position (i.e., side-lying, supine, or seated)	
6. Change position every 2–3 hours.	*Maintains skin integrity*
7. Apply splints to extremities, and perform active and passive ROM exercises.	*Prevents contractures and increases muscle strength*
8. Teach transfer, moving and positioning skills	*Prevents the risk of injury*
9. Encourage well-balanced, high-caloric diet. Instruct in tube feedings and feeding positions.	*Provides nutrition for proper growth, development and elimination*
10. Provide sensory stimulation through play therapy and during ROM exercises and ADLs.	*Promotes communication skills*
11. Support family in their attempts to care for the child.	*Encourages the family to comply with the treatment plan*

DOCUMENTATION

The following should be noted in the nursing note:

Child's general condition
Motor impairments
Adaptive appliances/devices needed
Diet, route of feeding, feeding intolerance
Site of feeding devices (i.e., gastrostomy tube)
Therapies performed and response to therapy
Developmental status
Presence of pain or discomfort during care
Family's interaction with child, knowledge of treatment plan, ability to change plan as needed, coping skills and teaching or instruction given to family
All caregiver teaching
   Topics to include in the teaching plan:
      safe and correct handling of equipment/supplies
      emergency procedures
      underlying disease pathology
      appropriate community resources and contact persons

INTERDISIPLINARY COLLABORATION:

The treatment plan for a child who is chronically ill is based on several therapies all working together with the family. These services include physical therapy, occupational therapy and speech language pathology working in collaboration with the home care team. Social services are essential to aid the family in acquiring community services that will support and aid them in caring for their child. [1, 5, 12, 13, 32]

PROCEDURE
Pain Management

DESCRIPTION

The pain experienced by children may be transient or chronic in nature. Sources of pain include surgical procedures, degenerative diseases, inflammatory disorders, fractures, malignancies, and medical procedures.

Since pain is a subjective experience, responses to pain are demonstrated by the child's developmental growth.

The management of pain includes the use of analgesic agents and nonpharmacologic interventions such as relaxation, diversion, play therapy, and massage.

PURPOSE
To provide adequate pain control through instruction on assessment, medication, and comfort measures

EQUIPMENT
Health Assessment forms
Pain log
Educational materials

OUTCOMES
The child/caregiver will:

▶ Be free of pain and able to continue with daily activities
▶ Exhibit normal vital signs for age
▶ Cope with the need to provide consistent pain management for the child

ASSESSMENT DATA
Question the child/caregiver about location of the pain
Use pain rating scale to determine intensity of the pain
Evaluate child's behavior in response to pain
Secure caregiver involvement to enlist cooperation of the child
Determine cause of pain
Evaluate child's response to intervention

RELATED NURSING DIAGNOSES
Activity intolerance
Anxiety
Knowledge deficit
Altered sleep pattern
Altered growth and development
Pain

SPECIAL CONSIDERATION:
Behavioral responses to pain are exhibited through the developmental growth of the child. The following behaviors are signs that the child may be experiencing pain:

▶ *Infants:* crying, irritability, grimacing, thrashing, refusal to eat, disturbed sleeping patterns, flexing of legs, generalized rigidity
▶ *Toddlers through school age:* screaming or loud crying, irritability, restlessness, complaints of pain or discomfort, clinging, rigid muscles in limb and body, gritting teeth, and refusal to move a body part or play
▶ *Adolescents:* able to verbally identify site, intensity, duration, and sensation of pain

The physiological signs of pain identified regardless of age include:

▶ Increased heart rate, blood pressure, respirations, diaphoreses, decreased oxygen saturation, dilated pupils, flushing, pallor, nausea, and muscle tension
▶ Behavioral changes are demonstrated through fear, anxiety, withdrawal, and regression.

TRANSCULTURAL CONSIDERATIONS

An interpreter will be needed for clients unable to speak English. Support and maintain the client's religious and cultural healthcare practices. Acquire healthcare materials written in the client's native language, if available. Consider use of AT&T Language Line. See also the Culturological Assessment procedure in Unit 2 for general overview of cultural considerations.

▶ INTERVENTIONS

1. Wash hands.	*Prevents transmission of microbes*
2. Assess child's response to pain.	*Establishes baseline*
3. Assess type, intensity, and duration of pain and record findings.	*Documents pain characteristics*
4. Ask child to describe pain by use of appropriate pain scale (see Display 5-3).	*Evaluates child's pain*
5. Evaluate caregiver/family's ability to respond to child's pain.	*Assesses caregiver's ability to care for the child*
6. Instruct caregiver to keep a log on frequency of pain, duration, therapy used, child's response to therapy, events around incidence of pain.	*Documents information to alert caregiver when pain therapy is needed. Informs physician of the effect of the plan of treatment*
7. Evaluate caregiver's knowledge on side effects of analgesics and ability to administer therapies that are nonpharmacological.	*Documents caregiver's ability to implement interventional strategies*
8. Collaborate with caregiver in planning strategies for treating pain before it becomes severe or in anticipation of a painful procedure.	*Mutually developed plans of care ensure compliance*

DOCUMENTATION

The following should be noted in the nursing note:

Child's verbal/nonverbal responses to pain
Cause of pain acute or chronic
Pain therapy used and child response to therapy
Pain and family coping skills related to pain management
Instruction given to caregiver/family on comfort measures or changes in plan of treatment to alleviate pain
All caregiver teaching:
    Topics to include in the teaching plan:
        safe and correct handling of equipment/supplies
        emergency procedures
        underlying disease pathology
        appropriate community resources and contact persons

INTERDISCIPLINARY COLLABORATION

Inform the physician on the effectiveness of the pain management plan. Whenever there is a change in the severity or frequency of the pain experienced, the physician should be notified. Members of the pain management team should be informed of changes as well. They may be able to offer suggestions that can be very helpful in relieving pain. [5, 12, 13, 21, 32]

Pain Rating Scales for Children

Faces Pain Rating Scale

This scale may be used for children as young as 3 years old.

Explain that the FACE 0 is a very happy face because there is no pain. FACE 1 hurts just a little bit. FACE 2 hurts a little bit more. FACE 3 hurts even more. FACE 4 hurts a whole lot. FACE 5 hurts very bad; it can make you cry.

Ask the child to choose the face that best describes the pain that is felt.

Numeric Scale

This scale can be used with children as young as 5 years old. 0 means no pain at all, 10 meaning the worst pain possible. Ask the child to choose on a scale from 0-10 the pain he is feeling.

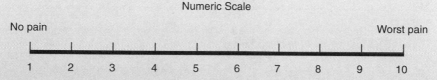

Word Graphic Rating Scale

This scale can be used with children from ages 4 years to 17 years. Ask the child to mark the line that best describes the pain you have. The more pain experienced the closer to 5 worst pain should be indicated

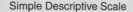
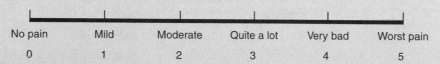

Faces Pain Rating Scale. Purdue Frederick Co., 100 Conneticut Ave., Norwalk, CT, 06856; 203-853-0123, ext 4010.
Numeric Scale. Wong, D. Wong and Whaley's Clinical Manual of Pediatric Nursing. St. Louis: Mosby, 1996.
Word Graphic Rating Scale from the Adolescent Pediatric Pain Study, University of California, School of Nursing. Department of Family Health Care Nursing. San Francisco, CA. 94143-0606; (415)-476-4040.

REFERENCES

1. Ahmann, E. *Home care for the high-risk infant: A family centered approach.* Gaithersburg, MD: An Aspen Publication, 1996.
2. Baker, SB, Baker, RD, & Davis, A, eds. *Pediatric enteral nutrition.* New York: Chapman & Hall, 1994.
3. Boswick, JA. *The Art and Science of Wound Care.* Rockland, MD: Aspen Publishers, 1987.
4. Brucker, JM, Wallin, KD, *Manual of pediatric nursing: Pediatric fact finder,* Boston: Little, Brown and Company, 1996.

5. Carpenito, LJ. *Nursing diagnosis: Application to clinical practice,* 7th, Edition. Philadelphia, PA: Lippincott, 1997.
6. *Coram healthcare corporation nursing orientation manual.* Denver, CO: The Corporation, 1995.
7. Glass, CA. *Home care management of ventilator-assisted patients.* Aliso Viejo: American Association of Critical-Care Nurses, 1998.
8. Gorski, LA. *High-tech home care manual.* Gaithersburg, MD: Aspen Publishers, Inc., 1997.
9. Gottschlich, MM, Matarese, LE, & Shronts, EP, eds. *Nutrition support dietetics core curriculum,* 2nd Edition. Silver Springs, MD: A.S.P.E.N., 1993.
10. Groh-Wargo, S, Thompson, M, Cox, JH, eds. *Nutritional care for high-risk newborns.* Chicago, IL: Precept Press, Inc., 1994.
11. Hodgson, BB & Kizior, RJ. *Saunders nursing drug handbook 1999.* Philadelphia, PA: WB Saunders Company, 1999.
12. Jaffe, MS, & Skidmore-Roth, L. *Home health nursing assessment and care planning.* St. Louis, MO: Mosby, 1997.
13. Johnson, JY, Smith-Temple, J., & Carr, P. *Nurses' guide to home health procedures.* Philadelphia, PA: Lippincott, 1998.
14. Keller, L & Weir, A. *The Skidmore-Roth outline series: pediatric nursing.* El Paso, TX: Skidmore-Roth Inc., 1993.
15. Kelley, CH, McBride, LH, & Randolph, SR, et al. *Home care management of the blood cell transplant patient.* Sudbury, MA: Jones and Bartlett Publishers, Inc. 1996.
16. Marks, *Broadribb's introductory pediatric nursing 5th ed.* Philadelphia, PA: Lippincott, 1998.
17. Martyn, JA. *Acute management of the burned patient.* Philadelphia, PA: WB Saunders, 1990.
18. McNeal, GJ. *Nursing care of the clients with burns.* In P. LeMone and K. Burke, Medical-Surgical Nursing: Critical Thinking in Client Care. California: Addison-Wesley Nursing. 1996, pp. 626–658.
19. Melko, M. *Pediatric formulas beyond infancy.* Building Block for Life—Ross Products Division Abbott Laboratories 1997; 21(3):1– 3, 7–8.
20. Melson, K & Jaffe, S., *Pediatric and postpartum home health nursing assessment and care planning,* St. Louis, MO: Mosby-Year Book Inc., 1997.
21. Nettina, SM, ed. *The Lippincott manual of nursing practice.* Philadelphia, PA: Lippincott, 1996.
22. *Nurses' handbook of home infusion therapy.* Springhouse, PA: Springhouse Home Care, 1997.
23. *Nurses' illustrated handbook of home health procedures.* Springhouse, PA: Springhouse Corporation, 1999.
24. *Nutrition assessment of pediatric patient and enteral and parenteral nutrition in the pediatric patient.* Coram Healthcare Corporation Policy and Procedure Clinical Manual. Denver, CO: The Corporation, 1997.
25. Powers, MA, ed. *Nutrition guide for professionals: diabetes education and meal planning.* Chicago, IL: American Dietetic Association and Alexandria, Va: American Diabetes Association, 1988.
26. Queen, PM, & Lang, CE., eds. *Handbook of pediatric nutrition.* Gaithersburg, MD: Aspen Publications, 1993.
27. Rice, R. *Procedures in home mechanical ventilation management.* Home Health Care Nurse. 13:73, 1995.
28. Richard, R, & Staley, M. *Burn care and rehabilitation: Principles and practice.* Philadelphia, PA: FA Davis, 1994.
29. Stanhope, M, & Knollmueller, RN. *Handbook of community and home health nursing.* St. Louis, MO: Mosby, 1996.
30. Sussman, C, & Bates-Jensen, B. *Wound care: A collaborative practice manual for physical therapists and nurses.* Gaithersburg, MD: Aspen Publishers, Inc., 1998.
31. *Pediatric manual of clinical dietetics.* Chicago, IL: American Dietetic Association, 1998.
32. Wong, D. *Wong and Whaley's clinical manual of pediatric nursing,* 4th ed. St Louis, MO: Mosby-Year Book Inc., 1996.

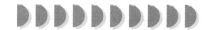

Appendices

Metric Units and Symbols

Quantity	Unit	Symbol	Equivalent
Length	millimeter	mm	1000 mm = 1 m
	centimeter	cm	100 cm = 1 m
	decimeter	dm	10 dm = 1 m
	meter	m	1000 m = 1 km
Volume	cubic centimeter	cc or cm³	1000 cc = 1 cm³ or liter
	milliliter	ml	1000 mL = 1 liter
	cu decimeter	dm³	1000 dm³ = 1 m³
	liter	L	1000 L = 1 m³
Mass	microgram	μg	1000 μg = 1 mg
	milligram	mg	1000 mg = 1 g
	gram	g	1000 g = 1 kg
	kilogram	kg	1000 kg = 1 metric ton (t)

Table of Metric and Apothecaries' Systems

(Approved *approximate* dose equivalents are enclosed in parentheses. Use exact equivalents in calculations.)

Conversion Factors

Metric	Apothecaries	Metric	Apothecaries
1 milligram (mg)	$\frac{1}{64}$ grain	3.888 cubic centimeters or grams	1 dram (4 cc or grams)
64.79 milligrams	1 grain (65 mg)	31.103 cubic centimeters or grams	1 ounce (30 cc or grams)
1 gram	15.43 grains (15 grains)	473.167 cubic centimeters	1 pint (500 cc)
1 cubic centimeter (cc)*	16 minims		

* Note: A cubic centimeter (cc.) is the approximate equivalent of a milliliter (ml.). The terms are used interchangeably in general medicine.

Celsius (Centigrade) and Fahrenheit Temperatures

Celsius (Centigrade) 0°	Fahrenheit 32°
36.0	96.8
36.5	97.7
37.0	98.6
37.5	99.5
38.0	100.4
38.5	101.3
39.0	102.2
39.5	103.1
40.0	104.0
40.5	104.9
41.0	105.8
41.5	106.7
42.0	107.6

CELSIUS

To convert degrees F. to degrees C.
Subtract 32, then multiply by 5/9

To convert degrees C. to degrees F.
Multiply by 9/5, then add 32

APPENDICES 5-1 ▶ Conversion tables

Blood Chemistries

These values are compiled from a review of current published literature, however, normal values vary with the analytic method used. If any doubt exists, consult your laboratory for its analytical method and normal range of values.

Determination	Conventional Units	SI Units	Determination	Conventional Units	SI Units
Acid phosphatase			Bilirubin (total)		
Newborn	7.4–19.4 U/ml	7.4–19.4 U/ml	Cord	<1.8 mg/dl	<30.6 µmol/L
2–13 yr	6.4–15.2 U/ml	6.4–15.2 U/ml	24 h		
Adult	M: 0.5–11 U/ml	0.5–11.0 U/ml	Preterm	≤8 mg/dl	≤103 µmol/L
	F: 0.2–9.5 U/ml	0.2–9.5 U/ml	Term	≤6 mg/dl	≤103 µmol/L
Alanine amino-			48 h		
transferase (ALT)			Preterm	<12 mg/dl	<137 µmol/L
Infants	<54 U/L	<54 U/L	Term	≤ 8 mg/dl	≤120 µmol/L
Children/adults	1–30 U/L	1–30 U/L	3–5 days		
Aldolase			Preterm	≤16 mg/dl	≤205 µmol/L
Adult	<8 U/L	<8 U/L	Term	≤12 mg/dl	<205 µmol/L
Children	<16 U/L	<16 U/L	1 mo-Adult	≤ 2 mg/dl	≤26 µmol/L
Newborn	<32 U/L	<32 U/L	Conjugated	≤ 1 mg/dl	≤9 µmol/L
Alkaline phosphatase			Calcium (total)		
Infant	150–420 U/L	150–400 U/L	Premature < 1 week	6–10 mg/dl	1.5–2.5 mmol/L
2–10 yr	100–320 U/L	100–300 U/L	Full-term < 1 week	7–12 mg/dl	1.75–3 mmol/L
11–18 yr			Child	8–10.5 mg/dl	2–2.6 mmol/L
Male	100–390 U/L	50–375 U/L	Adult	8.5–10.5 mg/dl	2.1–2.6 mmol/L
Female	100–320 U/L	30–300 U/L	Calcium (ionized)	4.4–5.4 mg/dl	0.1–1.35 mmol/L
Adult	30–120 U/L	30–100 U/L	Carbon dioxide		
Alpha-1-antitrypsin	2.1–5 gm/L		(CO$_2$ content)		
Alpha-fetoprotein	<10 mg/dl	<0.1 g/L	Cord blood	15–20 mmol/L	15–20 mmol/L
Ammonia nitrogen			Child	18–27 mmol/L	18–27 mmol/L
(venous sample:			Adult	24–35 mmol/L	24–35 mmol/L
heparinized			Carbon monoxide		
specimen in ice			(carboxyhemoglobin)		
water and analyzed			Nonsmoker	<2% of total	
within 30 min)				hemoglobin	
All ages	13–48 µg/dl	9÷34 µmol/L	Smoker	<10% of total	
Amylase				hemoglobin	
Newborn	5–65 U/L	5–65 U/L	Lethal	>60% of total	
> 1 yr	0–88 U/L	25–125 U/L		hemoglobin	
Arsenic	<10 µg/dl	<0.4 mmol/L	Carotenoids (carotenes)		
Aspartate			Infant	20–70 µg/dl	0.37–1.30 µmol/L
aminotransferase			Child	40–130 µg/dl	0.74–2.42 µmol/L
(AST)			Adult	60–200 µg/dl	1.12–3.72 µmol/L
Newborn/infant	25–75 U/L	25–75 U/L	Ceruloplasmin	23–58 mg/dl	1.32–3.83 µmol/L
Child/adult	0–40 U/L	0–40 U/L	Chloride	94–106 mEq/L	94–106 mmol/L
Bicarbonate			Cholesterol	See Lipids	
Premature	18–26 mEq/L	18–26 mmol/L	Copper		
Infant	20–26 mEq/L	20–26 mmol/L	0–6 mo	<70 µg/dl	<11 µmol/L
>2 yr	22–26 mEq/L	22–26 mmol/L	6 mo—5 yr	27–153 µg/dl	4.2–24.1 µmol/L
			5–17 yr	94–234 µg/dl	14.2–36.8 µmol/L
			Adult	70–155 µg/dl	11–24.4 µmol/L

(continued)

APPENDICES 5-2 ▶ Pediatric Laboratory Values

Blood Chemistries (continued)

Creatine Kinase (Creatine Phosphokinase)

Upper 95th Percentile (U/L)

Age	Males	Females
1 d	600	500
2–10 d	440	440
<1 yr	170	170
1–7 yr	109	100
7–9 yr	103	85
9–11 yr	109	88
11–13 yr	108	85
13–15 yr	129	85
15–17 yr	247	74
17–19 yr	190	68

Creatinine (serum)

Upper Limits, mg/dl (μmol/L)

Age (yr)	Males	Females
1	0.6 (53)	0.5 (44)
2–3	0.7 (62)	0.6 (53)
4–7	0.8 (71)	0.7 (62)
8–10	0.9 (80)	0.8 (71)
11–12	1.0 (88)	0.9 (80)
13–17	1.2 (106)	1.1 (97)
18–20	1.3 (115)	1.1 (97)
Adult	1.2 (106)	1.4 (124)

Ferritin		
Children	7–144 ng/ml	7–144 μg/L
Adult	F: 10–110 ng/ml	10–110 μg/L
	M: 30–265 ng/ml	30–265 μg/L
Fibrin degradation products		
Titer	1:50 = positive	
Fibrinogen	200–400 mg/dl	2–4 g/L
Folic acid (folate)	1.9–14 ng/L	4.3–23.6 nmol/L
Galactose		
Newborn	0–20 mg/dl	0–1.11 mmol/L
Thereafter	<5 mg/dl	<0.28 mmol/L
Gammaglutamyl transferase (GGT)		
Cord	19–270 U/L	19–270 U/L
Premature	56–233 U/L	56–233 U/L
0–3 wk	0–130 U/L	0–130 U/L
3 wk–3 mo	4–120 U/L	4–120 U/L
>3 mo		
M	5–65 U/L	5–65 U/L
F	5–35 U/L	5–35 U/L
1–15 yr	0–23 U/L	0–23 U/L
16 yr—Adult	0–35 U/L	0–35 U/L
Gastrin	<300 pg/ml	<300 ng/L
Glucose (serum)		
Premature	20–65 mg/dl	1.1–3.6 mmol/L
Full term	20–110 mg/dl	1.1–6.4 mmol/L
1 wk–16 yr	60–105 mg/dl	3.3–5.8 nmol/L
>16 yr	70–115 mg/dl	3.9–6.4 nmol/L
Haptoglobin*	400–1800 mg/L	0.4–1.8 g/L

* Detectable in only 10%–20 % of newborns.
† Use of oral contraceptives significantly raises both total serum cholesterol and serum triglyceride levels.

Iron

	Iron		Iron Binding Capacity		% Saturation
	(μg/dl)	(μmol/L)	(μg/dl)	(μmol/L)	(μg/dl)
Newborn	110–270	19.7–48.3	59–175	10.6–31.3	65%
4–10 mo	30–70	5.4–12.5	250–400	45–72	25%
3–10 yr	53–119	9.5–27.0	250–400	45–72	30%
Adult	72–186	12.9–33.3	250–400	45–72	35%

Ketones		
Qualitative	Negative	
Quantitative	up to 3 mg%	
Lactate		
Capillary blood		
Newborn	≤30 mg/dl	<3.0 mmol/L
Child	5–20 mg/dl	0.56–2.25 mmol/L
Venous	5–18 mg/dl	0.5–2.0 mmol/L
Arterial	3–7 mg/dl	0.3–0.8 mmol/L
Lactate dehydrogenase (37°C)		
Newborn	160–1500 U/L	160–1500 U/L
Infant	150–360 U/L	150–360 U/L
Child	150–300 U/L	150–300 U/L
Adult	100–250 U/L	100–250 U/L
Lactate dehydrogenase isoenzymes (% total)		
LD$_1$ Heart		24–34%
LD$_2$ Heart, erythrocytes		35–45%
LD$_3$ Muscle		15–25%
LD$_4$ Liver, trace muscle		4–10%
LD$_5$ Liver, muscle		1–9%
Lipase	20–180 U/L	20–180 U/L
Lipids		

Normal Upper Limits

	Total Serum Cholesterol mg/dl (mmol/L)		Serum Triglycerides mg/dl (g/L)	
Age	Males	Females†	Males	Females*
0–4 yr	203 (5.28)	200 (5.2)	99 (0.99)	112 (1.12)
5–9	203 (5.28)	205 (5.33)	101 (1.01)	105 (1.05)
10–14	202 (5.25)	201 (5.22)	125 (1.25)	131 (1.31)
15–19	197 (5.12)	200 (5.2)	148 (1.48)	124 (1.24)

	HDL-Cholesterol mg/dl (mmol/L)		Normal Upper Limits LDL mg/dl (mmol/L)		VLDL mg/dl (mml/L)	
Age	Males	Females	Males	Females	Males	Females
0–4	—	—	—	—	—	—
5–9	74 (1.91)	73 (1.89)	129 (3.34)	140 (3.62)	18 (0.47)	24 (0.62)
10–14	74 (1.91)	70 (1.81)	132 (3.41)	136 (3.52)	22 (0.57)	23 (0.59)
15–19	63 (1.63)	73 (1.89)	130 (3.36)	135 (3.49)	26 (0.67)	24 (0.62)

Magnesium	1.5–2 mEq/L	0.75–1 mmol/L
Manganese (blood)		
Newborn	2.4–9.6 μg/dl	2.44–1.75 μmol/L
2–18 yr	0.8–2.1 μg/dl	0.15–0.38 μmol/L
Methemoglobin	<0.3 g/dl or <3% of total Hb	<46.5 μmol/L
5′ Nucleotidase	2.2–15 U/L	2.2–15 U/L
Osmolality	285–295 mOsm/kg	270–285 mOsm/L plasma
Phenylalanine		
Premature	2.0–7.5 mg/dl	
Newborn	<4 mg/dl	<0.24 mmol/L
Child	<3 mg/dl	<0.18 mmol/L

Blood Chemistries (continued)

Phosphorus
Newborn	4.2–9.0 mg/dl	1.36–2.91 mmol/L
1 yr	3.8–6.2 mg/dl	1.23–2.0 mmol/L
2–5 yr	3.5–6.8 mg/dl	1.13–2.2 mmol/L
Adult	3.0–4.5 mg/dl	0.97–1.45 mmol/L
Porcelain	10–25 mg/dl	No SI conversion factor

Potassium
<10 days of age	3.5–6 mEq/L	3.5–6 mmol/L
>10 days of age	3.5–5 mEq/L	3.5–5 mmol/L

Prolactin
Newborn	<200 ng/ml	<200 µg/L
Adult	<20 ng/ml	<20 µg/L

Proteins Average (Range) in gr/dl

Age	Total	Albu-min	Globu-lin	Gamma Globu-lin
Premature	5.5 (4.0–7.0)	3.7 (2.5–4.5)	1.8 (1.2–2.0)	0.7 (0.5–0.9)
FT newborn	6.4 (5.0–7.1)	3.4 (2.5–5.0)	3.1 (1.2–4.0)	0.8 (0.7–0.9)
1-mo	6.6 (4.7–7.4)	3.8 (3.0–4.2)	2.5 (1.0–3.3)	0.3 (0.1–0.5)
3–12 mo	6.8 (5.0–7.5)	3.9 (2.7–5.0)	2.6 (2.0–3.8)	0.6 (0.4–1.2)
1–15 yr	7.4 (6.5–8.6)	4.0 (3.2–5.0)	3.1 (2.0–4.0)	0.9 (0.6–1.2)

Pyruvate   0.3–0.9 mg/dl   50–140 mmol/L

Sodium
Premature	130–140 mEq/L	130–140 mmol/L
Older	135–145 mEq/L	135–145 mmol/L

Transaminase (SGOT)	See Aspartate Aminotransferase (AST)	
Transaminase (SGPT)	See Alanine Aminotransferase (AT)	
Triglycerides	See Lipids	
Urea nitrogen	5–25 mg/dl	1.8–9 mmol/L

Uric acid
0–2 yr	2.0–7.0 mg/dl	0.12–0.42 mmol/L
2–12 yr	2.0–6.5 mg/dl	0.12–0.39 mmol/L
12–14 yr	2.0–7.0 mg/dl	0.12–0.42 mmol/L
14–adult		
M	3.0–8.0 mg/dl	0.18–0.48 mmol/L
F	2.0–7.0 mg/dl	0.12–0.42 mmol/L

Vitamin A (retinol)
0–1 yr	20–90 µg/dl	0.7–3.14 µmol/L
1–5 yr	30–100 µg/dl	1.05–3.50 µmol/L
5–16 yr	60–100 µg/dl	2.09–3.50 µmol/L
Adult	20–80 µg/dl	0.70–2.79 µmol/L
Vitamin B_1 (thiamine)	5.3–7.9 µg/dl	0.16–0.23 µmol/L
Vitamin B_2 (riboflavin)	3.7–13.7 µg/dl	98–363 mmol/L
Vitamin B_{12} (cobalamin)	130–785 pg/ml	96–579 pmol/L
Vitamin C (ascorbic acid)	0.2–2 mg/dl	11.4–113.6 µmol/L

Vitamin D (1.25 dihydroxy)
Newborn	21 ± 2 pg/ml	50 ± 4.8 nmol/L
Child	43 ± 3 pg/ml	103 ± 7.2 nmol/L
Adult	29 ± 2 pg/ml	69.6 ± 4.8 nmol/L
Vitamin E	5–20 µg/dl	8.4–23 µmol/L
Zinc	55–150 µg/dl	8.4–23 µmol/L

(From Johns Hopkins Hospital. The Harriet Lane Handbook. 13th ed. Chicago, Year Book Medical Pub, 1993)

Normal Values—Hematology

Age	Hgb (gm %) Mean (−2SD)	HCT (%) Mean (−2SD)	MCV (fl.) Mean (−2SD)	MCHC (gm/% RBC) Mean (−2SD)	Retic (%)	WBC/mm³ × 100 Mean (−2SD)	Plts (10³/mm³) Mean (±2SD)
26–30 wk gestation*	13.4 (11)	41.5 (34.9)	118.2 (106.7)	37.9 (30.6)	—	4.4 (2.7)	254 (180–327)
28 wk	14.5	45	120	31	(5–10)	—	275
32 wk	15.0	47	118	32	(3–10)	—	290
Term† (cord)	16.5 (13.5)	51 (42)	108 (98)	33 (30)	(3–7)	18.1 (9–30)‡	290
1–3 days	18.5 (14.5)	56 (45)	108 (95)	33 (29)	(1.8–4.6)	18.9 (9.4–34)	192
2 wk	16.6 (13.4)	53 (41)	105 (88)	31.4 (28.1)		11.4 (5–20)	252
1 mo	13.9 (10.7)	44 (33)	101 (91)	31.8 (28.1)	(0.1–1.7)	10.8 (5–19.5)	
2 mo	11.2 (9.4)	35 (28)	95 (84)	31.8 (28.3)			
6 mo	12.6 (11.1)	36 (31)	76 (68)	35 (32.7)	(0.7–2.3)	11.9 (6–17.5)	
6 mo—2 yr	12 (10.5)	36 (33)	78 (70)	33 (30)		10.6 (6–17)	(150–350)
2–6 yr	12.5 (11.5)	37 (34)	81 (75)	34 (31)	(0.5–1.0)	8.5 (5–15.5)	(150–350)
6–12 yr	13.5 (11.5)	40 (35)	86 (77)	34 (31)	(0.5–1.0)	8.1 (4.5–13.5)	(150–350)
12–18 yr							
Male	14.5 (13)	43 (36)	88 (78)	34 (31)	(0.5–1.0)	7.8 (4.5–13.5)	(150–350)
Female	14 (12)	41 (37)	90 (78)	34 (31)	(0.5–1.0)	7.8 (4.5–13.5)	(150–350)

* Values are from fetal samplings.
† Under 1 month, capillary Hgb exceeds venous: 1 h–3.6 gm difference; 5 days–2.2 gm difference; 3 wks–1.1 gm difference.
‡ Mean (95% confidence limits).
(From Johns Hopkins Hospital. The Harriet Lane Handbook. 13th ed. Chicago, Year Book Medical Pub, 1993)

APPENDICES 5-2 [CONTINUED] ▶ Pediatric Laboratory Values

Normal Serologic Reference Values

Determination	Value
Antinuclear antibody	<1:160
Anti-streptolysin	
O Titer*	
Preschool	<1:85
School ages and adults	<1:170
Older adults	<1:85
Anti-hyaluronidase	<1:256
Anti-nuclear Antibody	<1:160
C-reactive Protein	Negative
C_1 Esterase inhibitor	17.4–24 mg/dl
C_3	
1–6 mo	53–175 mg/dl
7–12 mo	75–180 mg/dl
1–5 yr	77–166 mg/dl
6–10 yr	88–199 mg/dl
Adult	83–177 mg/dl
C_4	
1–6 mo	7–42 mg/dl
7–12 mo	9.5–39 mg/dl
1–5 yr	9–40 mg/dl
6–10 yr	12–40 mg/dl
Adult	15–45 mg/dl
C_{H50}	75–160 U/ml
Rheumatoid factor	<20 negative
	20–40 suggestive
	≥80 positive
Rheumaton titer (modified Waaler-Rose slide test)	Negative
	≥10 may be significant
Total B cells	5%–20% of lymphocytes
Total T cells	50%–80% of lymphocytes
T helper cells	34%–56% of lymphoyctes
T suppressor cells	18%–32% of lymphocytes
Helper/suppressor ratio	1.1–2.5

* Significant if rising titer can be demonstrated at weekly intervals.
(From Johns Hopkins Hospital. The Harriet Lane Handbook. 13th ed. Chicago, Year Book Medical Pub, 1993)

Cerebrospinal Fluid Values

Determination	Value
Cell Count	
Preterm mean	9.0 (0–25.4 WBC/mm³) (57% PMNs)
Term mean	8.2 (0–22.4 WBC/mm³) (61% PMNs)
>1 mo	0–7 (0% PMNs)
Glucose	
Preterm	24–63 mg/dl (mean 50)
Term	34–119 mg/dl (mean 52)
Child	40–80 mg/dl
CSF Glucose/Blood Glucose (%)	
Preterm	55–105
Term	44–128
Child	50%
Lactic acid dehydrogenase	20 U/ml (range 5–30 U/ml)
Myelin basic protein	<4 ng/ml
Pressure (initial lumbar puncture)	
Newborn	80–110 (<110) mm H_2O
Infant	<200 (lateral recumbent position) mm H_2O
Child	
Respiratory movements	5–10 mm H_2O
Protein	
Preterm	65–150 mg/dl (mean 115)
Term	20–170 mg/dl (mean 90)
Children	
Ventricular	5–15 mg/dl
Cisternal	5–25 mg/dl
Lumbar	5–40 mg/dl

(From Johns Hopkins Hospital. The Harriet Lane Handbook. 13th ed. Chicago, Year Book Medical Pub, 1993)

Sample Conversions of Pounds and Ounces to Grams*

Pounds	Ounces															
	0	1	2	3	4	5	6	7	8	9	10	11	12	13	14	15
0	—	28	57	85	113	142	170	198	227	255	283	312	340	369	397	425
1	454	482	510	539	567	595	624	652	680	709	737	765	794	822	850	879
2	907	936	964	992	1021	1049	1077	1106	1134	1162	1191	1219	1247	1276	1304	1332
3	1361	1389	1417	1446	1474	1503	1531	1559	1588	1616	1644	1673	1701	1729	1758	1786
4	1814	1843	1871	1899	1928	1956	1984	2013	2041	2070	2098	2126	2155	2183	2211	2240
5	2268	2296	2325	2353	2381	2410	2438	2466	2495	2532	2551	2580	2608	2637	2665	2693
6	2722	2750	2778	2807	2835	2863	2892	2920	2948	2977	3005	3033	3062	3090	3118	3147

* 1 ounce = approximately 30 grams.
(From Avery GB. Neonatology. 4th ed. Philadelphia, JB Lippincott, 1994)

APPENDICES 5-2 [CONTINUED] ▶ Pediatric Laboratory Values

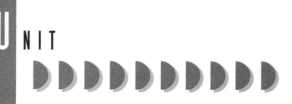

UNIT ▷▷▷▷▷▷▷▷▷▷

6 Adult Homecare

continued

1

Adult Respiratory System Procedures

Home Oxygen Administration

DESCRIPTION

With increasing frequency, the number of clients returning to the home setting with advanced pulmonary disease is growing significantly. Clients diagnosed with any of the following advanced lung conditions may be found in the home setting: pulmonary hypertension, chronic obstructive pulmonary disease, cystic fibrosis, and lung transplantation, to name a few. Depending on the severity of the pulmonary illness, clients may rquire oxygen administration in the home setting. The source of oxygen may be one of three types: the oxygen tank for short-term use, the liquid oxygen reservoir to fill a portable device, and the oxygen concentrator for long term use (Figure 6-1). The oxygen tank contains stored oxygen under pressure and typically holds enough oxygen to last for 1 to 3 hours depending on liter flow. The liquid oxygen reservoir is a system used for the more mobile client. The system permits the client to transfer oxygen from the reservoir to a refillable portable unit, which is worn over the shoulder. For more long-term therapy, an oxygen concentrator will be used to maintain a continuous source of oxygenation. The latter device works by concentrating the oxygen existing in ambient air to deliver the ordered liter flow [10, 19, 22, 41, 59].

PURPOSE

To improve oxygenation and prevent the development of atelectasis

EQUIPMENT

Oxygen tank/concentrator/reservoir
Flow meter
Pressure-reduction device if using a cylinder
Humidifier
Distilled water
Oxygen-in-use sign
Mask, cannula, trach collar, t-piece as appropriate
Tubing
Stethoscope
Suction equipment, if needed
Health Assessment forms

OUTCOMES

The client/caregiver will:

▸ Maintain adequate ventilation as determined by oximetry and physical assessment
▸ Demonstrate ability to perform procedure
▸ Verbalize understanding of procedure to follow in the event of equipment malfunction

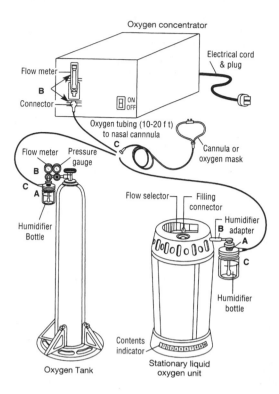

FIGURE 6-1 ▶ Three sources of oxygen.

ASSESSMENT DATA

Note signs and symptoms of hypoxemia
Record type and amount of oxygen therapy
Document respiratory rate and character
Review the prescribed medication therapy
Auscultate lung sounds and note abnormal sounds
Assess character of sputum
Assess client/caregiver's knowledge base regarding the procedure

RELATED NURSING DIAGNOSES

Impaired gas exchange
Altered breathing patterns
Ineffective airway clearance
Anxiety
Powerlessness

SPECIAL CONSIDERATIONS

Clients experiencing difficult breathing will often demonstrate signs of increased anxiety. Assisting the client to relax using correct breathing and relaxation techniques are priority nursing interventions. To safely maintain oxygen therapy in the home setting, see Unit 5 Management of Home Mechanical Ventilation, Pediatric. Be sure to inform the local fire department, electrical supplier, and the emergency medical service when oxygen is being used in the home.

TRANSCULTURAL CONSIDERATIONS

An interpreter will be needed for the client unable to speak or understand the English language

Obtain educational materials in the client's native language, if available

Contact the AT&T Language Line. See also the Culturological Assessment procedure in Unit 2 for general overview of cultural considerations

▶ INTERVENTIONS

1. Verify physician order.	*Reduces risk of error*
2. Wash hands.	*Prevents transmission of microbes*
3. Perform physical assessment.	*Establishes baseline information of physiological data findings*
4. Explain procedure.	*Allays anxiety*
5. Ensure safety of the home environment to support oxygen therapy.	*Oxygen supports the combustion of other materials and poses risk of fire*

For Portable Tank

1. Secure tank in designated stand.	*Prevents tank from falling*
2. Inspect tank for damage.	*Damage will cause malfunctioning of the equipment*
3. To open, turn outlet valve clockwise then close to bleed the tank.	*Bleeding blows out particulate matter*
4. Attach regulator and flowmeter per manufacture's recommendations.	*Ensures safe use*
5. Attach humidifier to flowmeter.	*Prevents drying of air passages*
6. Attach oxygen tubing to flowmeter and turn to ordered liter flow rate.	*Provides oxygen flow*
7. Apply appropriate oxygen delivery system (face mask, cannula, trach collar, t-piece) as ordered.	*Ensures oxygen delivery*
8. Check for visible and audible leaks in the system.	*Hazardous leaks pose risk of fire*
9. To close, turn outlet valve counterclockwise, turn flowmeter off, then on then off again, to bleed system.	*Prevents build up of pressure*
10. Instruct client to perform the procedure and permit return demonstration.	*Documents client's ability to perform ordered procedure*

For Oxygen Concentrator

1. Connect to three-pronged electrical outlet and never use an extension cord.	*Ensures adequate grounding of equipment*
2. Attach humidifier to flowmeter.	*Prevents drying of air passages*
3. Attach oxygen tubing to flowmeter and turn to ordered liter flow rate.	*Initiates oxygen flow*
4. Apply appropriate oxygen delivery system (face mask, cannula, trach collar, t-piece) as ordered.	*Ensures delivery of oxygen*

5. Check for signs of malfunction, if present, turn off the equipment and call the supplier.

6. Keep available supply of oxygen tanks for backup in case of power outage.

7. Instruct client to perform the procedure and permit return demonstration.

Malfunctioning equipment poses risk of fire

When electrical source fails, concentrator is rendered inoperable

Documents client's ability to perform ordered procedure

DOCUMENTATION
The following should be noted in the nursing note:

Client response to the procedure
Untoward responses reported to the physician
Interventions as a result of deviations from the norm
Respiratory physical assessment findings
All client/caregiver teaching:
    Topics to include in teaching plan:
        safe and correct equipment handling
        emergency procedures
        underlying disease pathology
        appropriate community resources and contact persons

INTERDISCIPLINARY COLLABORATION
Inform physician of presence of abnormal lung sounds, and compare with previous findings
Document interventions employed to treat untoward responses
Determine adequacy of supplies/equipment and need to initiate reorder from DME vendor or home health agency
Confer with respiratory therapist in the ordering/maintenance of respiratory equipment/supplies
Consult with social worker to determine client's eligibility for financial assistance/reimbursement for supplies and equipment, and to identify community resources [2, 6, 10, 15, 17, 19, 21, 22, 28, 33–35, 41, 57, 59]

PROCEDURE
Pulse Oximetry

DESCRIPTION
Pulse oximetry is a noninvasive monitoring technique designed to measure the arterial oxygen saturation of hemoglobin. The pulse oximeter device is composed of a monitor, cable, photodetector and connector. The device sends red and infrared light beams through body tissue that is highly perfused with arterial blood, and measures the relative amount of color absorbed by the arterial blood. The device also monitors pulse rate and amplitude. The monitor is preset with alarm limits, which, when exceeded, trigger a buzzing sound to alert the client and caregiver of the need for intervention [2, 4, 10, 41, 55].

PURPOSE
To evaluate adequacy of oxygenation

EQUIPMENT
Pulse oximeter
Sensor
Alcohol wipe
Nail polish remover
Health Assessment forms

OUTCOMES
The client/caregiver will:

▶ Maintain arterial oxygen saturation > 90%
▶ Demonstrate correct application of sensor
▶ Verbalize knowledge of factors that may affect accuracy of reading (displacement of probe, outside light, etc.)

ASSESSMENT DATA
Note signs and symptoms of hypoxemia
Record type and amount of oxygen therapy, if applicable
Document respiratory rate and character
Auscultate lung sounds and note abnormal sounds
Check quality of pulse and capillary refill proximal to selected sensor site

RELATED NURSING DIAGNOSES
Impaired gas exchange
Altered breathing patterns
Ineffective airway clearance
Anxiety
Powerlessness

SPECIAL CONSIDERATIONS
In the geriatric client, be aware of skin sensitivity to tape and pressure from the constant tension of the sensor. For the neonate or small infant, wrap the probe around the foot, and for the larger child select the great toe. If the client is wearing nail polish, use a polish remover to prevent obstruction of the light source. Trim long fingernails to permit proper positioning of the probe. Keep the client's hand positioned at the level of the heart while obtaining the reading to reduce possibility of venous pulsation. Be aware that clients with altered perfusion will have questionable readings secondary to poor circulation.

Review the client's medical record and note laboratory results for bilirubin, carboxyhemoglobin, or methemoglobin, if ordered. Elevated bilirubin may falsely lower the pulse oximeter reading, while elevated carboxyhemoglobin or methemoglobin levels will falsely elevate the reading. Be aware that ambient lighting may also interfere with the accuracy of the reading. If the room is too light, cover the probe. Observe for skin irritation at the probe site caused by adhesive tape, and consider the need to use nondisposable probes that do not require tape. Keep the monitoring site clean and dry to ensure accuracy of reading.

Generally, continuous monitoring of pulse oximetry readings is ordered to observe for periods of desaturation, as might occur during the night while the client is sleeping. Typically, pulse oximetry is performed intermittently to monitor client trends in oxygen saturation [2, 4, 10, 41, 55].

TRANSCULTURAL CONSIDERATIONS
For clients with dark pigmentation, be sensitive to the presence of keloids on earlobes. The thickness of these scars may interfere with accuracy of oximetric readings.

An interpreter may be needed for the client unable to speak or understand the English language. Obtain educational materials in the client's native language, if available. Consider use of AT&T Language Line. See also the Culturological Assessment procedure in Unit 2 for general overview of cultural considerations.

▶ INTERVENTIONS

1. Verify physician order.	*Prevents risk of error*
2. Wash hands.	*Reduces transfer of microorganisms*
3. Perform physical assessment.	*Establishes baseline information of physiological data findings*
4. Organize equipment.	*Promotes efficiency*
5. Explain procedure.	*Decreases anxiety and promotes cooperation*

For Finger Oximetry

1. Prepare site per agency protocol, cleanse the skin, remove nail polish.	*Removes debris and opaque nail coloring which may interfere with accuracy of reading*
2. Check capillary refill and pulse proximal to chosen site.	*Compromised circulation may yield false reading*
3. Apply sensor and turn to the "on" position.	*The photo detector will measure the amount of oxygenated hemoglobin*
4. Listen for the beep and note waveform.	*Each tone indicates detection of pulse*
5. Obtain reading for oxygen saturation and pulse rate.	*Changes in light or waveform indicates the strength of the pulse*
6. Instruct client in the common position changes that may trigger the alarm.	*Facilitates client participation in care*
7. Check alarm limits.	*Alarm limits should be set per physician order*
8. Teach client/caregiver to change position of sensor as needed or if circulation becomes impaired.	*Prevents tissue necrosis*
9. Allow client/caregiver to return demonstration.	*Documents client/caregiver's ability to perform procedure*

For Ear Oximetry

1. Massage the ear for several seconds with an alcohol pad.	*Produces a mild erythema to vascularize the area*
2. Attach probe to earlobe or pinna per manufacturer's recommendations. Turn on power.	*Variations in design models dictate the need to follow equipment-specific guidelines*
3. Follow steps 4–9 for finger oximetry above.	

DOCUMENTATION
The following should be noted in the nursing note:

Type and location of sensor
Presence of pulse and status of capillary refill
% of oxygen saturation
Rotation of sensor site according to guidelines
% of inspired oxygen
Interventions as a result of deviations from the norm
All client/caregiver teaching:
    Topics to include in teaching plan:
        safe and correct equipment handling
        emergency procedures
        underlying disease pathology
        appropriate community resources and contact persons

INTERDISCIPLINARY COLLABORATION
Inform physician of presence of abnormal readings, and compare findings with previous documentation

Determine adequacy of oxygen supply and need to order additional tanks from DME company

Consult with the physician to consider need for nebulizer therapy and consult with respiratory therapy to provide instruction

Consult with social worker to determine client eligibility for financial reimbursement/assistance and to assist in locating appropriate community resources [2, 4, 6, 10, 15, 21, 22, 41, 55, 59]

PROCEDURE
Nebulizer Therapy

DESCRIPTION
The nebulizer treatment is a respiratory therapeutic intervention that uses a device to deliver an aerosol mist to the air passages and lung tissue. During inhalation the nebulizer uniformly distributes the inhaled gases within the air passages to increase alveolar ventilation, humidify secretions, promote expectoration, humidify inspired oxygen and deliver inhalation medication. Various types of nebulizers may be used in the home setting: ultrasonic, large-volume, small-volume, or in-line (Figure 6-2). The ultrasonic nebulizer uses ultrasonic sound waves to form an aerated mist. The large-volume nebulizer is used to provide cooled or heated air for the client whose upper airway has been bypassed, as in the client with an endotracheal or tracheosotomy tube. The small-volume nebulizer is a handheld device used to deliver inhalation medication (see Figure 6-3). The in-line nebulizer is a component of the ventilator tubing and is used to provide intermittent nebulizer therapy for the client on continuous mechanical ventilation [25, 39, 41].

PURPOSE
To promote adequate gas exchange, humidify air passages, administer inhalation medication, and raise secretions

EQUIPMENT
Stethoscope
Suction equipment
Health Assessment forms

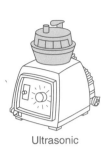

Ultrasonic

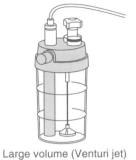

Large volume (Venturi jet)

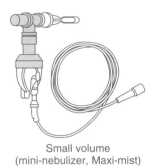

Small volume
(mini-nebulizer, Maxi-mist)

FIGURE 6-2 ▶ Types of nebulizers.

For Ultrasonic Nebulizer

Gas-delivery device
Oxygen tubing
Nebulizer compartment
Saline or inhalation medication as ordered

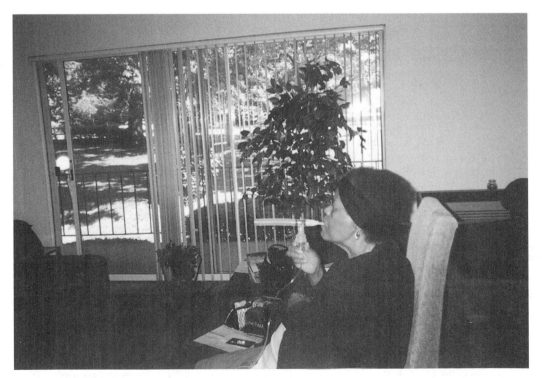

FIGURE 6-3 ▶ Client using small volume nebulizer.

For Large-volume Nebulizer

Pressurized gas
Oxygen tubing
Nebulizer canister
Sterile distilled water
Heater and in-line thermometer, if ordered
Saline or inhalation medication as ordered

For Small-volume Nebulizer

Pressurized gas
Flowmeter
Oxygen tubing
Nebulizer reservoir
Mouthpiece/mask
Saline or inhalation medication as ordered

For In-line Nebulizer

Pressurized gas
Flowmeter
Nebulizer reservoir
Saline or inhalation medication as ordered

OUTCOMES
The client/caregiver will:

▶ Maintain adequate ventilation
▶ Demonstrate ability to perform procedure
▶ Administer prescribed medication therapy
▶ Verbalize understanding of procedure to follow in the event of equipment malfunction

ASSESSMENT DATA
Note signs and symptoms of hypoxemia
Record type and amount of oxygen therapy, if applicable
Document respiratory rate and character
Auscultate lung sounds and note adventitious sounds
Assess character of sputum
Assess client/caregiver's knowledge base regarding the procedure

RELATED NURSING DIAGNOSES
Impaired gas exchange
Altered breathing patterns
Ineffective airway clearance
Anxiety
Powerlessness

SPECIAL CONSIDERATIONS
Clients experiencing difficult breathing will often demonstrate signs of increased anxiety. Assisting the client to relax using correct breathing and relaxation techniques are priority nursing interventions. In the neonatal and pediatric client, the nurse will need to observe for signs and symptoms of

overhydration from the mist formation. In all clients, the nurse must observe for the presence of mist during both inhalation and expiration. Bronchospasm and dyspnea may occur secondary to irritation of the bronchial passages caused by the nebulized particulate matter. When heating elements are used, the nurse must observe for the potential for airway burns. Equipment that is improperly cleaned between use may become contaminated with infectious microbes. As with all medication therapy, the nurse must observe for signs of adverse or allergic reactions to the prescribed inhalation medications. Lastly, universal precautions should be observed when administering inhalation medications. It may be necessary for the nurse to wear protective gear, use special nebulizer systems, and minimize risk of exposure to caregivers [25, 39, 41, 57].

TRANSCULTURAL CONSIDERATIONS

An interpreter will be needed for the client unable to speak or understand the English language

Obtain educational materials in the client's native language, if available. Consider use of AT&T Language Line. See also the Culturological Assessment procedure in Unit 2 for general overview of cultural considerations.

▶ INTERVENTIONS

1. Verify physician order.	*Reduces risk of error*
2. Wash hands.	*Prevents transmission of microbes*
3. Perform physical assessment.	*Establishes baseline information of physiological data findings*
4. Explain procedure.	*Allays anxiety*
5. Encourage the client to cough and expectorate; suction as needed.	*Clears airway*
6. Firmly attach mouthpiece, mask, tracheostomy tube, or in-line nebulizer to tubing per manufacturer's guidelines.	*Ensures tight air seal to system*
7. Add prescribed medication or saline to medication reservoir.	*Initiates drug administration*

For Ultrasonic Nebulizer

a. Fill the nebulizer compartment with the prescribed medication/solution	*Ensures medication administration*
b. Check the outflow port	*Ensures proper misting*

For Large-Volume Nebulizer

a. Attach the oxygen delivery device to the client	*Ensures adequate oxygenation*
b. Fill the canister with sterile distilled water and replace during therapy as needed	*Provides humidification*
c. If using a heating element, attach an in-line thermometer and instruct the client to report any discomfort	*Prevents overheating of the water and potential burning*

For Small-Volume Nebulizer

a. Draw up prescribed medication/saline and inject into nebulizer reservoir	*Promotes bronchodilation*

b. Attach flowmeter to gas source	*Initiates oxygen flow*
c. Attach nebulizer to flow meter	*Adjusts rate of oxygen flow*
d. Check outflow port	*Detects presence of mist*

For In-Line Nebulizer

a. Draw up medication/saline, remove nebulizer reservoir, and inject medication/saline into reservoir	*Promotes bronchodilation*
8. Turn machine on.	*Engages energy source*
9. Instruct client to breathe in taking slow deep breaths.	*Promotes optimal lung expansion*
10. Observe for signs and symptoms of complications.	*Provides early detection of un toward responses*
11. Assist with productive coughing and suction as needed.	*Raises sputum to upper air way and throat for expectoration and airway clearance*
12. At the completion of the nebulizer treatment, perform respiratory assessment.	*Evaluates effectiveness of therapy*
13. Clean and dry medication reservoir.	*Reduces transmission of microbes*
14. Instruct client to perform procedure and permit return demonstration.	*Documents client's ability to perform ordered procedure*
15. Wash hands.	*Prevents transmission of microbes*

DOCUMENTATION
The following should be noted in the nursing note:

Client response to the procedure
Untoward responses reported to the physician
Interventions as a result of deviations from the norm
Respiratory physical assessment findings
All client/caregiver teaching:
    Topics to include in teaching plan:
        safe and correct equipment handling
        emergency procedures
        underlying disease pathology
        appropriate community resources and contact persons

INTERDISCIPLINARY COLLABORATION
Inform physician of presence of untoward responses
Document interventions to treat untoward reactions
Determine adequacy of supplies/equipment and need to initiate reorder from DME vendor
Consult with respiratory therapist to provide supplement teaching, care for/maintain equipment, etc.
Consult with social worker to determine client's eligibility for financial assistance/reimbursement for supplies and equipment, and to identify community resources, such as asthma education and smoking-cessation programs (see Appendices 6-1, 6-2, and 6-3) [6, 13, 15, 21, 25, 39, 41, 57, 59].

Home Spirometry

DESCRIPTION
Recently a number of home electronic spirometry units have been designed to monitor clients with advanced pulmonary conditions. The most common electronic units contain a portable spirometer, digital display, keypad, disposable mouthpiece, tubing, printer, and modem. The keypad is used to input blood pressure, pulse, weight, symptoms, amount of exercise, and stress level. The client or caregiver downloads the data weekly using the unit's modem and a regular telephone-line hookup. The data are transmitted to the office of the primary care provider or to the home health agency for documentation and followup.

PURPOSE
To measure the volume and flow rates of expired gas to monitor pulmonary function parameters

EQUIPMENT
Electronic spirometer
Disposable mouthpiece
Tubing
Stethoscope
Health Assessment forms

OUTCOMES
The client/caregiver will:

▶ Demonstrate ability to perform procedure
▶ Verbalize understanding of procedure to follow for transmission of data to remote healthcare site

ASSESSMENT DATA
Note signs and symptoms of hypoxemia
Record type and amount of oxygen therapy
Document respiratory rate and character
Auscultate lung sounds and note abnormal sounds
Assess character of sputum
Evaluate pulmonary function parameters
Assess client/caregiver's knowledge base regarding the procedure

RELATED NURSING DIAGNOSES
Impaired gas exchange
Altered breathing patterns
Ineffective airway clearance
Anxiety
Powerlessness

SPECIAL CONSIDERATIONS
Electronic spirometry is used to measure the ability of the chest and lungs to adequately move air at the alveolar level. The electronic spirometry unit is used to calculate five pulmonary function parameters: forced vital capacity, forced expiratory volume, forced expiratory flow, midexpiratory flow, and peak expiratory flow rate. The forced vital capacity (FVC) is the total amount of air that

can be exhaled and measures lung capacity. The forced expiratory volume (FEV_1) is the amount of air that can be exhaled in 1 second and is reduced in the presence of airway restriction. The forced expiratory flow (FEF) and the midexpiratory flow (FEF 25–75%) serve as indicators of the performance of the medium and smaller airways. The peak expiratory flow rate (PEFR) measures the maximum airflow rate during forced expiration and is used to detect the narrowing of airways and helps monitor bronchoconstriction in asthma.

The unit stores data on vital signs, symptoms, and pulmonary measures for up to 8 days. The client is given instructions on how to download data. The mouthpiece is encoded with a serial number that is downloaded with the entered information, and documents how often the mouthpiece is changed. The client is taught to change the mouthpiece weekly or if damaged. The downloaded data are closely monitored and clients are contacted should changes in the treatment plan be required [3, 55, 59].

TRANSCULTURAL CONSIDERATIONS

An interpreter will be needed for the client unable to speak or understand the English language. Obtain educational materials in the client's native language, if available. Consider use of AT&T Language Line. See also the Culturological Assessment procedure in Unit 2 for general overview of cultural considerations.

INTERVENTIONS

Interventions	Rationale
1. Verify physician order.	*Reduces risk of error*
2. Wash hands.	*Prevents transmission of microbes*
3. Perform physical assessment.	*Establishes baseline information of physiological data findings*
4. Explain procedure.	*Allays anxiety*
5. Instruct client to sit straight and clear secretions.	*Maximizes positioning of the thoracic cage and clears airway*
6. Instruct client to inhale deeply, hold the breath, insert the mouthpiece and forcefully and rapidly exhale as much air as possible.	*Facilitates client's ability to inspire and expire at full lung capacity*
7. Instruct client to repeat steps 5 and 6 three times.	*Permits averaging of readings*
8. At completion of procedure, clean mouthpiece per manufacturer's recommendations.	*Reduces transmission of microbes*
9. Wash hands.	*Prevents transmission of microbes*
10. Review with the client procedure to download data via telephone line.	*Permits transmission of data to remote access site*
11. Allow client to return demonstration and document teaching.	*Evaluates client learning and ability to perform procedure*

DOCUMENTATION

The following should be noted in the nursing note:

Client response to the procedure
Untoward responses reported to the physician

Interventions as a result of deviations from the norm
Respiratory physical assessment findings
Record trends in pulmonary function test readings
All client/caregiver teaching:
    Topics to include in teaching plan:
        safe and correct equipment handling
        emergency procedures
        underlying disease pathology
        appropriate community resources and contact persons

INTERDISCIPLINARY COLLABORATION

Inform physician of presence of abnormal lung sounds, and compare with previous findings
Document interventions employed to treat untoward responses
Determine adequacy of supplies/equipment and need to initiate reorder from DME vendor
Consult with respiratory therapist in set-up, care, and maintenance of equipment
Consult with social worker to determine client's eligibility for financial assistance/reimbursement
    for supplies and equipment, and to identify community resources [3, 6, 15, 21, 25, 55, 59]

PROCEDURE

Obstructed Airway Management, Adult

DESCRIPTION

Insertion and/or maintenance of an artificial airway is a nursing procedure using any one of three of the following devices: oropharyngeal airway, nasopharyngeal airway, or transtracheal catheter. The ororpharyngeal airway is used for the unconscious client who is at risk for tongue obstruction of the posterior pharynx. The device, made of rubber or plastic to conform to the curvature of the palate, is intended for short-term use. The nasopharyngeal airway, also intended for short-term airway management, is used for the client requiring frequent nasotracheal suctioning; for the client with recent oral facial surgery/trauma; or, for the client with loose, cracked, or avulsed teeth. The device follows the normal curvature of the nasopharynx and is positioned at the posterior pharynx. The nasal end is flanged to prevent slippage and to facilitate nasotracheal suctioning. The transtracheal catheter, for long-term use, permits the delivery of oxygen via a tracheostoma, a surgical opening into the trachea [2, 22, 39, 41].

PURPOSE

To maintain a patent airway

EQUIPMENT

Suction apparatus and equipment
Stethoscope

For Nasopharyngeal Airway

Appropriately sized airway
Tongue blade
Water-soluble lubricant
Gloves
Resuscitation bag
Oxygen source, if ordered

For Oropharyngeal Airway

Appropriately sized airway
Padded tongue blade
Gloves
Resuscitation bag
Oxygen source, if ordered

For Transtracheal Catheter Care

Saline tracheal irrigant solution
Water-soluble lubricant
Cleaning rod
Nasal cannula
Oxygen source, if ordered
Cotton-tipped applicator

OUTCOMES
The client/caregiver will:

▶ Maintain a patent airway
▶ Maintain intact skin and membranes of the oral/nasal/tracheal mucosa
▶ Demonstrate ability to perform procedure

ASSESSMENT DATA
Note signs and symptoms of hypoxemia
Record type and amount of oxygen therapy
Document respiratory rate and character
Auscultate lung sounds and note adventitious sounds
Assess character of sputum
Assess client/caregiver's knowledge base regarding the procedure

RELATED NURSING DIAGNOSES
Impaired gas exchange
Altered breathing pattern
Ineffective airway clearance
Anxiety
Powerlessness
At risk for infection

SPECIAL CONSIDERATIONS
Remember that the nasopharyngeal and oropharyngeal airways are intended for short-term use only. Always observe the client's respiratory status and level of consciousness. Auscultate lung sounds frequently to determine adequacy of ventilation. Constantly observe for inadvertent dislodgment of the artificial airway. The presence of the airway in the oral and nasal passages may cause irritation and bleeding of the mucosa. Suction as needed to remove secretions or blood. An artificial nasal airway that is too long may enter the esophagus and cause gastric distension. The oral airway may cause tooth damage during insertion. An oral airway that is too long may press on the epiglottis and obstruct the larynx. To prevent tissue damage, ensure that the client's lips and tongue are not positioned between the client's teeth and the oral airway. When the client regains

consciousness and the natural patency of the airway is reestablished, remove the artificial airway [2, 39, 41].

The transtracheal catheter is surgically inserted to provide long-term airway patency. The transtracheal catheter site must be cleaned three times per day to prevent buildup of secretions, and the catheter should be irrigated frequently with a normal saline solution as ordered. The transtracheal catheter itself should be removed as ordered to permit thorough cleaning. The client and caregiver should be instructed to immediately insert a second transtracheal catheter after removal of the first catheter for cleaning [2, 39, 41].

TRANSCULTURAL CONSIDERATIONS

An interpreter will be needed for the client unable to speak or understand the English language. Obtain educational materials in the client's native language, if available. Consider use of AT&T Language Line. See also the Culturological Assessment procedure in Unit 2 for general overview of cultural considerations.

▶ INTERVENTIONS

1. Verify physician order.	*Reduces risk of error*
2. Wash hands.	*Prevents transmission of microbes*
3. Perform physical assessment.	*Establishes baseline information of physiological data findings*
4. Explain procedure.	*Allays anxiety*
5. Don gloves.	*Serves as protective barrier*
6. Suction the airway if needed.	*Optimizes visualization of the air passages*
7. Insert and/or remove appropriate type of airway.	*Maintains aritificial airway or reestablishes natural airway patency*

For Nasopharyngeal Airway

Used to facilitate clinician's ability to perform frequent nasotracheal suctioning

To insert:
    a. measure the diameter of the client's nostril and the distance from the tip of the nose to the earlobe, and select an airway that is slightly smaller in length and diameter
    b. lubricate the tip of the airway
    c. if not contraindicated, hyperextend the neck, and pass the airway through the nostril
    d. if resistance is met, remove the airway and gently advance again
    e. use a tongue blade to observe for tube placement at the back of the throat
    f. auscultate the lungs to confirm adequacy of ventilation

To remove:
    a. when the client's natural airway is reestablished, grasp the artificial airway and remove in one smooth motion
    b. if resistance is met, lubricate the tip of the airway and gently rotate while pulling out

For Oropharyngeal Airway

Used to prevent risk of airway occlusion by the client's tongue

To insert:
    a. lubricate the tip of the airway
    b. If not contraindicated, hyperextend the neck (Figure 6-4).
    c. insert the airway using the cross-finger technique [place thumb on client's lower teeth and index finger on upper teeth and push teeth apart] (Figure 6-5).
    d. insert the airway upside down, sliding over the tongue, and rotate the tip downward to position at the posterior wall of the pharynx (Figure 6-6).
    e. auscultate the lungs to assess adequacy of ventilation
    f. position the client on his or her side

To remove:
    a. when the client's natural airway is reestablished and the client is able to swallow, remove the airway by grasping the end and pulling downward and out
    b. test the client's cough and gag reflex

For Transtracheal Catheter Care

Used to maintain airway patency in presence of partial upper airway obstruction

Catheter Site Care

    a. clean around the catheter site with soap and water using a cotton-tipped applicator several times per day

To clean transtracheal catheter:
    a. if on continuous oxygen therapy, disconnect transtracheal catheter from oxygen source, apply nasal cannula and connect to oxygen source at ordered rate of flow
    b. instill 1–2 ml of normal saline solution into the catheter
    c. insert cleaning rod as far as it will go, then remove and reinsert three times
    d. instill 1–2 ml of normal saline solution
    e. reconnect transtracheal tube to oxygen source, if ordered and remove nasal cannula
    f. clean rod with antimicrobial soap and store in dry area

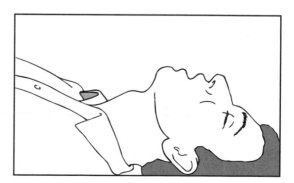

FIGURE 6-4 ▶ Hyperextend the neck.

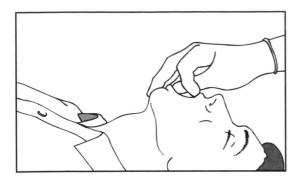

FIGURE 6-5 ▶ Using the cross-finger technique.

To remove transtracheal catheter:

⚡ **NOT TO BE PERFORMED UNTIL TRACT IS WELL HEALED**

a. if on continuous oxygen therapy, apply nasal cannula and connect to oxygen source at ordered rate of flow
b. twist and remove transtracheal catheter
c. immediately insert a second transtracheal catheter coated with a water soluble lubricant
d. secure in place
e. reconnect transtracheal tube to oxygen source, if ordered, and remove nasal cannula

To remove and clean transtracheal catheter:
a. remove as above
b. place catheter in ordered cleaning solution
c. use cleaning rod to clean interior surface of the catheter
d. rinse catheter well and allow to air dry
e. store in clean place
f. perform cleaning procedure weekly or as ordered
8. At the completion of the procedure, perform a respiratory assessment.

Evaluates adequacy of ventilation

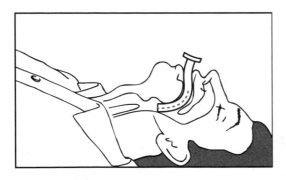

FIGURE 6-6 ▶ Oropharyngeal airway insertion.

9. Instruct the client and caregiver in performance of the procedure and permit return demonstration.

Documents client's/caregiver's ability to perform procedure

10. Wash hands.

Prevents transmission of microbes

DOCUMENTATION
The following should be included in the nursing note:

Client's response to the procedure
Untoward responses reported to the physician
Interventions instituted
Respiratory physical assessment findings
Record date and time of airway insertion, size of airway, condition of mucous membranes
Removal and cleaning of artificial airway
Oxygen source and type of delivery
All client/caregiver teaching:
  Topics to include in teaching plan:
    safe and correct equipment handling
    emergency procedures
    underlying disease pathology
    appropriate community resources and contact persons

INTERDISCIPLINARY COLLABORATION
Inform the physician of the presence of untoward responses and treatment plan followed
Determine adequacy of supplies/equipment and need to initiate reorder from DME vendor
Consult with respiratory therapist for set-up/maintenance of equipment
Consult with social worker to determine client's eligibility for financial assistance/reimbursement for supplies and equipment, and to identify appropriate community resources [2, 6, 15, 21, 22, 25, 39, 41]

PROCEDURE
Chest Drainage System Management

DESCRIPTION
Chest drainage systems are used to maintain negative pressure to reexpand the lung. The systems use either gravity or suction to remove air, fluid, or blood from the pleural cavity (Figure 6-7). Chest tubes are placed by the physician to enable lung reexpansion following the development of a pneumothorax, hemopneumothorax, or empyema. Placement depends on the severity of the condition and the amount of pleural space occupied. If the client has a small pneumothorax, a chest drain valve (Figure 6-8) may be used. For homecare management, a chest tube will be inserted and connected to a chest drainage system in the hospital setting. When the client stabilizes, he/she will discharged to home for care and maintenance of the system [2, 22, 29].

PURPOSE
To restore negative chest pressure and to remove fluid/air from the chest cavity

EQUIPMENT
Disposable chest drainage system
Suction apparatus
Gloves

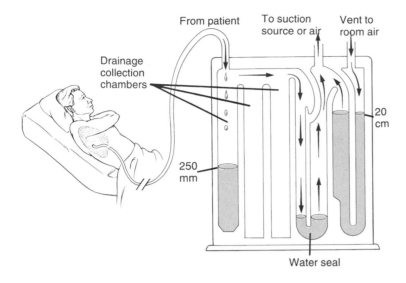

FIGURE 6-7 ▶ Disposable chest drainage system.

Sterile water
Funnel
Tape
Gauze

OUTCOMES

The client/caregiver will

▶ Maintain effective ventilation evidenced by respiratory rate, lung sounds, and color of mucus membranes
▶ Demonstrate ability to perform the procedure
▶ Verbalize understanding of the treatment plan

ASSESSMENT DATA

Note signs and symptoms of hypoxemia
Record type and amount of oxygen therapy
Document respiratory rate and character
Auscultate lung sounds and note adventitious sounds
Assess character of sputum
Review medical order for type of chest drainage system and amount of suction

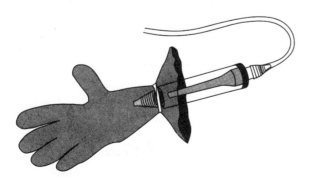

FIGURE 6-8 ▶ Heimlich valve.

Evaluate trending patterns of vital signs, blood gas or pulse oximetry results, and chest drainage
type and amount
Assess client/caregiver's knowledge base regarding the procedure

RELATED NURSING DIAGNOSES
Impaired gas exchange
Altered breathing pattern
Ineffective airway clearance
Anxiety
Powerlessness
Altered skin integrity
At risk for fluid volume deficit
At risk for injury
At risk for infection

SPECIAL CONSIDERATIONS
Agency policy will determine if and when the chest tube is to be clamped. To maintain patency of the
tube, the tube may be gently squeezed to facilitate drainage, or fluid may be allowed to drain by gravity into the collection chamber. Vigorous milking and/or stripping of the chest tube are controversial
interventions which can create excessive negative pressure causing trauma to the lung tissue. If not
contraindicated, encourage ambulation to facilitate lung reexpansion. It is imperative that the client
and caregiver understand that at no time should the chest drainage system be positioned above the
level of the client's chest, and that the tubes must be free of kinks or blockage [2, 22, 39].

TRANSCULTURAL CONSIDERATIONS
An interpreter will be needed for the client unable to speak or understand the English language.
Obtain educational materials in the client's native language, if available. Consider use of AT&T
Language Line. See also the Culturological Assessment procedure in Unit 2 for general overview of
cultural considerations.

▶ INTERVENTIONS

1. Verify physician order.	*Reduces risk of error*
2. Wash hands.	*Prevents transmission of mi-crobes*
3. Perform physical assessment.	*Establishes baseline informa-tion of physiological data findings*
4. Explain procedure.	*Allays anxiety*
5. Don gloves.	*Serves as protective barrier*
6. Follow manufacturer's recommendation for care and management of chest drainage system.	*Reduces risk of error*

To Change Disposable Chest Drainage System

Protocol to follow when system becomes damaged or when collection chamber becomes full

a. open package maintaining sterile technique
b. remove cap from tube of water-seal chamber and use funnel to fill to the 2-cm level using
sterile water or saline as ordered
c. remove the cap from the suction chamber and fill to the –20-cm level using sterile water or
saline as ordered

  d. hang drainage unit from side of bed or place in floor stand
  e. have client take deep breath and bear down while holding breath
  f. quickly disconnect old drainage system and connect tube of collection chamber to the chest tube maintaining sterility
  g. if ordered, connect tubing of suction chamber to suction source and adjust flow regulator to effect gentle bubbling

For Disposable Drainage System Maintenance

Protocol to follow in routine care and maintainence of system

  a. observe water-seal chamber for gentle oscillation of water level, if bubbling is present suspect possible air leak or note that pneumothorax has not yet resolved
  b. note amount, color, consistency of chest drainage and record
  c. monitor bubbling of suction chamber and fill as needed to maintain −20-cm level
  d. if drainage slows or stops, gently milk tube per agency policy and observe for blockage
  e. observe chest tube dressing for drainage
  f. if ordered, change soiled dressings being careful to maintain jelly gauze seal at chest tube insertion site
  g. if the drainage system is accidentally overturned, reestablish the water seal and evaluate client's status
  h. if the drainage system malfunctions or breaks, disconnect from chest tube and place open end of chest tube in a sterile saline solution, obtain new disposable drainage system and set up as above
  i. keep drainage system below level of client's chest at all times
  j. observe for tension hemo/pnuemothorax
  k. excessive drainage and changes in the client's condition must be immediately reported to the physician

For Chest Drainage Valve Maintenance

Protocol to follow for routine care and maintainence of chest valve drainage system

  a. ensure that valve is patent and maintains flutter
  b. if fluttering stops, check for obstruction, if cause is not found or is not correctable inform the physician

7. At the completion of the procedure, perform a respiratory assessment.

Evaluates adequacy of ventilation

8. Obtain body temperature several times per day.

Febrile state may indicate presence of infection

9. Instruct the client and caregiver in performance of the procedure and permit return demonstration.

Documents client's/caregiver's ability to perform procedure

10. Wash hands.

Prevents transmission of microbes

DOCUMENTATION
The following should be included in the nursing note:

Client's response to the procedure
Untoward responses reported to the physician

Interventions instituted
Respiratory physical assessment findings
Record chest drainage amount, color, and consistency
Record status of water-seal, suction and drainage chambers
All client/caregiver teaching:
   Topics to include in teaching plan:
      safe and correct equipment handling
      emergency procedures
      underlying disease pathology
      appropriate community resources and contact persons

INTERDISCIPLINARY COLLABORATION

Inform the physician of the presence of untoward responses and treatment plan followed
Determine adequacy of supplies/equipment and need to initiate reorder from DME vendor
Consult with social worker to determine client's eligibility for financial assistance/reimbursement for
    supplies and equipment, and to identify appropriate community resources [2, 6, 19, 21, 22, 25, 39]

PROCEDURE

Management of Home Mechanical Ventilation, Adult

DESCRIPTION

A wide variety of home mechanical ventilation devices are currently on the market to assist the client in the maintenance of adequate oxygenation. These devices fall into three main categories: invasive/noninvasive positive-pressure ventilators, noninvasive negative-pressure devices, and diaphragmatic augmentation devices.

    For in-depth discussion of special considerations, see Unit 5, Management of Home Mechanical Ventilation, Pediatric [2, 6, 10, 16, 17, 41, 49, 54, 59].

PURPOSE

To maintain adequate ventilation

EQUIPMENT

Home ventilator equipment and supplies, as appropriate
Oxygen equipment and related supplies
Tracheostomy equipment and related supplies
Personal communication aid
Health Assessment forms
Stethoscope
Resuscitation bag
Suction equipment

OUTCOMES

The client/caregiver will:

▶ Maintain adequate ventilation
▶ Demonstrate ability to perform procedure
▶ Verbalize understanding of procedure to follow in the event of equipment malfunction

ASSESSMENT DATA

Note signs and symptoms of hypoxemia
Record type and amount of oxygen therapy

Document respiratory rate and character
Auscultate lung sounds and note abnormal sounds
Assess character of sputum
Evaluate client for evidence of cardiopulmonary compromise
Review prescribed medication therapy
Assess client/caregiver's knowledge base regarding the procedure

RELATED NURSING DIAGNOSES

Impaired gas exchange
Altered breathing patterns
Ineffective airway clearance
Anxiety
Powerlessness
At risk for ineffective family coping

SPECIAL CONSIDERATIONS

Client's experiencing difficult breathing will often demonstrate signs of increased anxiety. Assisting the client to relax using correct breathing and relaxation techniques are priority nursing interventions. The caregiver should be thoroughly trained in the ability to manage the client on home ventilator therapy. Prior to discharge from the acute care setting, the caregiver should be allowed to spend at least 48 hours with the client demonstrating an ability to safely care for and manage the client on home ventilator therapy.

TRANSCULTURAL CONSIDERATIONS

An interpreter will be needed for the client unable to speak or understand the English language
Obtain educational materials in the client's native language, if available. Consider use of AT&T
Language Line. See also the Culturological Assessment procedure in Unit 2 for general
overview of cultural considerations.

▶ INTERVENTIONS

1. Verify physician order.	*Reduces risk of error*
2. Wash hands.	*Prevents transmission of microbes*
3. Perform physical assessment.	*Establishes baseline information of physiological data findings*
4. Explain procedure.	*Allays anxiety*
5. Perform safety check of equipment.	*Assures proper functioning of equipment*

    inspect for evidence of excessive wear
    check connections for tightness
    perform routine cleaning per manufacturer's
      recommendations

For Invasive Positive-Pressure Devices

See Unit 5, Management of Home Mechanical Ventilation, Pediatric.

For Noninvasive Positive Pressure Ventilation

See Unit 5, Management of Home Mechanical Ventilation, Pediatric.
- a. full-mask mechanical ventilation [FMMV]
- b. nasal intermittent positive-pressure ventilation [NIPPV]
- c. continuous positive airway pressure [CPAP]
- d. BiPAP—is a bilevel respiratory system that maintains a constant level of positive airway pressure. The inspiratory pressure level provides the client with a pressure boost, while the expiratory pressure level maintains positive end expiratory pressure to keep the alveoli open and facilitate gas exchange (see Figure 6-9)
  1. Ensure that mask fits tightly over nose or mouth as ordered.   *Maintains tight airseal*

For Noninvasive Negative Pressure Devices

See Unit 5, Management of Home Mechanical Ventilation, Pediatric.
- a. NU MO Suit

For Diaphragmatic Augmentation Devices

- a. The *Rocking Bed Unit* alternates between placing the client in the Trendelenburg or Reverse Trendelenburg positions to force and release pressure on the abdominal contents to stimulate diaphragmatic movement
  1) Place client onto bed and set to run per manufacturer's recommendations   *Ensures accuracy of application*

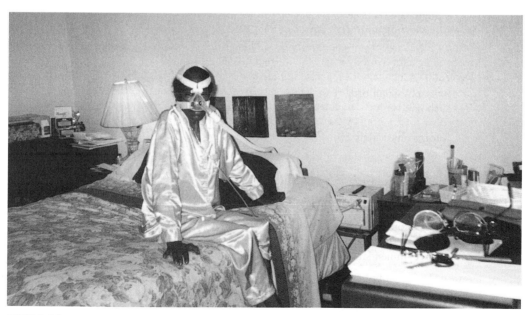

FIGURE 6-9 ▶ Client using BiPAP airway management system.

b. The *Insufflation Belt* is wrapped around the waist and intermittently inflates a balloon which places pressure on the abdominal contents to push against the diaphragm to effect exhalation and reverses the process during inhalation.

   1) Apply belt per manufacturer's recommendations   *Ensures accuracy of application*

6. Instruct client/caregiver in home mechanical ventilation procedure and permit return demonstration.   *Documents client's/caregiver's ability to implement ordered procedure*

7. Notify local emergency medical system and power supply company for priority of service.   *Initiates emergency preparedness protocol*

DOCUMENTATION

The following should be noted in the nursing note:

Client response to the procedure
Untoward responses reported to the physician
Interventions as a result of deviations from the norm
Respiratory physical assessment findings
Ventilator settings
Client/caregiver coping strategies
All client/caregiver teaching:
    Topics to include in teaching plan:
        safe and correct equipment handling
        emergency procedures
        underlying disease pathology
        appropriate community resources and contact persons

INTERDISCIPLINARY COLLABORATION

Inform physician of presence of abnormal lung sounds and compare with previous findings
Document interventions employed to treat untoward responses
Determine adequacy of supplies/equipment and need to initiate reorder from DME vendor
Consult with social worker to determine client's eligibility for financial assistance/reimbursement for supplies and equipment, and to identify community resources
Consult with respiratory therapist for set-up/maintenance of equipment and supplies [2, 6, 10, 15–17, 21, 41, 49, 54, 59]

PROCEDURE
Use of Manual Self-Inflating Resuscitation Bag

DESCRIPTION

The manual self-inflating resuscitation bag is used to provide emergency ventilation for the client who is ventilator dependent or who is at risk for demonstrating signs of cardiopulmonary deterioration. The bag must remain at all times at the bedside of the client who is on ventilatory assistance or who has an artificial airway [2, 41].

PURPOSE

To provide ventilation

EQUIPMENT
Oxygen
Face mask or airway adapter
Tubing
Stethoscope
Suction equipment
Health Assessment forms

OUTCOMES
The client/caregiver will:

▶ Maintain adequate ventilation
▶ Demonstrate ability to perform procedure
▶ Verbalize understanding of procedure to follow in the event of equipment malfunction

ASSESSMENT DATA
Note signs and symptoms of hypoxemia
Record type and amount of oxygen therapy
Document respiratory rate and character
Auscultate lung sounds and note abnormal sounds
Assess character of sputum
Assess client/caregiver's knowledge base regarding the procedure

RELATED NURSING DIAGNOSES
Impaired gas exchange
Altered breathing patterns
Ineffective airway clearance
Anxiety
Powerlessness

SPECIAL CONSIDERATIONS
Client's experiencing difficult breathing will often demonstrate signs of increased anxiety. Assisting the client to relax using correct breathing and relaxation techniques are priority nursing interventions.

TRANSCULTURAL CONSIDERATIONS
An interpreter will be needed for the client unable to speak or understand the English language. Obtain educational materials in the client's native language, if available. Consider use of AT&T Language Line. See also Culturological Assessment procedure in Unit 2 for general overview of cultural considerations.

▌ INTERVENTIONS

1. Verify physician order.	*Reduces risk of error*
2. Wash hands.	*Prevents transmission of microbes*
3. Perform physical assessment.	*Establishes baseline information of physiological data findings*
4. Explain procedure.	*Allays anxiety*

5. Attach bag to oxygen source.	*Permits oxygen to flow through bag*
6. Disconnect client from ventilator, and attach resusitation bag.	*Permits manual ventilation*
7. Assess breathing pattern.	*Establishes baseline*
8. Encourage client to relax.	*Facilitates manual ventilation*
9. Manually deliver deep breaths gradually slowing rate to equal rate frequency set on ventilator.	*Reestablishes synchronized rhythm*
10. Evaluate lung sounds.	*Assesses adequacy of ventilation*
11. Suction airway if indicated.	*Maintains patency of airway*
12. Return to ventilator and observe breathing pattern.	*Indicates relief of respiratory distress*
13. Wash hands.	*Prevents transmission of microbes*
14. Instruct caregiver on implementing the procedure and permit return demonstration	*Documents caregiver's ability to perform ordered procedure*

DOCUMENTATION
The following should be noted in the nursing note:

Client response to the procedure
Untoward responses reported to the physician
Interventions as a result of deviations from the norm
Respiratory physical assessment findings
Ventilator settings
Client/caregiver coping strategies
All client/caregiver teaching:
    Topics to include in teaching plan:
        safe and correct equipment handling
        emergency procedures
        underlying disease pathology
        appropriate community resources and contact persons

INTERDISCIPLINARY COLLABORATION
Inform physician of presence of adventitious lung sounds, and compare with previous findings
Document interventions employed to treat untoward responses
Determine adequacy of supplies/equipment and need to initiate reorder from DME vendor
Consult with respiratory therapist for maintenance of equipment
Consult with social worker to determine client's eligibility for financial assistance/reimbursement for supplies and equipment, and to identify community resources [2, 6, 15–17, 21, 41, 49, 54]

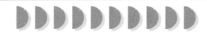

Adult Cardiovascular System Procedures

2

Ambulatory ECG Monitoring

DESCRIPTION

Ambulatory ECG monitoring can be performed using any one of three electronic devices: Holter monitor, telemetry monitor or transtelephonic monitor. The Holter monitor is a type of hardwire monitoring system that records and stores electrocardiographic data on a taped recording that is played back at a later time for analysis. The lightweight unit is attached to the client's belt so that s/he is free to conduct normal daily activity while the device records electrical cardiac activity. The unit can store up to 3 days worth of electrocardiographic data. The telemetric monitoring system allows the client's electrocardiagraphic data to be constantly monitored by a wireless device and directly viewed by the nurse in the home setting for immediate feedback. The small device is comfortably worn by the client and permits the direct observation of the ECG tracing via a monitoring window located on the device itself. The transtelephonic monitoring system stores the client's electrocardiographic data in a small computerized device that is worn on the wrist. Data retrieval can be downloaded into a computerized medical record, or transmitted over telephone lines to a remote location for analysis of the ECG tracing [17, 29–37, 41].

PURPOSE

To record cardiac electrical activity for diagnostic or documentation purposes

EQUIPMENT

Electrodes
Leads
Monitoring unit
Battery
Stethoscope
Sphygmomanometer
Thermometer
Health Assessment forms
Diary/log

OUTCOMES

The client will:

► Correctly maintain lead placement
► Document activity in event diary
► Verbalize understanding of procedure

ASSESSMENT DATA

Assess for signs and symptoms of alteration in cardiac status
Auscultate heart sounds and document findings
Review prescribed medication therapy
Obtain history of cardiac disease
Determine client's knowledge base regarding procedure

RELATED NURSING DIAGNOSES

At risk for altered cardiac output
At risk for altered tissue perfusion
Powerlessness
At risk for pain
Anxiety

SPECIAL CONSIDERATIONS

Most ambulatory monitoring units are battery operated. Ensure that the battery has been newly installed. While the client will not be able to shower with the device attached, he or she will be able to engage in all other ADLs. The client should be instructed to record all activity and untoward sensations/feelings in the accompanying diary.

TRANSCULTURAL CONSIDERATIONS

An interpreter will be needed for the client unable to speak or understand the English language. Obtain educational materials in the client's native language, if available. Consider use of AT&T Language Line. See also Culturological Assessment procedure in Unit 2 for general overview of cultural considerations.

▶ INTERVENTIONS

1. Verify physician order.	*Reduces risk of error*
2. Wash hands.	*Prevents transmission of microbes*
3. Perform physical assessment.	*Establishes baseline information of physiological data findings*
4. Explain procedure.	*Allays anxiety*

For Holter Monitoring

1. Insert battery into the unit per manufacturer's recommendations.	*Ensures accuracy and supplies power source*
2. Connect electrodes to lead wires and place at standard lead sites per manufacturer's recommendation.	*Site selection will depend on chest configuration and skin integrity*
3. Prepare skin surface by cleaning with soap and water, and shaving if necessary.	*Allows for adequate transmission of electrical impulses*
4. Abraid the skin with a washcloth.	*Removes dead skin cells*
5. Remove backing and apply electrode to skin.	*Initiates contact*
6. Turn on device.	*Establishes energy source*
7. Begin diary entry.	*Documents activity*

8. Instruct client in the procedure and permit return demonstration.	*Documents client's ability to perform the procedure*

For Telemetric Monitoring

1. Connect electrodes to lead wires per manufacturer's recommendations.	*Ensures accuracy of application*
2. Follow instructions provided by manufacturer to set up continuous electronic monitoring and transmission of tracing to dysrhythmia detection service or to physician office.	*Device uses telecommunication technology to transmit electronic graphic record of cardiac activity*
3. Place call to dysrhythmia service to verify telemetry transmission.	*Ensures that electronic connection has been established*
4. Instruct client in procedure to apply leads and troubleshoot monitoring device, and permit return demonstration.	*Documents client's ability to implement the procedure*

For Transtelephonic Monitoring

1. Apply wrist recorder per manufacturer's instructions.	*Ensures accuracy of application*
2. If applicable, instruct client to press event button when symptomatic.	*Initiates the memory feature of the device to record events 2 minutes prior*
3. Instruct client in the procedure to transmit ECG data and permit return demonstration.	*Documents client's ability to perform the procedure*

DOCUMENTATION
The following should be noted in the nursing note:

Client response to the procedure
Untoward responses reported to the physician
Interventions as a result of deviations from the norm
Cardiovascular physical assessment findings
Interpretation of ECG tracing
All client/caregiver teaching:
    Topics to include in teaching plan:
      safe and correct equipment handling
      emergency procedures
      underlying disease pathology
      appropriate community resources and contact persons

INTERDISCIPLINARY COLLABORATION
Inform physician of presence of abnormal heart sounds, and compare with previous findings
Document interventions employed to treat untoward responses
Determine adequacy of supplies/equipment and need to initiate reorder from DME vendor
Consult with social worker to determine client's eligibility for financial assistance/reimbursement
    for supplies and equipment [6, 15, 17, 21, 25, 28–37, 41, 42]

12-Lead Electrocardiogram

DESCRIPTION
The 12-lead electrocardiogram (ECG) is used to provide electrocardiographic data from 12 different views of the heart. It is used to identify the location of a myocardial infarction, axis deviation, conduction defect, cardiac hypertrophy, dysrhythmias, and the effects of drugs and electrolytes on the heart's electrical system.

PURPOSE
To record cardiac electrical activity for diagnostic or documentation purposes

EQUIPMENT
Electrodes
Leads
Electrocardiogram
Stethoscope
Sphygmomanometer
Thermometer
Health Assessment forms

OUTCOMES
The client will:

▶ Tolerate the procedure
▶ Verbalize understanding of procedure

ASSESSMENT DATA
Assess for signs and symptoms of alteration in cardiac status
Auscultate heart sounds and document findings
Review prescribed medication therapy
Obtain history of cardiac disease
Determine client's knowledge base regarding procedure

RELATED NURSING DIAGNOSES
At risk for altered cardiac output
At risk for altered tissue perfusion
Powerlessness
At risk for pain
Anxiety

SPECIAL CONSIDERATIONS
Depending on the type of ECG used, the nurse will be able to transmit the recording of the 12-lead ECG either by faxing the hardcopy to the client's physician, or by transmitting the recording electronically from a computerized ECG machine over the client's telephone line. The client's home outlet will need to be three-pronged to maintain proper grounding.

TRANSCULTURAL CONSIDERATIONS
An interpreter will be needed for the client unable to speak or understand the English language. Obtain educational materials in the client's native language, if available. Consider use of AT&T

Language Line. See also Culturological Assessment procedure in Unit 2 for general overview of cultural considerations.

▶ INTERVENTIONS

1. Verify physician order.	*Reduces risk of error*
2. Wash hands.	*Prevents transmission of microbes*
3. Perform physical assessment.	*Establishes baseline information of physiological data findings*
4. Explain procedure.	*Allays anxiety*
5. Connect electrodes to lead wires and apply electrodes to standard lead sites.	*Site selection may depend on chest configuration and skin integrity*
6. Expose limbs and chest.	*Permits unobstructed view of lead site locations*
7. Prepare skin surface by cleaning with soap and water and shaving if necessary.	*Allows for adequate transmission of electrical impulses*
8. Abraid the skin with a washcloth.	*Removes dead skin cells*
9. Remove backing and apply electrode to skin.	*Initiates contact*
10. Check the wiring for evidence of damage.	*Maintains safety*
11. Plug unit into three-pronged outlet.	*Establishes energy source*
12. Correctly connect electrodes to lead wires.	*Provides for accurate identification leads and interpretation of electrocardiographic data*
13. Turn on the power.	*Establishes energy source*
14. Press run button to record tracing assessing quality.	*Determines clarity of tracing*
15. Disconnect equipment and remove excess gel.	*Gel can be irritating to skin surfaces*
16. Wash hands.	*Prevents transmission of microbes*

DOCUMENTATION
The following should be noted in the nursing note:

Client response to the procedure
Untoward responses reported to the physician
Interventions as a result of deviations from the norm
Cardiovascular physical assessment findings
Interpret ECG rhythm and record interpretation
All client/caregiver teaching:
    Topics to include in teaching plan:
        safe and correct equipment handling
        emergency procedures
        underlying disease pathology
        appropriate community resources and contact persons

INTERDISCIPLINARY COLLABORATION

Inform physician of presence of abnormal heart sounds and abnormal ECG changes, and compare with previous findings

Document interventions employed to treat untoward responses

Determine adequacy of supplies/equipment and need to initiate reorder from DME vendor [2, 6, 13–15, 17, 21, 25, 29, 31–33, 36, 37, 39]

PROCEDURE
Automatic Implantable Cardioverter Defibrillator Care

DESCRIPTION

Research has shown that the most common cause of sudden cardiac death is believed to be ventricular tachycardia, which converts to ventricular fibrillation. Early detection and treatment have significantly improved survival rates. The automatic implantable cardioverter defibrillator (AICD) is a device that monitors heart rate and rhythm, and delivers an electrical shock when a lethal dysrhythmia is detected. The device consists of a battery-run electrical generator with epicardial or transvenous leads. For epicardial lead placement, the device is surgically implanted using a lateral thoracotomy, medial thoracotomy or subxiphoid approach (Figure 6-10). The transvenous lead system is implanted using a nonthoracotomy approach. The generator is typically positioned in a subcutaneous or submuscular pocket in the upper-left abdominal quadrant. The current third-generation AICDs are able to provide antitachycardia and bradycardia pacing, cardioversion and defibrillation depending on the dysrhythmia detected. Clients may be managed concomitantly with pharmacologic agents [22, 39, 41, 44].

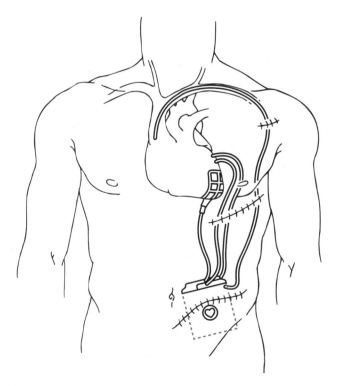

FIGURE 6-10 ▶ Automatic implantable cardioverter defibrillator.

PURPOSE
To maintain constant monitoring of cardiac activity and to terminate lethal dysrhythmias

EQUIPMENT
Dressing supplies as ordered
Gloves
Event diary
Health Assessment forms

OUTCOMES
The client/caregiver will:

▶ Maintain adequate cardiac output and regain skin integrity
▶ Be free of signs and symptoms of infection
▶ Verbalize understanding of AICD maintenance and emergency management

ASSESSMENT DATA
Record cardiovascular and respiratory clinical findings
Observe for evidence of infection
Monitor effects of cardiac pharmacologic agents
Review ECG tracings
Document client/caregiver understanding of and ability to perform procedure

RELATED NURSING DIAGNOSES
At risk for altered cardiac output
Impaired skin integrity
Knowledge deficit
Anxiety
Loss
Powerlessness

SPECIAL CONSIDERATIONS
Caregivers must be able to perform cardiopulmonary resuscitation in the event of circulatory collapse. Because of the level of anxiety and apprehension often associated with the fear of recurrent episodes of sudden cardiac death, the client may be unable to process information during the first home visit. Reinforcement of all teaching may be needed by repeating information at subsequent visits until the client and caregiver are able to demonstrate understanding. The client should be given information regarding how to obtain a medic alert bracelet, and the local emergency medical system should be informed that the client has received an AICD.

The client and caregiver must understand that the device does not prevent ventricular dysrhythmias from occurring, but rather delivers a countershock to reestablish cardiac rate and rhythm The teaching plan should include a basic description of AICD function, the implantation procedure, symptoms of infection, and indicators of device malfunction. The client and caregiver should keep an event diary to document symptoms correlating with AICD countershocks. Caregivers should be aware that during the delivery of an electrical shock, they may feel a harmless, weak sensation if they are touching the client. The physician should be notified when countershocks occur, and followup visits must be maintained to assess the function of the device, status of the battery, and client response to therapy. The client and caregiver should be aware that electromagnetic sources may disrupt AICD functioning, rendering the device inoperable. The client will hear tones emanating from the device when in contact with an electromagnetic field. The tones signal deactivation of the device and must be reported immediately [22, 39, 41, 44].

The client and caregiver should be aware that during the delivery of shock the client may experience vertigo or syncope and may feel a slight jolt or shock when the device fires. At the onset of feelings of lightheadedness, the client should be instructed to sit or lie down to prevent injury during a fall.

Both clients and caregivers may experience fear and anxiety of possible death, fear of the device malfunctioning, and fear of being alone during an episode. Allowing the client to ventilate concerns and to verbalize feelings will assist in alleviating anxiety over time [22, 39, 41, 44].

TRANSCULTURAL CONSIDERATIONS

An interpreter will be needed for the client unable to speak or understand the English language. Obtain educational materials in the client's native language, if available. Consider use of AT&T Language Line. See also the Culturological Assessment procedure in Unit 2 for general overview of cultural considerations.

▶ INTERVENTIONS

Intervention	Rationale
1. Verify physician order.	*Reduces risk of error*
2. Wash hands.	*Prevents transmission of microbes*
3. Perform physical assessment.	*Establishes baseline information of physiological data findings*
4. Reinforce teaching initiated in the hospital setting.	*Facilitates retention of information*
5. Don gloves.	*Serves as protective barrier*
6. Observe incision site and note evidence of drainage, redness, swelling, tenderness, warmth, and approximation of incision line.	*Documents wound healing*
7. Cleanse wound as ordered.	*Removes debris*
8. Examine device pocket and remind client to avoid wearing tight-fitting clothing.	*Prevents skin chafing over generator site*
9. Review signs and symptoms of lethal dysrhythmias and remind client to sit or lie down during episodes.	*Reduces risk of injury from falling*
10. Review CPR and procedure to alert EMS with caregivers.	*CPR will maintain perfusion and ventilation until the EMS team arrives*
11. Review event diary.	*Documents symptoms correlating with AICD countershock*
12. Assess the home for environmental safety and electromagnetic interference.	*Contact with electromagnetic sources will deactivate the AICD device*
13. Instruct the client to wear medic alert bracelet.	*Provides others with information during emergency assistance*
14. Instruct the client and caregiver in performance of the procedure and permit return demonstration.	*Documents client's/caregiver's ability to perform procedure*
15. Wash hands.	*Prevents transmission of microbes*

DOCUMENTATION

The following should be noted in the nursing note:

Client response to the procedure
Untoward responses reported to the physician
Interventions instituted
Cardiac physical assessment findings
Condition of incision site and generator pocket
Evaluation of client responses to AICD shocks and accuracy of the device's dysrhythmia detection
All client/caregiver teaching:
   Topics to include in teaching plan:
     safe and correct equipment handling
     emergency procedures
     underlying disease pathology
     appropriate community resources and contact persons

INTERDISCIPLINARY COLLABORATION

Inform the physician of the presence of untoward responses and treatment plan followed
Determine adequacy of dressing supplies/equipment and need to initiate reorder from DME vendor
Consult with social worker to determine client's eligibility for financial assistance/reimbursement
   for dressing supplies and equipment, and to identify appropriate community resources [6, 15,
   21, 22, 25, 39, 41, 44]

PROCEDURE
Hemodynamic Monitoring in the Home Setting

DESCRIPTION

Noninvasive measurement of blood flow using thoracic electrical bioimpedance permits hemodynamic surveillance in the home setting of parameters typically monitored in the traditional ICU: cardiac output, index, stroke volume, systemic vascular resistance, heart rate, ejection fraction, end diastolic volume, and mean arterial pressure. The procedure enables the close monitoring of end-stage cardiac clients and allows for the safe titration of inotropic infusions in the home environment [17].

PURPOSE

To monitor hemodynamic parameters

EQUIPMENT

Electrodes
Leads
Hemodynamic surveillance computer
Stethoscope
Sphygmomanometer
Thermometer
Health Assessment forms

OUTCOMES

The client/caregiver will:

▶ Tolerate the procedure
▶ Verbalize understanding of procedure
▶ Maintain hemodynamic parameters as ordered

ASSESSMENT DATA

Assess for signs and symptoms of alteration in cardiac status
Auscultate heart sounds and document findings
Review prescribed medication therapy
Obtain history of cardiac disease
Determine client's knowledge base regarding procedure

RELATED NURSING DIAGNOSES

At risk for altered cardiac output
At risk for altered tissue perfusion
Powerlessness
At risk for pain
Anxiety

SPECIAL CONSIDERATIONS

The hemodynamic surveillance system uses three-dimensional computer signal averaging to compute parameters. Electrodes must be correctly positioned onto the thorax to measure the pulsatile changes associated with thoracic blood flow. The client's home outlet will need to be three-pronged to maintain proper grounding [17].

TRANSCULTURAL CONSIDERATIONS

An interpreter will be needed for the client unable to speak or understand the English language. Obtain educational materials in the client's native language, if available. Consider use of AT&T Language Line. See also the Culturological Assessment procedure in Unit 2 for general overview of cultural considerations.

▶ INTERVENTIONS

Intervention	Rationale
1. Verify physician order.	*Reduces risk of error*
2. Wash hands.	*Prevents transmission of microbes*
3. Perform physical assessment.	*Establishes baseline information of physiological data findings*
4. Explain procedure.	*Allays anxiety*
5. Connect electrodes to lead wires and apply to lead sites.	*Site selection will depend on chest configuration and skin integrity*
6. Prepare skin surface by cleaning with soap and water, and shaving if necessary.	*Allows for adequate transmission of electrical impulses*
7. Remove backing and apply electrodes/impedence strips to skin per manufacturer's recommendation.	*Initiates electrical contact*
8. Check the wiring for evidence of damage.	*Maintains safety*
9. Plug unit into three-pronged outlet.	*Establishes energy source*
10. Turn on the power.	*Establishes energy source*
11. Follow manufacturer's instructions to compute hemodynamic parameters.	*Ensures accuracy of data findings*
12. Complete the procedure and obtain printout of hemodynamic readings.	*Documents data findings*
13. Wash hands.	*Prevents transmission of microbes*

DOCUMENTATION
The following should be noted in the nursing note:

Client response to the procedure
Untoward responses reported to the physician
Interventions as a result of deviations from the norm
Cardiovascular physical assessment findings
Record hemodynamic pressure readings
All client/caregiver teaching:
    Topics to include in teaching plan:
        safe and correct equipment handling
        emergency procedures
        underlying disease pathology
        appropriate community resources and contact persons

INTERDISCIPLINARY COLLABORATION
Inform physician of presence of adventitious heart sounds, and compare with previous findings
Document interventions employed to treat untoward responses
Determine adequacy of supplies/equipment and need to initiate reorder from DME vendor
Confer with social worker to determine client eligibility for reimbursement/financial assistance for equipment/supplies and to identify appropriate community resources. [6, 15, 17, 21]

PROCEDURE
Phlebotomy

DESCRIPTION
Phlebotomy refers to the removal of blood through a vein for the purpose of reducing blood viscosity and relieving symptoms of polycythemia. The term also refers to the technique of venipuncture, used to extract small amounts of blood from peripheral vessels, for the purpose of obtaining specimens for laboratory analysis. Discussion in this section will focus on the technique used to reduce circulating blood volume.

PURPOSE
To reduce circulating blood volume

EQUIPMENT
Phlebotomy donor set
Alcohol pads
IV insertion kit
Biohazard container

OUTCOMES
The client will:

▶ Avoid strenuous activity, smoking, or ingestion of alcoholic beverages for 3 hours post-procedure
▶ Increase fluid intake for 2 days following procedure
▶ Eat a snack and drink a sweetened beverage following the procedure

ASSESSMENT DATA

Assess baseline vital signs prior to initiating procedure
Assess hydrational status and confirm that client has eaten an adequate meal prior to initiating the procedure
Observe for untoward reactions to procedure

RELATED NURSING DIAGNOSES

At risk for fluid volume deficit
At risk for decreased cardiac output
At risk for infection
At risk for ineffective coping
Anxiety
Knowledge deficit

SPECIAL CONSIDERATIONS

Be aware that sensitivity to changes in fluid volume will be heightened in the geriatric and mal-nourished client populations

TRANSCULTURAL CONSIDERATIONS

An interpreter will be needed for the client unable to speak or understand the English language. Obtain educational materials in the client's native language, if available. Consider use of AT&T Language Line. See also the Culturological Assessment procedure in Unit 2 for general overview of cultural considerations.

▶ INTERVENTIONS

Intervention	Rationale
1. Wash hands.	*Prevents transmission of microbes*
2. Verify physician order.	*Reduces risk of error*
3. Perform physical assessment.	*Establishes baseline information physiological findings*
4. Organize equipment.	*Facilitates efficiency*
5. Explain procedure.	*Alleviates anxiety*
6. Don gloves.	*Serves as protective barrier*
7. Prep insertion site and insert phlebotomy needle as described in IV-insertion procedure.	*Maintains aseptic technique*
8. Withdraw amount of blood per physician order.	*The amount of blood to be withdrawn to achieve therapeutic effect is specified by physician order*
9. Remove needle from IV site, cover with gauze, and apply pressure.	*Reduces risk of bleeding at site*
10. Elevate arm above head for 2 minutes.	*Reduces risk of bleeding at site*
11. Dispose of blood products and used supplies per state regulations and agency protocol.	*Secures biohazardous waste products*
12. Encourage oral intake of snack and sweetened beverage.	*Increases blood glucose and fluid volume*
13. Monitor vital signs for 30 minutes post-phlebotomy.	*Permits early detection of untoward reactions*

DOCUMENTATION

The following should be included in the nursing note:

Date time and amount of blood withdrawn
Pre- and post-phlebotomy serum specimens obtained
Client's tolerance to the procedure
Untoward reactions and interventions employed to reverse untoward reactions
All client/caregiver teaching:
   Topics to include in teaching plan:
      safe and correct equipment handling
      emergency procedures
      underlying disease pathology
      appropriate community resources and contact persons

INTERDISCIPLINARY COLLABORATION

Notify the physician if unable to complete the procedure or if reaction occurs
If blood is to be donated notify the blood bank for instructions regarding collection and storage
   [6, 15, 21, 25, 39]

PROCEDURE
Managing Infusion Therapy

DESCRIPTION

Home infusion therapy is used to administer antibiotics, parenteral nutrition, immunosuppressive agents, analgesics, inotropic agents, hydrational fluids, and blood products. When provided in the home, infusion therapy can reduce hospitalization for clients with a variety of acute and critical illnesses. Infusions may be administered via any one of several routes of administration: intrathecal, intraarterial, intraperitoneal, or intravenous. The common sites for long-term vascular access devices are peripheral, tunneled/nontunneled central, and vascular access port (Figure 6-11). Several types of catheters may be used, see Display 6-1. Continuous infusions are regulated with electronic pumps. See Appendix 6-4, Infusion Access Devices for detailed description of access devices [1, 2, 17, 22, 40, 41, 48, 62].

PURPOSE

To control pain, provide nutrition/hydration, reduce infection, suppress the immune system, improve cardiac output, or replace blood components

EQUIPMENT

Prescribed medication in appropriate infusion system
Administration set
Tubing
Gloves
Saline flush
Health Assessment forms
Consent form
Thermometer
Stethoscope
Protective gear
Alcohol pads

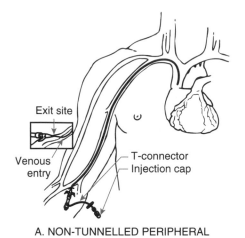

A. NON-TUNNELLED PERIPHERAL

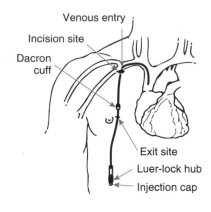

B. TUNNELLED

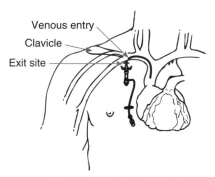

C. NON-TUNNELLED CENTRAL

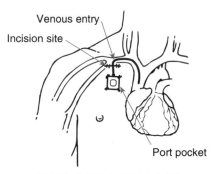

D. VENOUS ACCESS PORT

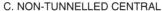

FIGURE 6-11 ▶ Common sites for long-term venous access devices. **A.** Non-tunneled peripheral. **B.** Tunneled. **C.** Non-tunneled central. **D.** Venous access port.

Tape
Pole or hanger
Labels
Infusion device
Appropriate size needles or needleless device

OUTCOMES
The client/caregiver will:

▶ Maintain infusion at ordered rate
▶ Exhibit stable vital signs, urine output, and respiratory status
▶ Identify adverse reactions to report

Types of Tunneled Catheters

Groshong catheter
- Silicone rubber
- Approximately 35″ (89 cm) long
- Closed end with pressure-sensitive, two-way valve
- Polyester fiber (Dacron) cuff
- Single lumen or multilumen

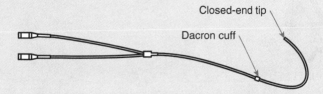

Closed-end tip

Dacron cuff

Triple-lumen Hickman catheter
- Silicone rubber
- Approximately 35″ (89 cm) long
- Open-ended with clamp
- Dacron cuff
- Single lumen or multilumen

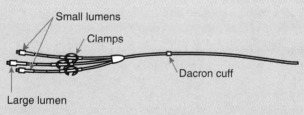

Small lumens

Clamps

Dacron cuff

Large lumen

Broviac catheter
- Identical to Hickman, but with smaller diameter

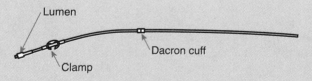

Lumen

Dacron cuff

Clamp

- Demonstrate ability to perform procedure, if appropriate and depending on complexity of the system used
- Verbalize understanding of procedure

ASSESSMENT DATA
Assess the client's nutritional status
Evaluate the client's blood chemistries, blood count, and profiles
Obtain history of allergies, cellulitis, and thrombosis

Perform physical assessment and record clinical findings

Observe for signs and symptoms of fluid/electrolyte imbalance, body weight, fluid balance, and mucus membranes

Evaluate appearance of access site

Complete an environmental assessment

Determine ability of client/caregiver to maintain therapy as ordered

RELATED NURSING DIAGNOSES

At risk for infection

Altered skin integrity

Anxiety

Fluid volume excess/deficit

Altered nutrition, less than body requirements

Pain

SPECIAL CONSIDERATIONS

Most infusion solutions containing admixtures will be prepared by the pharmacist and shipped to the home for storage in the refrigerator at ordered temperature ranges, to maintain potency and reduce risk of spoiling. Remove the solution from refrigeration at least 30 to 60 minutes prior to administration. Inspect the container for any evidence of drug incompatibility, particulate matter, cloudiness, cracks, or solution separation. Read the label and note the date of expiration, name of solution and drug admixtures, client name, date of preparation, name of pharmacist, and infusion rate. Verify with the medical order. If additional admixtures are to be added in the home, prepare the medications, add to the solution, and label the infusion bag appropriately. Have the client maintain a clean work area for preparation of the infusion [1, 2, 17, 22, 40, 41, 48, 62].

Home Infusion Pumps—Infusion therapy pump devices are available as either external or implantable infusion systems. External systems include peristaltic pumps and elastomeric balloon pumps. Peristaltic pumps are lightweight and can be worn in a pouch attached to a belt. Several models are available as computerized programmable units that use a peristaltic mechanism to compress the administration tubing at a predetermined rate of delivery. Elastomeric units are spring operated, disposable, and available in several shapes and sizes. These pumps contain an inner balloon reservoir and pumping mechanism that forces the medication through the delivery tubing at a slow rate. The accuracy of the rate of flow depends upon environmental temperature and viscosity of the solution being delivered. Flow rate will increase in warmer environments and will tend to infuse at a slower rate with thick, more concentrated solutions. With implantable infusion systems there are no external components. The pump can be surgically implanted in the subcutaneous tissue of the abdomen, and an attached silicone outlet catheter is then tunneled to the intraaterial, intrathecal, or intraperitoneal infusion site for regional infusion of medications. For systemic intravenous infusion, the pump may be implanted in the subcutaneous tissue near the subclavian vessels, and an attached silicone outlet catheter is then tunneled into the subclavian vena cava [1, 2, 17, 22, 40, 41, 48, 62].

An environmental assessment of the home will establish the adequacy of the home electrical system to support the use of electronic infusion pumps. Additionally, clients and caregivers should be instructed to maintain backup power systems (generators, batteries as appropriate) and additional infusion pumps in the event of power or equipment failure.

TRANSCULTURAL CONSIDERATIONS

An interpreter will be needed for the client unable to speak or understand the English language. Obtain educational materials in the client's native language, if available. Consider use of AT&T

Language Line. See also the Culturological Assessment procedure in Unit 2 for general overview of cultural considerations.

▶ INTERVENTIONS

1. Verify physician order.	*Reduces risk of error*
2. Wash hands.	*Prevents transmission of microbes*
3. Perform physical assessment.	*Establishes baseline information of physiological data findings*
4. Assess the home for environmental safety.	*Establishes suitability of the home setting*
5. Explain procedure.	*Allays anxiety*
6. Evaluate client/caregiver's ability to perform the procedure.	*Ensures client/caregiver's ability to manage the therapy as prescribed*
7. Don gloves.	*Serves as protective barrier*
8. Assess access site.	*Detects presence of drainage, redness, swelling, tenderness, warmth, or occlusion*
9. Set up infusion per agency guidelines and/or manufacturer's recommendations.	*Reduces risk of error*

To Prepare the Infusion

Initiates fluid therapy as ordered
   a. place the infusion on a flat surface
   b. open administration set, close all clamps, and remove protective cap
   c. remove protective cap and spike the bag using sterile technique
   d. hang the bag and fill the drip chamber half full
   e. prime the line
   f. If an inline filter is needed, follow manufacturer's recommendations
   g. completely fill the line with solution and clamp
   h. obtain infusion device and follow manufacturer's recommendations for setup
   i. turn on power
   j. program the setting
   k. clean the end of the access site with alcohol pad
   l. connect infusion to access device
   m. open the clamp to infusion set
   n. start the infusion
   o. disconnect at completion of infusion

For a Continuous Infusion

Establishes fluid maintainence therapy
   a. clean capped port of access site with alcohol pad
   b. flush catheter with flush solution as ordered
   c. initiate infusion as above
   d. tape over all non-luer lock connections to secure in place
   e. maintain infusion at ordered rate

For Secondary Administration

Secondary set up facilitates intermittent fluid therapy administration without disruption of primary infusion

  a. obtain secondary administration set
  b. spike infusion bag and prime line
  c. ensure compatibility of primary and secondary infusions
  d. cleanse Y port of primary line or capped lumen of multilumen catheter with alcohol pad
  e. insert needle or needleless access device into port of capped lumen
  f. infuse as above

Changing the Tubing and Solution

Initiates start of new infusion maintaining aseptic handling of solution and tubing

  a. follow agency policy for changing of lines and solutions
  b. when possible change lines and solutions at the same time
  c. obtain new solution, spike the bag and prime the line
  d. stop the infusion
  e. clamp the catheter with an inline clamp, do not use hemostat which will crack the hub or catheter
  f. if the catheter does not have an inline clamp, have the client perform Valsalva's maneuver during changing of the tubing
  g. at the needle or catheter hub site quickly disconnect the old tubing and attach the newly primed line using sterile technique
  h. adjust rate as above

Flushing the Catheter

Maintains patency of catheter

  a. all catheters must be routinely flushed per agency policy
  b. use only the flush solution ordered
  c. clean the capped lumen with alcohol pad
  d. allow to air dry
  e. inject the ordered flush solution
  f. after flushing maintain pressure on the plunger of the syringe while withdrawing to prevent blood backup and clot formation in the catheter.

Changing the Injection Cap

Reduces risk of infection

  a. follow agency policy for frequency of cap changing
  b. clean the connection with alcohol or providone-iodine swab as ordered
  c. have the client perform Valsalva's maneuver and clamp the catheter
  d. quickly disconnect old cap and replace with new cap using sterile technique

10. Instruct the client and caregiver in performance of the procedure, if appropriate, and permit return demonstration

Documents client's/caregiver's ability to perform procedure

11. Wash hands

Prevents transmission of microbes

DOCUMENTATION
The following should be included in the nursing note:

Date and time of medication/infusion administration
Condition of access site
Document dressing, tubing, and solution changes
Any difficulty in performing the procedure
Client's response to therapy
Document client/caregiver's ability to maintain infusion and safety of environment
All client/caregiver teaching:
>   Topics to include in teaching plan:
>   safe and correct equipment handling
>   emergency procedures
>   underlying disease pathology
>   appropriate community resources and contact persons
>   complications of infusion therapy

INTERDISCIPLINARY COLLABORATION
Confer with physician regarding the development of any complications
Consult with the pharmacist regarding the preparation and storage of infusion solutions
Consult with the social worker to identify client's eligibility for financial assistance/reimbursement for supplies, and to identify appropriate community resources
Anticipate need to order equipment/supplies from DME vendor [1, 2, 6–8, 15, 17, 20–22, 40, 41, 48, 52, 57, 62]

PROCEDURE
Superficial Peripheral Intravenous Insertion

DESCRIPTION
Insertion of a peripheral intravenous line is performed to provide a superficial venous access site. The nurse determines the type and size of catheter depending on condition of the client's veins and the kinds of fluids to be infused. The procedure is performed by cannulating a superficial vein using an intravenous start kit and an appropriate-size catheter.

PURPOSE
To provide a peripheral venous access site for the administration of IV fluids, medications, blood products, and nutritional supplements

EQUIPMENT
IV start kit
Appropriate size needles
Small/large gauge catheters
Alcohol wipes
Gauze
Gloves

IV solution
IV tubing
Tape
Antiseptic ointment, if ordered

OUTCOMES
The client/caregiver will:

▶ Verbalize understanding of purpose of procedure
▶ Experience minimal discomfort

ASSESSMENT DATA
Assess the client's hydrational and nutritional status
Observe for signs and symptoms of fluid/electrolyte imbalance
Assess condition of peripheral veins
Obtain history of allergies, vascular disease, placement of shunts/fistulas
Review results of electrolyte profile and complete blood count

RELATED NURSING DIAGNOSES
Fluid volume deficit/excess
At risk for infection
Altered nutrition, less than body requirements
Anxiety
Knowledge deficit

SPECIAL CONSIDERATIONS
It may be difficult for the nurse to visualize the veins of the pediatric, geriatric, dehydrated, or mal-nourished client. The application of a warm compress prior to initiating the procedure will effect vasodilatation to facilitate visualization of the superficial veins. Do not attempt to insert an intra-venous catheter into an extremity with poor lymphatic drainage, with placement of a shunt or fis-tula for hemodialysis, or with severe scarring, cellulitis, or phlebitis.

TRANSCULTURAL CONSIDERATIONS
An interpreter will be needed for the client unable to speak or understand the English language. Obtain educational materials in the client's native language, if available. Consider use of AT&T Language Line. See also the Culturological Assessment procedure in Unit 2 for general overview of cultural considerations.

▶ INTERVENTIONS

Intervention	Rationale
1. Verify physician order.	*Reduces risk of error*
2. Explain procedure.	*Allays anxiety*
3. Wash hands.	*Prevents transmission of mi-crobes*
4. Prepare IV solution as ordered and prime IV tubing.	*Maintains patency of IV line*
5. Don gloves.	*Serves as protective barrier*
6. Apply tourniquet and observe for venous engorgement.	*Increases venous pressure per-mitting visualization of vein*
7. Select a vein and cleanse site per agency protocol.	*Decreases number of skin mi-crobes*

8. Puncture skin at 45-degree angle with bevel facing up needle held parallel to vein.

Facilitates entry of needle into the vein

9. Slowly insert needle into vein and observe for retrograde flow of blood.

Ensures that needle has entered blood vessel

10. Release tourniquet.

Reduces risk of rupturing the vein

11. Advance catheter using appropriate procedure depending on needle type.

For Catheter over Needle Insertion Set

Needle sits within the lumen of the catheter and must puncture the vein before catheter can be advanced
   a. with stylet held firmly in place slide catheter over stylet and puncture the vein
   b. remove stylet while holding hub of catheter securely
   c. connect end of primed IV tubing to catheter hub
   d. initiate intravenous infusion and observe for evidence of infiltration
   e. tape catheter in place

For Catheter Through Needle Insertion Set

Catheter sits within the lumen of the needle and can only be advanced after the needle punctures the vein
   a. hold the hub of the stylet and advance catheter while simultaneously pulling needle back
   b. withdraw the needle out of the catheter while applying pressure to site to secure catheter
   c. remove catheter sleeve and flow control plug
   d. connect end of primed IV tubing to catheter hub
   e. initiate intravenous infusion and observe for evidence of infiltration
   f. apply needle guard slipping needle and catheter into groove of needle guard then snap closed
   g. tape catheter in place

For Multilumen Peripheral Catheter Insertion Set

Enables the simultaneous administration of more than one kind of peripheral intravenous solution
   a. flush the proximal port with NSS
   b. enter the vein and advance both catheter and needle simultaneously
   c. advance catheter over the stylet and remove needle while holding stylet hub
   d. connect primed IV tubing to distal port
   e. obtain blood return from proximal port to check placement
   f. connect second primed IV tubing to proximal port
   g. initiate infusions
   h. tape catheter in place

12. Apply IV dressing per agency protocol using aseptic technique.

Retards growth of microbes at IV site

13. Regulate infusion as ordered.

Ensures accuracy of rate of fluid administration

14. Label dressing with date, time, catheter gauge and length, and initial.

Documents date of insertion
.

15. Discard used supplies appropriately.	*Maintains universal precautions*
16. Wash hands.	*Prevents transmission of microbes*

DOCUMENTATION

The following should be included in the nursing note:

Date and time of insertion
Insertion site
Type, length, and gauge of catheter used
Any difficulty in performing the procedure
All client/caregiver teaching:
    Topics to include in teaching plan:
        safe and correct equipment handling
        emergency procedures
        underlying disease pathology
        appropriate community resources and contact persons

INTERDISCIPLINARY COLLABORATION

Confer with physician regarding the development of any complications of the therapy
Consult with the pharmacist regarding the preparation of solutions requiring admixtures
Consult with the social worker to identify client's eligibility for financial assistance/reimbursement for supplies
Confer with DME vendor for ordering of supplies [1, 2, 6, 7, 17, 48, 62]

PROCEDURE

Insertion, Care, and Removal of Peripheral Central Venous Catheter

DESCRIPTION

The peripherally inserted central venous catheter (PICC) is inserted by the specially trained critical care nurse to establish a long-term venous access site. The catheter is advanced via venipuncture of the basilic, medial cubital, or cephalic vein. Once inserted via an arm vein, the catheter is advanced until the tip is positioned in the lower end of the superior vena cava (Figure 6-12). The PICC is used to avoid the complications associated with neck and chest insertion sites: catheter sepsis, air emboli, and injury to veins from trauma associated with repeated venipuncture.

PURPOSE

To provide central venous access for the administration of intravenous solutions, drug therapy, TPN, antiomicrobials, chemotherapy, and blood sampling

EQUIPMENT

Measuring tape/adhesive tape
Sterile barrier and fenestrated drape
Sphygmomanometer
Protective eyewear

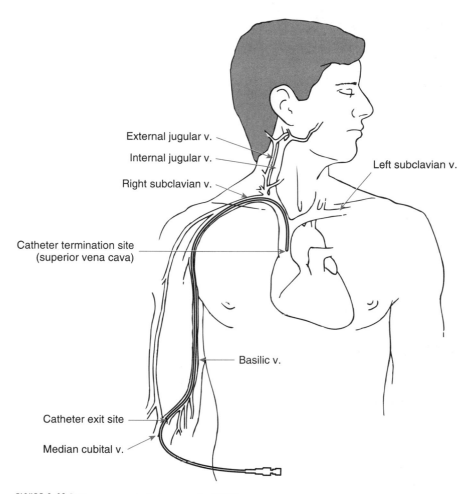

FIGURE 6-12 ▶ Recommended placement of PICC.

Cap or head covering
Sterile gown, gloves, saline solution
TB syringe
Catheter of choice with guide wire
Gauze
Suture removal/dressing change kit
Scissors
Alcohol swabs
Packet of steri strips
Saline flush kit
10-cc syringes for flushing as ordered
IV solution
IV tubing

Infusion pump
Client consent form

OUTCOMES
The client will:

▶ Verbalize understanding of purpose of procedure
▶ Experience minimal discomfort
▶ Be free of symptoms of infection

ASSESSMENT DATA
Assess the client's hydrational and nutritional status
Observe for signs and symptoms of infection
Obtain baseline physical assessment findings
Assess vasculature of the antecubital spaces
Obtain history of allergies, disease progression, vascular surgery, and contraindications for use of arm
Review results of electrolyte profile, complete blood count, culture and sensitivity reports

RELATED NURSING DIAGNOSES
At risk for injury
Infection
Altered body temperature
Anxiety
Knowledge deficit

SPECIAL CONSIDERATIONS
This procedure should only be performed by nurses who have received certification in the insertion of PICC lines. State boards of nursing will need to be consulted to ensure that the performance of this procedure is within the scope of nursing practice.

TRANSCULTURAL CONSIDERATIONS
An interpreter will be needed for the client unable to speak or understand the English language. Obtain educational materials in the client's native language, if available. Consider use of AT&T Language Line. See also the Culturological Assessment procedure in Unit 2 for general overview of cultural considerations.

▶ INTERVENTIONS

1. Verify physician order.	*Reduces risk of error*
2. Explain procedure.	*Allays anxiety*
3. Wash hands.	*Prevents transmission of microbes*
4. Perform physical assessment.	*Establishes baseline*
5. Measure from insertion site to lower one-third of superior vena cava.	*Ensures proper catheter tip placement*
6. Measure mid-arm circumference.	*Establishes baseline for assessment of venous occlusion*
7. Place arm on sterile field.	*Prevents contamination*

8. Don gloves, face mask, head covering, gloves. — *Serves as protective barrier*
9. Scrub the client's arm from mid-forearm to mid-upper arm with antiseptic solution. — *Removes microbes*
10. Cover the client's arm with sterile towel. — *Protects from contamination*
11. Nurse removes old gloves and scrubs own hands and forearms for 5 minutes with antiseptic soap. — *Prevents contamination*
12. Don sterile gown and gloves. — *Maintains aseptic technique*
13. Place all needed sterile supplies on sterile field. — *Maintains aseptic technique*
14. Measure catheter and cut to size using sterile scissors. — *Ensures correct positioning*
15. Position the arm at 45 to 90 degrees extension from the body. — *Facilitates advancement of catheter*
16. Scrub arm with antiseptic solution as ordered. — *Prevents contamination*
17. Place fenestrated drape over the arm leaving venipuncture site exposed. — *Maintains aseptic technique*
18. Apply tourniquet. — *Promotes vasodilation of vein for ease of access*
19. Remove old gloves and apply new sterile gloves. — *Maintains sterility*
20. Perform venipuncture per manufacturer's guidelines. — *Ensures accuracy*
21. Insert catheter. — *Establishes venous access*
22. Release tourniquet. — *Vasodilation not needed to advance catheter*
23. Have client turn head toward the cannulated arm and drop chin to shoulder. — *Prevents malpositioning of catheter in jugular vein*
24. Advance the remainder of the catheter and observe for evidence of cardiovascular compromise. — *Cardiac dysrhythmia may occur as catheter advances to the heart*
25. Have client turn head to opposite side. — *Prevents respiratory contamination*
26. Measure length of catheter outside of body and reposition to predetermined length. — *Ensures proper positioning of catheter*
27. Remove guidewire. — *Prevents recoiling of wire*
28. Attach 10-cc syringe filled with NSS and flush catheter, apply luer lock injection cap. — *Luer lock system secures catheter connections*
29. Flush with heparin lock solution per orders maintaining positive pressure to prevent blood backflow. — *Maintains patency of catheter*
30. Secure catheter with steri strips. — *Prevents migration of catheter*
31. Apply sterile dressing. — *Prevents contamination*
32. Obtain chest x-ray to ensure placement. — *Verifies catheter placement*
33. Discard protective gear appropriately and wash hands. — *Prevents transmission of microbes*

Site Care

1. Wash hands. — *Prevents transmission of microbes*
2. Don face mask, eyewear, and gloves. — *Serves as protective barrier*
3. Remove dressing and discard. — *Maintains universal precautions*
4. Inspect site for evidence of inflammation, infection, damage. — *Detects onset of complications*

5. Remove gloves and discard.	*Maintains universal precautions*
6. Don sterile gloves.	*Serves as protective barrier*
7. Cleanse insertion site per agency protocol using concentric circles moving from insertion site to surrounding tissue.	*Removes debris from skin and prevents contamination*
8. Apply transparent dressing.	*Permits direct visualization of insertion site*
9. Secure the catheter hub with tape.	*Prevents inadvertent catheter dislodgment*
10. Loop tubing to the arm.	*Provides slack to prevent undo pulling on insertion site*
11. Discard gloves.	*Maintains universal precautions*
12. Wash hands.	*Prevents transmission of microbes*

Removal of PICC line

1. Wash hands.	*Prevents transmission of microbes*
2. Establish sterile field.	*Prevents transmission of microbes*
3. Open suture removal kit, if applicable.	*Permits cutting of sutures to free catheter*
4. Open dressing change kit maintaining aseptic technique.	*Prevents transmission of microbes*
5. Turn off infusion.	*Discontinues the flow of intravenous fluid*
6. Don gloves.	*Serves as protective barrier*
7. Remove PICC dressing and discard in appropriate receptacle.	*Maintains universal precautions*
8. Remove gloves and don a clean pair.	*Serves as protective barrier*
9. Cleanse catheter site per agency protocol.	*Prevents contamination*
10. Remove sutures or steri strips.	*Frees catheter for ease in removal*
11. Grasp end of catheter and pull in outward direction.	*Fascilitates catheter removal*

    Instruct client to hold his/her breath (for the vent-dependent client remove during expiration)
    Grasp the PICC line at the insertion site and slowly remove
    Cover site with a sterile gauze and apply pressure for several minutes until bleeding stops
    Apply gauze dressing and cover with sterile gauze pad, assess length of catheter
    Secure dressing with tape
        if the resistance is met, apply warm compress to site, per agency protocol, and retry; if still having difficult notify physician

12. Discard gloves.	*Maintains universal precautions*
13. Wash hands.	*Prevents transmission of microbes*

DOCUMENTATION
The following should be included in the nursing note:

Date and time of insertion, catheter make, lumen, length
Insertion site
Method of securing catheter
Mid-upper arm circumference
Date and time of catheter removal
Informed consent obtained
Client response to procedure
Results of monitoring laboratory studies
Untoward reactions and interventions employed
All client/caregiver teaching:
    Topics to include in teaching plan:
        safe and correct equipment handling
        emergency procedures
        underlying disease pathology
        appropriate community resources and contact persons

INTERDISCIPLINARY COLLABORATION
Confer with physician regarding the development of any complications of the therapy
Consult with the pharmacist regarding the preparation of solutions requiring admixtures
Consult with the social worker to identify client's eligibility for financial assistance/reimbursement
    for supplies [1, 2, 6, 7, 15, 17, 21, 22, 39, 40, 41, 62]

PROCEDURE
Accessing/Deaccessing Implanted Ports

DESCRIPTION
The implanted port is surgically placed in an outpatient setting under local anesthesia. It is inconspicuously placed under the skin in a subcutaneous pocket and is accessed for the administration of infusion therapy or to obtain blood specimens (Figure 6-13). See also procedure on Managing Infusion Therapy.

PURPOSE
To permit infusion of solutions or withdrawal of blood specimens for laboratory analysis

EQUIPMENT
Sterile barrier
Gloves, sterile/non-sterile
Povidone-iodine/alcohol swab sticks per agency protocol
Gauze
Huber needle appropriate size
10-cc syringes
20-g 1-inch needles or needleless access devices
NSS for injection
Transparent dressing
Tape
Alcohol preps
Ordered IV solution

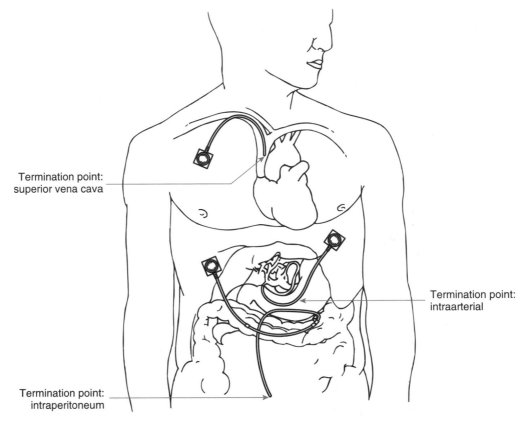

Termination point:
superior vena cava

Termination point:
intraarterial

Termination point:
intraperitoneum

FIGURE 6-13 ▶ Termination sites for implanted infusion ports.

Heparin lock solution
Injection cap
Male luer-lock adapter

OUTCOMES
The client/caregiver will:

▶ Verbalize understanding of the procedure
▶ Experience minimal discomfort

ASSESSMENT DATA
Observe for signs of infection
Assess for altered skin integrity at site

RELATED NURSING DIAGNOSES
At risk for infection
At risk for altered skin integrity
Anxiety
Knowledge deficit

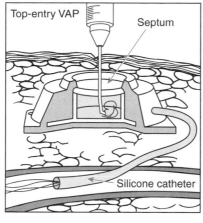

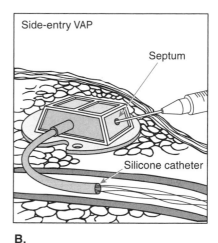

A. **B.**

FIGURE 6-14 ▶ Vascular access ports. **A.** Top-entry VAP. **B.** Side-entry VAP.

SPECIAL CONSIDERATIONS

Only a noncoring Huber needle is used to access the site (Figure 6-14). Use of any other type needle will damage the silicone septum. Refer to agency policy and manufacturer recommendations for protocol to follow for flushing of access device.

TRANSCULTURAL CONSIDERATIONS

An interpreter will be needed for the client unable to speak or understand the English language. Obtain educational materials in the client's native language, if available. Consider use of AT&T Language Line. See also the Culturological Assessment procedure in Unit 2 for general overview of cultural considerations.

▶ INTERVENTIONS

To Access Implanted Port for Instillation of Infusion

1. Verify physician order.	*Reduces risk of error*
2. Wash hands with antiseptic solution.	*Prevents transmission of microbe*
3. Perform physical assessment.	*Establishes baseline information of physiological data findings*
4. Explain procedure.	*Allays anxiety*
5. Create a sterile field adding Huber needle, 20-g needles or vial access devices, 10-cc syringes, and gauze to field.	*Accessing is performed as a sterile procedure*
6. Cleanse top of NSS vial with alcohol prep.	*Maintains sterility*
7. Don one sterile glove.	*Maintains sterility*
8. Attach 20-g 1-inch needle to 10-cc syringes and fill with NSS.	*Prepares syringe*
9. Don other sterile gloves.	*Maintains sterility*
10. Using concentric circles prep the site using povidone-iodine or alcohol then allow to air dry per agency protocol.	*Reduces microbes*

11. Remove needle from syringe and connect to Huber needle administration set and instill NSS system leaving syringe intact.	*Primes the line*
12. Palpate for location of silicone septum within port.	*Verifies position of port*
13. Stabilize the port with thumb and index finger.	*Pressure cannot be applied if port is not firmly positioned*
14. Use forefinger to guide insertion of Huber needle into port septum until the needle lodges within the port reservoir.	*Prevents deflection of needle*
15. Pull back on syringe to withdraw blood, slowly inject the NSS and remove syringe.	*Confirms placement*
16. Connect Huber administration set to an injection cap or intravenous infusion and seal connection with tape, start infusion. If not starting infusion, administer ordered heparin flush solution.	*Initiates intravenous therapy*
17. Apply steri-strips, tape, or sterile transparent dressing.	*Provides support to Huber needle*
18. Remove gloves.	*Remainder of procedure does not require sterility*
19. Form loop with the Huber administration set tubing and secure to chest with tape.	*Reduces tension and prevents accidental dislodgment*
20. Discard used supplies appropriately.	*Maintains universal precautions*
21. Wash hands.	*Prevents transmission of microbes*

To Deaccess Implanted Port

1. Verify physician order.	*Reduces risk of error*
2. Wash hands with antiseptic solution.	*Prevents transmission of microbes*
3. Perform physical assessment.	*Establishes baseline data*
4. Explain procedure.	*Allays anxiety*
5. Don gloves.	*Serves as protective barrier*
6. Create sterile field.	*Prevents contamination*
7. Cleanse NSS vial with alcohol prep and withdraw 5 cc–10 cc as ordered, recap needle, and set on field.	*Maintains sterility*
8. Cleanse heparin lock vial with alcohol prep and withdraw 3 cc–5 cc as ordered of heparin solution, recap and set on field.	*Maintains sterility*
9. Clamp extension tubing, remove injection cap or tubing.	*Prevents backflow*
10. Cleanse access port of extension tubing attached to Huber point needle with alcohol prep.	*Prevents transmission of microbes*
11. Flush access port with NSS.	*Clears port*
12. Remove transparent dressing.	*Facilitates removal of Huber needle*
13. Remove gauze, tape, steri-strips.	*Facilitates visualization of Huber needle*
14. Flush the port with heparin lock solution using a pulsative action to prevent backflow of blood, then stabilize the port and grasp the hub of the Huber needle removing needle at a perpendicular angle.	*Deaccesses port*
15. Apply pressure to site until bleeding stops.	*Prevents hematoma formation*

16. Apply bandage to site.   *Prevents contamination*
17. Discard used supplies appropriately.   *Maintains universal precautions*

18. Remove gloves and wash hands.   *Prevents transmission of microbes*

DOCUMENTATION
The following should be included in the nursing note:

Date and time of procedure
Type of infusion, rate of administration, size and length of huber needle used to access port
Amount and concentration of heparin flush solution
Skin integrity
Ease of insertion/de-accessing of Huber needle
Patency of port
Presence or absence of blood return
Signs of extravasation
Client's tolerance of the procedure
Clinical findings
Clients/caregiver's ability to perform procedure
All untoward responses and interventional strategies initiated
All client/caregiver teaching:
    Topics to include in teaching plan:
        safe and correct equipment handling
        emergency procedures
        underlying disease pathology
        appropriate community resources and contact persons

INTERDISCIPLINARY COLLABORATION
Notify physician of any evidence of infection, occlusion, altered skin integrity, or protrusion of
    port
Confer with DME vendor for reordering of supplies
Consult with the pharmacist for ordering of medication [1, 2, 6, 7, 15, 17, 21, 39–41, 48, 62]

PROCEDURE

Home Inotropic Infusion Therapy: Prototype Dobutamine

DESCRIPTION
Various positive inotropic agents are used for the home management of end-stage congestive heart failure (CHF), in clients who have not responded to digitalis, diuretics, or vasodilators. A variety of cardiac diseases and disorders cause the deterioration of cardiac pump function that leads to chronic CHF.

Congestive heart failure involves a cycle of compensatory responses. Decreased cardiac output leads to compensatory increases in catecholamines, angiotensin II, and argine vasopressin. Vasoconstriction out of proportion to what is needed to balance the deficit increases afterload and further impairs cardiac output. The cycle then starts over. Compensatory mechanisms then lose their effect on cardiac output, and lead to systemic cardiac and pulmonary congestion. Once the heart cannot keep pace, signs and symptoms of CHF become apparent.

Most clients referred for home inotropic therapy have severe CHF. Except in the case of maintaining a client awaiting heart transplantation, intravenous inotropic therapy is administered as a form of palliative therapy in order to improve the client's quality of life. The client's functional capacity can be measured by the New York Heart Association Functional Classification System of Persons with CHF (see Appendix 6-5). Clients with Class III or IV may be candidates for home inotropic therapy. Functional ability may improve while a client is maintained on home inotropic therapy. Shortness of breath and an improvement in minimal physical activity may be seen.

Dobutamine is a potent inotrope with mild positive chronotropic and vasodilating actions. Its action directly enhances myocardial contractility, stroke volume, and cardiac output. Because dobutamine is the primary parenteral inotropic agent used in home care, this discussion will focus on its use as a prototype.

This improved function, combined with appropriate interventions to prevent or reverse drug-related problems, may reduce the need for hospitalizations [5, 8, 17, 38, 40, 45, 53].

PURPOSE
To improve cardiac output

EQUIPMENT
Venous access kit
Infusion pump
Compatible intravenous set
Inotropic infusion, as ordered
Weight scale

OUTCOMES
The client/caregiver will be able to:

▶ Demonstrate the ability to administer and maintain dobutamine infusion
▶ Show improvement in cardiac output as evidenced by mental status improvement, increased urine output, decreased edema, shortness of breath, and absent S3 Gallop
▶ Verbalize understanding of signs and symptoms of worsening CHF or fluid overload
▶ Verbalize understanding of drug side effects
▶ Identify signs of infection related to infusion through central venous access
▶ Understand the prognosis related to end-stage CHF

ASSESSMENT DATA
Observe for signs and symptoms of altered cardiac and renal status: tachycardia, hypertension, ectopy, chest pain, diminished urinary output.
Compare baseline vital signs with vital signs obtained during each visit
Monitor electrolytes and CBC weekly
Note fluid status, observe for weight gain or loss.
Identify signs of infection related to infusion through venous access device

RELATED NURSING DIAGNOSIS
Alteration in cardiac output
Altered perfusion
At risk for infection
Knowledge deficit
Anxiety
Anticipatory grieving

SPECIAL CONSIDERATIONS

Clients should be stabilized in the hospital with several days of continuous infusion therapy, or at least one course of intermittent infusion therapy, prior to being admitted to homecare service. A responsible adult must be in attendance during the time of inotropic infusion. A nurse must be present for the first home dose to observe for complications or side effects and to remaining until the client is stable.

Tolerance to dobutamine is a well-defined problem commonly associated with long-term therapy. Unlike in the acute care setting, escalating doses of dobutamine are not needed. It has been shown that tolerance and dysrhythmia development can be minimized by limiting the dose of outpatient infusions to 5 mcg/kg/min. In practice dosages up to 7.5 mcg/kg/min are often seen without tachycardia or dysrhythmia.

It has been found that the benefits of dobutamine seem to last after the drug has been discontinued. This conditioning effect is the basis for the intermittent dobutamine therapy for clients less severely incapacitated by CHF. Intermittent therapy typically takes the form of administering a 48-hour infusion of the inotropic followed by a drug-free interval of 1 day or more [5, 8, 17, 38, 40, 45, 53].

TRANSCULTURAL CONSIDERATIONS

An interpreter will be needed for the client unable to speak or understand the English language. Obtain educational material in the client's native language, if available. Consider use of AT&T Language Line. See also the Culturological Assessment procedure in Unit 2 for general overview of cultural considerations.

▶ INTERVENTIONS

1. Verify physician orders for dose/hour, concentration, duration of infusion, type of venous access, parameters for blood pressure, heart rate, weight range, and laboratory specimens to be obtained.

    Reduces risk of error

2. Maintain strict handwashing procedures and the maintenance of universal precautions.

    Prevents the transmission of microbes and spread of infection.

3. Perform a physical assessment and record clinical findings.

    Documenting baseline data elements of physiological findings is imperative to evaluate outcome criteria.

4. Provide client and family teaching regarding procedures.

    Allays anxiety.

5. Gather the intravenous solution, equipment, administration set, don gloves, prepare the infusion, connect to infusion pump, access the intravenous site, and initiate infusion (see Managing Intravenous Therapy).

    An organized approach ensures efficiency and maximizes time utilization

6. Instruct and document client/caregiver in aseptic intravenous infusion procedure and permit return demonstration.

    Documents client's/caregiver's ability to implement the procedure

7. Instruct client/caregiver in self-monitoring procedures: temperature, blood pressure, heart rate, daily weight, intake and output.

    Promotes client self-sufficiency

8. Assess client response to treatment and document presence of side effects or evidence of drug tolerance.

    Indicates effectiveness of treatment

For Management of Drug Intolerance

Promotes early detection of untoward medication reactions

1. Establish baseline parameters. Vital signs and weights.
2. Evaluate fluid status. Monitor intake and output.
3. Detect presence of fluid volume overload. Assess lung sounds, abdominal girth, extremity edema, skin turgor.
4. Monitor for electrolyte imbalance.
5. Facilitate self sufficiency by instructing client/caregiver in self-monitoring procedures.

For Management of Fluid Volume Overload

See procedure for Loop Diuretic Infusion Therapy.

For Management of Dysrhythmias

Promotes early detection of cardiac rhythm disturbance

1. Establish baseline cardiac rate and rhythm prior to initiating therapy.
2. Detect presence of fluid overload by observation of decreased cardiac output.
3. Monitor potassium and magnesium levels to avoid predisposing client to dysrhythmias.
4. Document client's ability to perform pulse-taking technique.
5. Document client's understanding of signs and symptoms of fluid overload.
6. Establish baseline cardiac rhythm by obtaining an ECG.

DOCUMENTATION

The following information should be included in the nursing note:

Dose, concentration, rate, and duration of infusion
Type of IV access
Clinical findings
Client response to therapy
Presence of drug side effects
Clients/caregiver's ability to perform procedure
All untoward responses and interventional strategies initiated
All client/caregiver teaching:
    Topics to include in teaching plan:
        safe and correct equipment handling
        emergency procedures
        underlying disease pathology
        appropriate community resources and contact persons

INTERDISCIPLINARY COLLABORATION

Inform the physician of 5% increase/decrease in weight, abnormal laboratory results or vital signs. Evaluate need for supplemental oxygen and confer with physician. Consult with social worker to identify community support groups for assistance in coping with end stage of disease progression. Integrate nutritional consultation regarding prescribed dietary restrictions. Consult physical therapy to maximize physical activity with minimal increase in myocardial oxygen demands. Confer with pharmacist for ordering and delivery of infusion. Anticipate need to reorder supplies and infusion equipment from DME vendor [1, 5, 6, 8, 11, 13–15, 17, 20, 21, 38, 40, 41, 45, 48, 53, 62].

PROCEDURE
Home Loop Diuretic Intravenous Therapy: Prototype Furosemide Injection

DESCRIPTION
Loop diuretics inhibit the reabsorption of sodium and chloride in the proximal and distal tubules, resulting in the excretion of sodium chloride, and, to a lesser degree, potassium and bicarbonate ions. These agents are used to treat fluid volume excess. Because furosemide is the most common parenteral loop diuretic agent used in the home, this discussion will focus on its use as a prototype.

PURPOSE
To reduce fluid volume

EQUIPMENT
Venous access kit
Furosemide injection
Peripheral IV catheter, butterfly, or permanent venous access with injection cap

OUTCOMES
The client/caregiver will:

▶ State improvement in symptoms of fluid overload
▶ Verbalize understanding of signs and symptoms of adverse and side effects of furosemide therapy
▶ Verbalize signs and symptoms of fluid overload/deficit
▶ Identify signs of infection at insertion site
▶ Maintain body weight per physician guidelines

ASSESSMENT DATA
Note baseline laboratory results screening for impairment of renal or liver function
Monitor response to therapy assessing hydrational status, respiratory status, vital signs and symptoms of electrolyte imbalance (weakness, muscle cramps, confusion)
Observe for ototoxicity (tinnitus, hearing loss, vertigo)
Document trends in daily weights
Observe for signs of infection at intravenous site

RELATED NURSING DIAGNOSES
Ineffective breathing patterns
Decreased cardiac output
Fluid volume excess
Impaired gas exchange
Potential for altered skin integrity
Anxiety
Anticipatory grieving
Knowledge deficit
Altered urinary elimination

SPECIAL CONSIDERATIONS

Furosemide is the most common parenteral diuretic therapy used in the home. Clients with severe volume overload are typically managed with loop diuretic therapy in the home setting. Generally, this therapy is used in the client with Class III–IV congestive heart failure (see Home Inotropic Infusion Therapy: Prototype Dobutamine). A combination of both intravenous and oral diuretic agents may be used. The nurse should monitor for profound diuresis and/or electrolyte imbalance. Either continuous infusions or intermittent bolus intravenous injections may be used to treat overload.

Use of furosemide in pregnant or lactating women is not recommended.

Monitor laboratory results for evidence of potassium depletion and confer with physician regarding need to add potassium supplements to the treatment plan. Note potential for ototoxicity when used concomitantly with aminoglycosides. Consider dosing in the morning to avoid diuresis during the night and potential for sleep pattern disturbance.

TRANSCULTURAL CONSIDERATIONS

An interpreter will be needed for the client unable to speak or understand the English language. Obtain educational materials in the client's native language, if available. Consider use of AT&T Language Line. See also the Culturological Assessment procedure in Unit 2 for general overview of cultural considerations.

▶ INTERVENTIONS

1. Verify physician.	*Reduces risk of error*
2. Wash hands.	*Prevents transmission of microbes*
3. Perform physical assessment.	*Establishes baseline information*
4. Explain procedure.	*Reduces anxiety*
5. Access existing primary line or insert heparin lock via peripheral IV site, and flush with NSS per protocol.	*Establishes patency*
6. Draw up ordered dose of medication and infuse slowly via heparin lock or Y-port of primary line after temporarily stopping primary infusion.	*Dosage should not exceed 4 mg/min*
7. Flush hep lock with NSS and heparin if ordered.	*Maintains patency of heparin lock*
8. Observe for diuresis.	*Indicates drug effectiveness*
9. Instruct client to obtain and record daily weights and to maintain intake and output record.	*Promotes client self-sufficiency*
10. Instruct client to take potassium supplements as ordered and to increase intake of potassium-rich foods.	*Prevents development of hypokalemia*

DOCUMENTATION

The following should be included in the nursing note:

Medication dosage and rate and method of administration
Type of IV access
Condition of access site
Client's response to therapy
Presence of side effects or adverse reactions and interventions employed

All client instruction and verbalization of understanding
All client/caregiver teaching:
Topics to include in teaching plan:
safe and correct equipment handling
emergency procedures
underlying disease pathology
appropriate community resources and contact persons

INTERDISCIPLINARY COLLABORATION

Inform physician of persistent edema, weight gain/loss > 2 lb per day, respiratory difficulty, poor urinary response, vital signs, and laboratory results. Evaluate need for oxygen therapy and confer with physician.

Consult with social worker to identify community support groups for end-stage disease progression. Consult nutritionist to assist with menu planning for dietary and fluid restrictions. Consult physical therapy to maximize physical activity with minimal increase in myocardial oxygen demands. Consult with pharmacist in the preparation and delivery of medication to the home [6, 15, 17, 20, 21, 33, 41, 48, 62].

PROCEDURE
Home Anticoagulant Infusion Therapy: Prototype Heparin

DESCRIPTION

Heparin is an anticoagulant that acts by inhibiting the conversion of prothrombin to thrombin and fibrinogen to fibrin. The drug is used to prevent the formation or extension of an existing clot. The continuous or intermittent parenteral administration of heparin in the home setting is typically used to treat the pregnant client who is predisposed to developing thromboembolic activity. Nonobstetric clients diagnosed with deep vein thrombosis are also candidates for home heparin infusion.

PURPOSE
To prevent the formation of blood clots

EQUIPMENT
Infusion pump
Intravenous set
Heparin infusion

OUTCOMES
The client/caregiver will:

▶ Demonstrate ability to administer/maintain heparin infusion
▶ Maintain APTT at 1.5 to 2.5 times the control
▶ Verbalize understanding of drug side effects, signs of bleeding, and need to avoid injury

ASSESSMENT DATA
Observe for evidence of bleeding: hematuria, melena, hematoma, ecchymosis, epistaxis, hematemesis, hemoptysis
Monitor APTT, clotting times, and platelet counts as ordered
Monitor electrolytes and CBC weekly
Note fluid status

RELATED NURSING DIAGNOSES
Decreased cardiac output
Altered tissue perfusion
Fatigue
Knowledge deficit

SPECIAL CONSIDERATIONS
Anticoagulation with heparin is contraindicated in the client with a history of hypersensitivity to pork, beef, or other animal products. The risk of complication increases as the course of therapy lengthens. Menstruating females will need to observe and report any evidence of excessive vaginal bleeding. All clients should be taught to avoid use of over-the-counter medications unless ordered by their physician.

TRANSCULTURAL CONSIDERATIONS
An interpreter will be needed for the client unable to speak or understand the English language. Obtain educational materials in the client's native language, if available. Consider use of AT&T Language Line.

A client of the Jehovah Witness faith may be unwilling to accept blood transfusion should hemorrhaging develop.

See also the Culturological Assessment procedure in Unit 2 for general overview of cultural considerations.

▶ INTERVENTIONS

1. Verify physician orders for dose/hour, concentration, duration of infusion, type of venous access parameters for blood pressure, heart rate, weight range, and laboratory results.	*Ensures client specific care*
2. Wash hands.	*Prevents transmission of microbes*
3. Perform physical assessment.	*Establishes baseline information of physiological data findings*
4. Explain procedure.	*Allays anxiety*
5. Establish intravenous site.	*Prepares route of administration*
6. Instruct client/caregiver in aseptic parenteral infusion procedure and permit return demonstration. See managing infusion therapy.	*Documents client/caregiver's ability to implement procedure*
7. Instruct client/caregiver in self-monitoring procedures: temperature, blood pressure, heart rate, signs of bleeding, intake and output.	*Promotes client self-sufficiency*
8. Assess client response to treatment and document presence of side effects.	*Indicates effectiveness of treatment*

DOCUMENTATION
The following should be included in the nursing note:

Dose, concentration and duration of infusion
Type of access site

Results of clotting times
Clinical findings
Client response to therapy
Presence of drug side effects
Client/caregiver's ability to perform procedure
All untoward responses and interventional strategies initiated
All client/caregiver teaching:
    Topics to include in teaching plan:
        safe and correct equipment handling
        emergency procedures
        underlying disease pathology
        appropriate community resources and contact persons

INTERDISCIPLINARY COLLABORATION

Inform physician of bleeding tendency, abnormal vital signs, or laboratory results
Consult with DME vendor to reorder supplies as needed
Consult with pharmacy to reorder infusion as needed [1, 6, 15, 17, 20, 21, 40, 41, 62]

PROCEDURE
Home Antibiotic Infusion Therapy

DESCRIPTION

Home antibiotic infusion therapy is used to administer drugs used in the treatment of serious infection: antibacterial, antiviral, antifungal, and antiprotozoal agents. Throughout home antibiotic infusion therapy, intense monitoring of renal function, drug levels, hearing loss, bone marrow suppression, and other assessment parameters must be routinely performed depending on drug used. At times it may be necessary to administer two or more antibiotic agents during the same course of treatment.

PURPOSE

To destroy or inhibit the growth of pathogenic organisms

EQUIPMENT

IV start kit if access site has not been established (see procedures on inserting peripheral intravenous lines)
Saline flush kit
10-cc syringes for flushing as ordered
Appropriate size needles or needleless access devices
Small/large gauge catheters
Alcohol wipes
Gauze
Gloves
IV antibiotic infusion as ordered
IV tubing
Infusion pump
Tape

OUTCOMES

The client/caregiver will:

▶ Verbalize understanding of purpose of procedure
▶ Experience minimal discomfort

▶ Be free of symptoms of infection and complications of intravenous therapy
▶ Demonstrate ability to implement the procedure

ASSESSMENT DATA

Assess the client's hydrational and nutritional status
Observe for signs and symptoms of infection
Assess condition of peripheral veins or central access site
Obtain history of allergies, and disease progression
Review results of electrolyte profile, complete blood count, creatinine, liver function studies, and culture and sensitivity reports

RELATED NURSING DIAGNOSES

Fluid volume deficit/excess
Infection
Altered body temperature
Anxiety
Knowledge deficit

SPECIAL CONSIDERATIONS

The first dose of the antibiotic therapy may be administered in a well-monitored setting: hospital or outpatient setting, physician office. If agency policy permits the first dose to be administered in the home, determine that the community resources include emergency service teams, the client has a functioning telephone line, and that client has not had an allergic response to medication therapy in the past. The nurse must have access to an anaphylaxis kit and physician orders for its use.

TRANSCULTURAL CONSIDERATIONS

An interpreter will be needed for the client unable to speak or understand the English language. Obtain educational materials in the client's native language, if available. Consider use of AT&T Language Line. See also the Culturological Assessment procedure in Unit 2 for general overview of cultural considerations.

▶ INTERVENTIONS

1. Verify physician order.	*Reduces risk of error*
2. Explain procedure.	*Allays anxiety*
3. Wash hands.	*Prevents transmission of microbes*
4. Perform physical assessment.	*Establishes baseline*
5. Don gloves.	*Serves as protective barrier*
6. Access existing IV site or insert peripheral line (see procedure on insertion of superficial intravenous or PICC line).	*Establishes patency of access site*
7. Instruct client/caregiver in the aseptic administration of antibiotic therapy and permit return demonstration.	*Documents client/caregiver's ability to maintain sterility and implement procedure*

For Routine Antibiotic Infusion

Protocol to initiate intermittent infusion

a. wash hands
b. obtain IV antibiotic solution from refrigerator 30 minutes prior to infusion

    c. check to insure that solution is clear and that bag is
       intact

    d. note expiration date of solution

    e. spike the IV bag, prime the IV line, clamp tubing, and
       hang bag

    f. connect to infusion pump

    g. cleanse venous access site

    h. flush site per agency protocol

    i. remove protective cap and insert into access site

    j. tape to secure in place

    k. turn on pump, open clamp, and initiate infusion

    l. infuse over time period ordered by physician

    m. at completion of infusion disconnect from medication
        delivery system and flush line with saline and heparin
        as ordered

    n. cleanse access site with alcohol wipe

    o. dispose of used supplies in appropriate container

    p. wash hands

1. Review signs and symptoms of infection and review   *Ensures client understanding*
   emergency protocol.

For Anaphylaxis in the Adult: Mild Reaction

Protocol must specifically indicate nursing interventions for mild allergic reaction

1. Stop infusion.
2. Report to physician.
3. Administer Benadryl per protocol.
4. Monitor vital signs and symptoms.
5. Document interventions.

For Anaphylaxis in the Adult: Severe Reaction

Protocol must specifically indicate nursing interventions for severe allergic reaction

1. Stop infusion.
2. Administer epinephrine per protocol.
3. Mobilize community EMS team.
4. Ensure patency of airway.
5. Initiate CPR as indicated.
6. Administer IV fluids per protocol.
7. Monitor vital signs frequently.
8. Notify physician when paramedic team arrives.

DOCUMENTATION

The following should be included in the nursing note:

Date and time of insertion
Insertion site
Client response to therapy
Results of monitoring laboratory studies

Untoward reactions and interventions employed
Medication, infusion rate, dose, delivery system
All client/caregiver teaching:
    Topics to include in teaching plan:
        safe and correct equipment handling
        emergency procedures
        underlying disease pathology
        appropriate community resources and contact persons

INTERDISCIPLINARY COLLABORATION

Confer with physician regarding the development of any complications of the therapy
Consult with the pharmacist regarding the preparation of solutions requiring admixtures
Consult with the social worker to identify client's eligibility for financial assistance/reimbursement
    for supplies
Anticipate need to reorder supplies/equipment from DME vendor [1, 6, 7, 15, 17, 20, 21, 40, 41,
    48, 62]

PROCEDURE
Home Total Parenteral Nutrition (TPN) Therapy, Adult

DESCRIPTION

Home total parenteral nutrition (TPN) is used for both short-term and long-term management of malnutritious states. Through venous access devices, nutritional intravenous solutions are administered via central veins. Typically, the client is stabilized in the hospital setting, then discharged to home for long-term therapy. The composition of the TPN solution is determined by the client's need for calories, protein, fat, vitamins, trace minerals, and fluid. The TPN solution may be administered continuously over 24 hours or intermittently over a 10–12 hour period with or without tapering. See also Unit 5, Home Total Parenteral Nutrition Therapy, Pediatric.

PURPOSE

To provide nutritional requirements by maintaining or restoring weight, and promoting tissue healing and growth when use of oral and/or enteral supplements cannot be used.

EQUIPMENT

Ordered TPN solution
Infusion pump
IV tubing with .22 micron filter for solution without lipids; tubing with 1.2 micron filter when
    lipid infusion is added to the solution (3 in 1 solution)
Medication additives
Alcohol wipes
Urine or glucose monitoring equipment
Equipment to access central line
Refrigerator

OUTCOMES

The client/caregiver will:

▶ Be independent in the administration of TPN solution and care of access site
▶ Verbalize knowledge of signs and symptoms of infection and potential side effects related to
    TPN therapy

ASSESSMENT DATA

Record results of urine or blood glucose levels
Observe for signs and symptoms of hyper/hypoglycemia
Record daily weights
Monitor blood chemistries as ordered
Evaluate client/caregiver for knowledge of safety measures
Observe for evidence of fluid volume overload/deficit
Observe skin surfaces and access sites for evidence of infection
Evaluate nutritional status

RELATED NURSING DIAGNOSES

At risk for infection
Altered nutrition, less than body requirements
At risk for fluid volume deficit/overload
Knowledge deficit
Altered skin integrity
At risk for ineffective family coping

SPECIAL CONSIDERATIONS

For clients with 3 in 1 solutions, instruction must include the need to inspect the solution for "oiling out" or cracking, which occurs when the fat emulsion separates or falls out of solution state
See also Unit 5, Home Total Parenteral Nutrition Therapy, Pediatric

TRANSCULTURAL CONSIDERATIONS

An interpreter will be needed for the client unable to speak or understand the English language. Obtain educational materials in the client's native language, if available. Consider use of AT&T Language Line. See also the Culturological Assessment procedure in Unit 2 for general overview of cultural considerations.

▶ INTERVENTIONS

1. Verify physician order. — *Reduces risk of error*
2. Wash hands. — *Prevents transmission of microbe*

3. Perform physical assessment. — *Establishes baseline data*
4. Explain procedure. — *Allays anxiety*
5. Prepare a clean table top surface, wipe with antiseptic solution per agency protocol. — *Reduces presence of microorganisms during solution preparation*

6. Remove TPN solution from the refrigerator at least 2 hours prior to administration per agency protocol. — *Decreases vasoconstriction*

7. Instruct the client to perform catheter care using aseptic technique. — *Decreases risk of infection*

8. Instruct client on administration of TPN solution, permit return demonstration. — *Documents client's ability to perform ordered procedure*

9. Instruct client on self-monitoring activities (temperature, daily weights, symptoms of infection hypo/hyperglycemia, urine or blood glucose testing). — *Ensures client's understanding of complications of therapy*

10. Observe for side effects of TPN therapy and follow agency protocol for management.

For Catheter-Related Infections

Preventative measures will reduce risk of infection
  a. follow good handwashing technique prior to initiating all procedures
  b. perform regular access site care and inspection per agency protocol
  c. use aseptic technique when changing IV lines, infusion solution, and dressings
  d. change IV tubing every 24 hours
  e. change TPN solution every 24 hours
  f. observe for signs and symptoms of infection
  g. record temperature readings daily
  h. culture all purulent exudate and report immediately to physician

For Metabolic Complications

Maintaining blood chemistries/fluid balance within ordered parameters enhances physiological tolerance
  a. Blood glucose: Maintain fingerstick blood glucose (FSBS) levels between 100–250 mg/dl or per physician order obtain FSBS prior to initiating TPN, every 8 hours for continuous infusion, and 1 hr after discontinuation of TPN as ordered. Initiate a taper up at the start of therapy and a taper downtime for all cyclic TPN infusions as ordered
  b. Fluid excess/deficit:
     Obtain daily weight
     Record intake and output
     Monitor serum electrolytes
  c. Electrolyte imbalance: Monitor the following blood studies as ordered: electrolyte levels, liver function test results, CBC with platelet count, BUN, cholesterol, PT, proteins, phosphorous, magnesium, calcium, and creatinine

DOCUMENTATION
The following should be noted in the nursing note:

Untoward responses reported to the physician
Interventions employed as a result of deviations from the norm
Cardiovascular, respiratory, and nutritional assessment findings
Pump settings
Client/caregiver verbalized understanding of all self-monitoring activities
Ability to perform the procedure using aseptic technique
Ability to prepare solution, inject additives, access/deaccess site, perform site care, operate the
     pump, connect/disconnect tubing
All client/caregiver teaching:
   Topics to include in teaching plan:
      safe and correct equipment handling
      emergency procedures
      underlying disease pathology
      appropriate community resources and contact persons

INTERDISCIPLINARY COLLABORATION

Inform the physician of weight gain or loss, blood chemistry results, untoward reactions

Consult with pharmacist and nutritionist for recommendations for change to formula consistent with laboratory findings.

Confer with social worker to determine client eligibility for reimbursement/financial assistance for all equipment/supplies, and to identify appropriate community resources

Anticipate need to reorder supplies from DME vendor [1, 2, 6, 7, 17, 18, 20–22, 25, 39, 40, 51, 61, 62]

PROCEDURE
Home Blood Component Therapy

DESCRIPTION

Transfusion therapy is implemented to increase hemoglobin stores and improve the blood's oxygen-carrying capacity, to restore clotting factors, and to reduce risk of infection in the neutropenic client (see Table 6-1). Prior to administration, the client will be typed and crossmatched to ensure compatibility and reduce risk of transfusion reaction. Blood is tested for ABO blood typing and crossmatching, Rh typing, human leukocyte antigens (HLA), the direct antiglobin test, and the antibody screening test. Additionally, the blood is routinely screened for hepatitis B, syphilis, human immunodeficiency virus (HIV), and cytomegalovirus.

PURPOSE

To restore blood components for therapeutic purposes

EQUIPMENT

Nonsterile gloves
Emergency drug kit
Stethoscope
Syphgmomanometer
Thermometer
Blood administration set with filter
Biohazardous waste container
Sharps container
IV start kit

TABLE 6-1 Home Blood Component Therapy

Blood Product	Volume*	Action and Uses
Packed Red Blood Cells (RBCs)	250 ml	increase red cell mass
Leukocyte-poor RBCs	200 ml	prevent febrile non-hemolytic transfusion reactions
White Blood Cells	150 ml	for chronic malignant conditions
Cryoprecipitate	10–20 ml/bag	replacement of clotting factors
Platelets	30–60 ml/unit	restore platelet count in clients with thrombocytopenia
Albumin 5% (buffered saline)	250 ml	treat chronic hypoproteinemia
Albumin 25% (salt-poor)	50 ml	treat chrnoic hypoproteinemia
Gamma globulin	100–500 mg/kg	provide passive immunity against infection

*verify duration of transfusion and frequency of administration with physician order

Transfusion consent form
Normal saline IV solution
Flush solution

OUTCOMES
The client/caregiver will:

▶ Provide informed consent for transfusion
▶ Verbalize signs and symptoms of potential long-term transfusion reactions
▶ Inform nurse of development of allergic reactions
▶ Assist the nurse in verifying blood tag label with the blood bank ID bracelet

ASSESSMENT DATA
Obtain transfusion history, transfusion order, and verify signed consent form
Obtain baseline vital signs and vital signs throughout procedure per agency protocol
Check verbally with the caregiver the client's name with medical record, bracelet and blood tag, component expiration time/date, and any special component orders
Assess for signs of transfusion reaction (circulatory overload, fever, rash, wheezing, chest pain, dyspnea, allergic reaction, sepsis, acute hemolytic reaction)
Evaluate client for 30–60 minutes post-transfusion, per agency policy
Obtain serum specimen for appropriate laboratory studies (CBC with differential, etc.) as ordered

RELATED NURSING DIAGNOSES
Altered tissue perfusion
Fluid volume deficit
Decreased cardiac output
Knowledge deficit

SPECIAL CONSIDERATIONS
Clients selected to receive home transfusion therapy should have a stable cardiopulmonary system and have no history of blood transfusion reactions in the past. The maximum amount of blood that can be infused in the home cannot exceed two units per day. Typing and crossmatching should have been performed within 48 hours prior to transfusion. The client's home environment must safely support the administration of blood: functioning telephone line, access to an EMS team, physician availability during the transfusion, and a responsible adult able to initiate emergency protocol [7, 17, 22, 40, 41].

Elderly clients have decreased cardiac functioning, and therefore require a slower rate of infusion and less volume of solution. Age-related slowing of the immune system places the elderly client at risk for infection, and at risk for delayed response to transfusion reactions. Pediatric transfusions are usually given on a pump, prepared in half-unit packages, and infused via a smaller gauge catheter. The transfusion should be initiated as soon as possible after the unit has been received from the blood bank. Rapid infusion of cold blood products through a central line can result in ventricular dysrhythmias. Some types of blood components have specific infusion sets to be used for administration and may be supplied by the blood bank [7, 17, 22, 40, 41].

Regulations governing the administration of blood products in the home are established by the American Association of Blood Banks, American Red Cross, and state and agency guidelines. The nurse should be familiar with the rules governing state practice acts and agency procedures. The blood must be obtained from the blood bank no more than 30 minutes prior to the start of the infusion. Before accepting the blood unit, check the blood bag label for the client's full name and social security or identification number, ABO and Rh type, product to be infused, and expiration date. Follow state and federal regulations to maintain temperature of the unit, which will be delivered in a special shipping container. Open the shipping container only when ready to initiate the transfusion. Once opened, the blood must be used within 4 hours. [7, 17, 22, 40, 41]

Prior to administration, verify the client's name, identification number against ID bracelet, and check with another responsible adult in the home. Notify the blood bank of any discrepancies and do not administer the blood. Inspect the blood unit for evidence of contamination, discoloration, agglutination, or gas bubbles. If present, return the unit to the blood bank [7, 17, 22, 40, 41].

Blood filters should be used on all blood products to avoid the infusion of fibrin clots. The standard blood administration set comes with a leukocyte-removal filter. If administering more than one unit of blood, check with agency policy regarding changing of tubing and inline filter [7, 17, 22, 40, 41].

TRANSCULTURAL CONSIDERATIONS

Some religions prohibit followers from receiving blood or blood products. Ensure that the client has given informed consent.

Obtain educational materials in the language of the client, if available. Consider use of AT&T Language Line. See also the Culturological Assessment procedure in Unit 2 for general overview of cultural considerations.

▶ INTERVENTIONS

1. Verify physician order.	*Reduces risk of error*
2. Wash hands.	*Prevents transmission of microbes*
3. Perform physical assessment.	*Establishes baseline data*
4. Explain procedure.	*Allays anxiety*
5. Organize equipment.	*Promotes efficiency*
6. Remove blood component from ice 20 minutes prior to reinfusing.	*Reduces risk of transfusion-lated dysrhythmias*
7. Verify the product and identify the client with a person considered to be qualified according to agency policy and obtain a co-signature.	*Reduces risk of error*
8. Administer premedication as ordered.	*Helps reduce possible transfusion reaction*
9. Open blood administration set and clamp tubing.	*Prevents accidental spilling of blood*
10. Don gloves.	*Serves as protective barrier*
11. If using Y-tubing set, perform procedure as follows	*Y-set enables the simultaneous administration of saline and blood product*
a. turn roller clamps to off position	
b. spike the normal saline bag, hang the solution, and open clamp between unit and drip chamber	
c. fill chamber with NSS, cover filter	
d. prime tubing	
e. close clamp	
f. gently invert the blood component 2–3 times	
g. spike the blood unit, hang the unit, and open clamp between unit and drip chamber	
h. fill chamber with blood, cover filter	
12. Take vital signs.	*Establishes baseline*

13. Establish or access venous site, cleanse site, and flush with saline per agency policy.	*Maintains patency of line*
14. Attach primed tubing to venous access site using direct connection.	*Initiates infusion*
15. Unclamp blood tubing and allow to infuse at rate of 2 ml/min for first 15 minutes.	*Most reactions occur within the first 15 minutes*
16. Monitor vital signs for first 15 to 30 minutes and frequently thereafter per agency policy.	*Permits early detection of untoward reactions*
17. Adjust drip rate to infuse per physician order.	*Infuse blood over a period of time not to exceed 4 hours to prevent risk of bacterial growth*
18. After transfusion is complete, clamp tubing leading to blood unit.	*Prevents formation of air emboli in the intravenous line*
19. Unclamp tubing leading to normal saline solution and flush tubing thoroughly.	*Infuses remainder of blood in distal tubing*
20. Reclamp and disconnect from client.	*Discontinues infusion*
21. Flush access site with normal saline solution and cap with new injection cap.	*Maintains patency of access site*
22. Complete transfusion tag.	*Documents completion or discontinuance of blood product*
23. Remain with client for 30–60 minutes post-transfusion.	*Permits assessment of post-transfusion reactions*
24. Provide client with post-transfusion instructions.	*Allows client to identify symptoms of untoward reaction (allergic reaction, low back pain, nausea and vomiting, angina, hematuria, anuria)*
25. Draw post-transfusion lab work as ordered.	*Monitors client response to therapy*

If a Reaction Occurs, Follow Emergency Protocol

1. Turn off blood transfusion and disconnect blood tubing from access site.	*Stops further infusion of blood product*
2. Obtain new IV tubing, spike new bag of normal saline, prime line, and infuse.	*Prevents client from receiving any blood that may be remaining in old IV line*
3. Infuse saline at prescribed rate per emergency protocol.	*Ensures patency of catheter*
4. Obtain urine and two blood specimens, and return to blood bank with unused blood product.	*Determines presence of hemolysis*
5. Complete forms for transfusion reaction.	*Documents reaction and interventions employed*
6. Obtain vital signs until stable.	*Monitors cardiopulmonary status*
7. Arrange for transportation to hospital.	*Transfusion reactions require medical intervention*

If Shock Occurs	
1. Administer IV fluids per emergency protocol.	*Treats hypovolemic reaction*
2. Monitor vital signs.	*Detects further cardiopul-monary collapse*
3. Administer oxygen if available.	*Corrects hypoxia*
4. Initiate CPR in event of respiratory/cardiac arrest.	*Maintains ventilation and circulation*
5. Initiate EMS service.	*Mobilizes community emergency team*

DOCUMENTATION

The following should be noted in the nursing note:

Date, time, and description of procedure including the transfusion component, rate, and amount infused

Client's tolerance of the procedure

Any untoward reactions and interventions to counteract reactions

Name of person verifying client information in the home

All client/caregiver teaching:

   Topics to include in teaching plan:

      safe and correct equipment handling

      emergency procedures

      underlying disease pathology

      appropriate community resources and contact persons

INTERDISCIPLINARY COLLABORATION

Inform physician of all untoward reactions and interventions employed.

Consult with blood bank to coordinate blood delivery to the home

Consult with DME vendor for acquisition of supplies

Confer with social worker to determine client's eligibility for financial assistance/reimbursement for blood products/supplies. [6, 7, 15, 17, 21, 22, 40, 41]

3 Adult Immune System Procedures

PROCEDURE
Organ Transplant Care and Management, Adult

DESCRIPTION
Transplantation refers to the procedure used to transfer living tissue from human to human, from animal to human, or from one part of the body to another in the same individual. Commonly transplanted organs include: kidney, heart, lung, liver, bone marrow, skin, cornea, and pancreas. Several types of graft tissue are used in transplantation: *autograft*, a transplant of the client's own tissue; *isograft*, a transplant of tissue from an identical twin; *allograft*, a transplant of tissue from a human donor; and, *xenograft*, a transplant of tissue from an animal species [17, 23, 25, 40].

Bone marrow transplantation is a treatment option for clients with certain kinds of cancer. The client may be infused with the bone marrow acquired from a donor (allogeneic marrow transplantation), an identical twin (syngeneic), or may receive his or her own bone marrow (autologous marrow transplantation) harvested prior to the initiation of intensive therapy. Bone marrow may be obtained from the iliac crest, sternum, or ribs. A newer technique permits the obtaining of bone marrow cells through an apheresis procedure that separates the cells from the circulating blood. See also Pediatric Immune System Procedures [17, 23, 25, 40].

PURPOSE
To decrease incidence of complications associated with organ transplantation

EQUIPMENT
Health assessment forms
Stethoscope
Syphygmomanometer
Thermometer
Infusion equipment and supplies as indicated
Venipuncture supplies
Weight scale

OUTCOMES
The client/caregiver will:

▶ Verbalize knowledge of signs and symptoms of complications
▶ Be free of infection and complication of therapy
▶ Demonstrate ability to perform all procedures as ordered
▶ Use aseptic technique for all procedures
▶ Verbalize protocol for emergency intervention and demonstrate ability to implement

▶ Maintain adequate oxygenation, hydration, nutrition, and hemodynamic stability
▶ Control nausea and vomiting
▶ Control pain

ASSESSMENT DATA
Obtain history of current illness
Monitor and document vital signs
Assess nutritional status
Monitor fluid losses and gains
Assess level of pain experienced
Document trends in body weight
Assess client/caregiver's ability to implement procedures
Monitor trends in blood chemistries and other laboratory studies as ordered

RELATED NURSING DIAGNOSES
Anxiety
Altered bowel/bladder elimination
Caregiver role strain
At risk for injury
At risk for altered perfusion
Pain
Fatigue
Fluid volume excess/deficit
At risk for altered skin integrity
At risk for infection
At risk for altered body image
Altered nutrition, less than body requirements

SPECIAL CONSIDERATIONS
A constant concern throughout the post-transplant period is the potential for organ rejection. There are three potential phases of rejection: hyperacute, acute, and chronic. In the hyperacute phase, tissue rejection occurs in 2–3 days following the transplant. During this phase, rejection may even be evident before the transplant procedure is completed. The organ will suddenly become cyanotic, and the client will demonstrate symptoms of rejection. In the acute phase, which occurs between 4 days and 3 months, the client will manifest the following symptoms of rejection: fever, redness and tenderness at the graft site, elevated blood chemistries (BUN, creatinine, liver enzymes, bilirubin, cardiac enzymes) and signs of cardiac failure. Lastly, in the chronic phase, which occurs from 4 months to years after the transplantation, the client will experience a gradual deterioration of the transplanted organ [17, 23, 25, 40].

A potentially fatal complication of bone marrow transplant is graft-versus-host disease (GvHD). The disease occurs when immunocompetent cells in the grafted tissue recognize the host cells as foreign and begin to attack the host cells. If the host cells are immunocompromised, they will be unable to destroy the graft cells. Acute GvHD occurs within the first 100 days following the transplant. The skin, liver, and gastrointestinal tract are primarily affected. The client develops abdominal pain, nausea, melanotic diarrhea, and a generalized pruritic rash, which leads to desquamation [17, 23, 25, 40].

TRANSCULTURAL CONSIDERATIONS
An interpreter will be needed for the client unable to speak or understand the English language.

Obtain educational materials in the client's native language, if available. Consider use of the AT&T Language Line. See also the Culturological Assessment procedure in Unit 2 for general overview of cultural considerations.

▶ INTERVENTIONS

Pre-Transplant Assessment

1. Wash hands.	*Prevent transmission of microbes*
2. Perform a physical assessment.	*Establishes baseline information of physiological data findings*
3. Obtain history of current illness.	*Assists in the development of an individualized plan of care*
4. Obtain a nutritional assessment.	*Determines metabolic nutritional requirements*
5. Determine the client's psychosocial needs.	*Assists in anticipating social service intervention*
6. Obtain specimens for baseline laboratory analysis.	*Monitors trends in laboratory studies*
7. Perform environmental assessment.	*Determines suitability of the home setting and ability of client/caregiver to maintain a clean, aseptic environment*
8. Evaluate client/caregiver's ability to perform necessary procedures.	*Documents client/caregiver's ability to implement procedures as ordered*

Post-Transplant Assessment

1. Wash hands.	*Prevents transmission of microbes*
2. Maintain adequate nutrition and hydration. a. monitor intake and output b. administer parentera/enteral feedings as ordered c. obtain and record daily weights d. provide dietary counseling	*Prevents development of malnutrition and dehydration*
3. Manage nausea and vomiting. a. administer antiemetics as ordered b. hold po intake c. administer parenteral nutrition as ordered	*Prevents fluid and electrolyte imbalance*
4. Evaluate functioning of the renal system. a. obtain and record intake and output b. assess character of urine c. hydrate until urine is clear	*Monitors renal perfusion*
5. Manage pain. a. administer analgesia as ordered b. encourage diversional activity c. use guided imagery	*Controls discomfort*
6. Control infection. a. administer anti-infectives as ordered b. monitor vital signs c. be aware that the immunocompromised client may not exhibit typical symptoms of infection	*Prevents growth of infectious organisms*

    d. observe for purulent drainage/exudate

    e. maintain aseptic care of all indwelling catheters

    f. perform respiratory toileting

    g. encourage strict mouth care

    h. observe for immunocompromise

    i. culture all exudate

    j. maintain neutropenic precautions [avoid crowds, persons with colds, fresh fruit and flowers]

Prepare to administer, if ordered, the following:

Biological Agent: Immune Globulin IV (IGIV)

Provides passive immunity against infection

    a. monitor body temperature

    b. used to prevent GvHD in the client with bone marrow transplant

    c. first dose must be given in controlled setting

    d. premedicate with acetaminophen, hydrocortisone, diphenhydramine as ordered

    e. infuse intravenously via pump

    f. observe for adverse reactions

    g. observer for evidence of anaphylaxis, have epinephrine and hydrocortisone injection at bedside, train caregiver to administer

    h. monitor CBC, IgG, IgM, IgA, IgE, liver function tests

7. Monitor laboratory studies.   *Documents trends in labora-*

    a. routinely obtain, per agency protocol, CBC, blood   *tory data*

       chemistries, urinalysis, T-cell count

    b. perform complete physical assessment

    c. obtain pulse oximetry twice per week per agency protocol

8. Maintain immunosuppression   *Prevents tissue rejection*

Prepare to administer, if ordered, the following:

Cytotoxic Agents: Imuran, Cytoxan, Cyclosporine

Used to promote immunsuppression

    a. monitor CBC and platelet counts, renal and liver function tests

    b. increase fluids to maintain hydration

    c. observe for bleeding tendency

    d. use strict handwashing technique

    e. instruct client to avoid exposure to infection

    f. administer per physician order

Monoclonal Antibody: Muromonab-CD3 (OKT3)

Used to promote immunosuppression

    a. obtain chest x-ray prior to initiating therapy to document that no congestion is present

    b. premedicate with hydrocortisone, acetaminophen, and diphenhydramine as ordered

    c. ensure that test dose has been administered in a controlled setting and that no untoward reaction has occurred

    d. administer by IV push over 1–2 minutes

    e. monitor CBC

    f. assess for evidence of infection

    g. observe for evidence of anaphylaxis, have epinephrine and hydrocortisone injection at bedside, train caregiver to administer

    h. observe for adverse side effects: fever, chills, tachycardia, hypo/hypertension, nausea, vomiting, diarrhea, angina, wheezing

Antilymphocyte Globulins: ATG, ALG

Used to promote immunosuppression

    a. perform skin test for hypersensitivity prior to administering first dose, do not give and notify physician if positive skin test results are obtained

    b. observe for evidence of anaphylaxis, have epinephrine and hydrocortisone injection s at bedside train caregiver to administer

    c. administer by IV infusion over 4–6 hours

    d. monitor VS hourly

    e. observe for adverse side effects: chills, fever, erythema, and pruritus

    f. monitor CBC

    g. assess renal function

    h. observe for signs of infection

9. Instruct client/caregiver in all related procedures and permit return demonstration.

     Documents client/caregiver's ability to implement procedure

DOCUMENTATION

The following should be noted in the nursing note:

Physical assessment clinical findings
Client/caregiver's ability to implement all related procedures
All untoward reactions and interventional strategies instituted
Client response to and compliance with medication regime
All client/caregiver teaching:
    Topics to include in teaching plan:
        safe and correct equipment handling
        emergency procedures
        underlying disease pathology
        appropriate community resources and contact persons

INTERDISCIPLINARY COLLABORATION

Inform the physician of the presence of drug-related side effects, abnormal laboratory values, untoward reactions
Consult with nutritionist for dietary recommendations related to anorexia, weight loss, etc.
Consult with social worker to identify community support groups

Consult with pharmacist regarding evidence of drug side effects, reordering of all pharmacy supplies

Confer with DME vendor to reorder supplies as needed [2, 6, 7, 15, 17, 20, 21, 23, 25, 40]

PROCEDURE
Home Chemotherapy Continuous Infusion

DESCRIPTION

Chemotherapy refers to the treatment process which uses cytotoxic and chemical agents to disrupt various phases of the cell cycle thereby interrupting cell metabolism or replication. Phase-specific agents act during critical phases or subphases of the cell cycle, while non–phase-specific agents act throughout the cell cycle. Chemotherapeutic agents are often given in combination, interfering with cell function at different times throughout the cell cycle to stop the abnormal growth of malignant cells. Chemotherapeutic drugs are classified as: alkylating agents, antimetabolites, cytotoxic antibiotics, plant alkaloids, hormones and hormone antagonist, and miscellaneous [17, 39, 40, 43, 48].

PURPOSE

Chemotherapy is used to prevent or treat suspected metastases, reduce the size of tumors, or effect a cure of some cancers.

EQUIPMENT

Latex/chemotherapy gloves
Gown, moisture resistant with elastic cuffs
Chemo spill kit
Ambulatory infusion pump
Extravasation equipment
Central line dressing kit
Chemotherapeutic agent in infusion bag
Mask, goggles, face shield as needed
Saline for pre- and post-transfusion flushing
Biohazard waste containers
Sharps containers
Heparin for post-infusing flushing, if ordered
10-cc syringes for flushing procedure, if ordered
Chemical waste container

OUTCOMES

The client/caregiver will:

▶ Verbalize an understanding of the signs and symptoms of infection, side effects of the agent(s) used
▶ Demonstrate ability to perform catheter dressing change procedure
▶ Demonstrate ability to troubleshoot the infusion pump
▶ Verbalize understanding of chemo spill procedure
▶ Verbalize understanding of disease process
▶ Assess IV access site for complications

ASSESSMENT DATA

Observe for response to therapy
Note development of side effects to ordered agent
Assess for signs of infection at access site

Monitor lab values for maintenance of values within ordered parameters
Assess access site for possible complications

RELATED NURSING DIAGNOSES
Fatigue
Anxiety
Pain
Altered body image
Altered skin integrity
Caregiver role strain
Ineffective coping
Altered nutrition, less than body requirements
At risk for infection
Knowledge deficit
At risk for altered perfusion
At risk for fluid volume deficit

SPECIAL CONSIDERATIONS
When teaching the client and caregiver to manage home chemotherapy, include the following points in the discussion: adverse effects of drugs; signs and symptoms to be reported to the physician; safety maintainence in the home environment, especially considering children and pet access to equipment and contaminated items; wearing of protective gear during tubing changes, medication administration and disposal; safe handling of drugs for child-bearing woman; infection prevention; pain management; equipment use and troubleshooting; and body-fluid precautions—double-flushing of toilet, double-laundering of soiled linens, and wearing of gloves when handling body fluids and soiled items. Chemo agents are excreted in the bile and urine up to 48 hours post-administration. Nurses and caregivers must wear latex gloves when handling stool, vomitus, urine, and blood for 48 hours post-administration. [17, 39, 40, 43, 48]

All admixing and compounding of chemo agents are conducted under a laminar flow hood by a pharmacist or specially trained oncology-certified nurse, as defined by the Occupational Safety and Health Administration (OSHA). If laminar flow is not available, prepare the infusion in a well-ventilated work space, away from heating or cooling vents, refrigerators, and other people. The health professional preparing the infusion should don long-sleeved gown, two pairs of latex chemotherapy gloves, face shield or goggles and face mask, shoe protectors, and obtain chemo-absorbent disposable pads and covers for the work area, spill kit, and disposable dustpan and scraper to clean up broken glass. See Chemotherapy Spill Protocol.

The gloves should be changed every 30 minutes while preparing infusion, taking care to wash hands between glove changes. If the drug comes in contact with the skin, wash thoroughly with soap and water. If the drug splashes into the eye, wash immediately with water or isotonic eye wash for 15 minutes and obtain a medical evaluation as soon as possible. [17, 39, 40, 43, 48]

TRANSCULTURAL CONSIDERATIONS
An interpreter will be needed for the client unable to speak or understand the English language.

Obtain educational materials in the client's native language, if available. Consider use of AT&T Language Line. See also the Culturological Assessment procedure in Unit 2 for general overview of cultural considerations.

▶ INTERVENTIONS

1. Verify physician order.	*Reduces risk of error*
2. Wash hands.	*Prevents transmission of microorganisms*

3. Perform physical assessment.	*Establishes baseline*
4. Explain procedure.	*Allays anxiety*
5. Don appropriate protective gear.	*Decreases risk of exposure to cytotoxic agents*
6. Explain procedure.	*Reduces anxiety*
7. Turn off pump and disconnect current intravenous infusion.	*Terminates previous infusion*
8. Attach infusion administration set to chemo IV bag/ cassette to infusion device, prime line, clamp catheter.	*Secures connection sites and assess for leakage*
9. Program the pump and verify settings against pharmacy prescription.	*Ensures accuracy of drug delivery*
10. Cleanse site port with alcohol wipe.	*Reduces risk of contamination*
11. Attach administration tubing to central access device, open clamp, and initiate infusion.	*Establishes rate of administration*
12. Instruct client in procedure and permit return demonstration.	*Documents client's ability to perform procedure*
13. Dispose of all used supplies in chemo waste container.	*Prevents exposure to cytotoxic agents*
14. Instruct client in use of chemo spill kit.	*Emergency procedure education decreases risk of prolonged exposure to chemo agent*
15. Instruct client to inspect central access insertion site frequently during infusion.	*Permits early detection of infection or signs of infiltration*
16. Instruct client in self-monitoring activities (weight, I&O, vital signs).	*Promotes independence in managing therapy*
17. Obtain appropriate serum, urine, sputum, and other laboratory specimens as ordered.	*Monitors client trends in laboratory findings*
18. Confirm written orders for needed antiemetics, fluids, diuretics, or electrolytes that may need to be administered prior to, during, or following the chemotherapy infusion.	*Restores fluid/electrolyte losses during therapy*

Extravasation Management

1. Stop the infusion.	*Prevents client from receiving additional chemotherapeutic agent*
2. Aspirate as much drug as possible from access site.	*Extracts chemo agent from the site*
3. Institute physician protocol for antidotes for vesicant/ irritants as ordered (See Table 6-2).	*Retards injury to surrounding tissue*
4. Notify physician.	*To obtain emergency orders*
5. Record in clinical record.	*Documents reactions and interventional strategies used*
6. Provide followup care per agency protocol.	*Monitors client response*

Side-Effects Management

Early detection and intervention slows the development of untoward medication reactions

1. Myelosuppression
   a. obtain CBC with diff 24–48 hours prior to administration of chemo agent

TABLE 6-2 Management of an Extravasation

Chemotherapeutic Agent	Local Antidote	Method of Administration
Dacarbazine (DTIC) Dactinomycin (Actinomycin D) Mitomycin C (Mutamycin) Mechlorethamine (nitrogen mustard)	Isotonic sodium thiosulfate 10% Mix 4 ml of sodium thiosulfate 19% with 6 ml of sterile water for injection	1. Inject 5–6 ml of mixture through the existing line and SQ in divided doses into the extravasated site with multiple injections. Repeat SQ dosing over several hours 2. Apply cold compresses for 6–12 hrs after the extravasation
Vinblastine (Velban) Vincristine (Oncovin) Teniposide (Vm26) Etoposide (VePesid) Streptozocin (Zanosar) Mithramycin (Mithracin)	Hyaluronidase (Wydase) 150 units/ml Add 1 ml USP NaCl	1. Inject 1–6 ml (150–900 units) SQ into extravasated site with multiple injections 2. Apply warm compresses
Daunorubicin (Cerubidine) Doxorubicin (Adriamycin) Mitoxantrone (Navantrone) Amasacrine (m-AMSA)	Hydrocortisone 50–100 mg/ml	1. Inject 0.5 ml (50–100 mg) IV through the existing line and SQ into the extravasated site with multiple injections. Total dose not to exceed 100 mg 2. Apply cold compresses for 15 min four times in a 24-hour period
Carmustine (BCNU)	Sodium bicarbonate (0.5 mEq/ml)	1. Inject 2–6 ml of mixture (1.0–3.0 mEq) IV through the existing IV line and into the extravasated site with multiple injections 2. Total dose not to exceed 10 ml of 0.5 mEq/ml solution (5.0 mEq) 3. Apply cold compresses. Do not apply pressure
Paclitaxel (Taxol)	None	1. Apply warm compresses to the extravasation site for 24 hours

Source: Lippincott Manual of Nursing Practice, 6th Ed. Philadelphia: Lippincott. p. 110

b. hold the drug if neutrophil count drops below physician-established parameter and inform the client's physician
c. instruct client to avoid crowds and exposure to infections
d. observe for bleeding tendency
2. Nausea and vomiting
a. administer antiemetics as ordered
b. correct electrolyte imbalance and fluid volume deficit if present
3. Stomatitis
a. instruct client in mouth-care routine
b. if severe, obtain order for anti-inflammatory or antifungal agents
4. Alopecia
Encourage client to wear wigs, hats, scarves, etc. to maintain body image.
5. Sun sensitivity
Limit exposure to sunlight.
6. Anxiety and depression
a. provide psychosocial support

   b. encourage use of effective coping mechanisms
   c. identify community support groups
7. Neurological effects
   a. observe for ototoxicity, paresthesias, constipation, paralytic ileus, muscle flaccidity
   b. encourage intake of high-fiber diet, promote adequate bowel/bladder function
   c. instruct client to report numbness/tingling of extremities

---

DOCUMENTATION
The following should be noted in the nursing note:

All client/caregiver instructions
Client/caregiver's ability to program and troubleshoot infusion pump, implement tubing change and flushing procedure, perform aseptic central line dressing change
All untoward reactions and interventional strategies instituted
Medications administered, side effects and adverse reactions noted
All client/caregiver teaching:
   Topics to include in teaching plan:
      safe and correct equipment handling
      emergency procedures
      underlying disease pathology
      appropriate community resources and contact persons

INTERDISCIPLINARY COLLABORATION
Inform the physician of the presence of drug-related side effects, abnormal laboratory values, untoward reactions
Consult with nutritionist for dietary recommendations related to anorexia, weight loss, etc.
Consult with social worker to identify community cancer support groups, and to determine client eligibility for financial assistance/reimbursement for cost of supplies
Consult with pharmacist regarding evidence of drug side effects, preparation and delivery of medication
Anticipate need to reorder supplies from DME vendor [6, 7, 15, 17, 20, 21, 27, 39, 40, 43, 48]

PROCEDURE
Chemotherapy Spill Protocol

DESCRIPTION
Chemotherapeutic agents are extremely cytotoxic. If accidentally spilled in the home setting, the potential to cause exposure to others in the home must be minimized. For small spills, the following procedure should be used. For large spills, the nurse should remove the client and others from the immediate area and refer to the agency policy/state regulations for further direction [7, 17, 40].

PURPOSE
To provide the safe and effective removal of spilled chemotherapeutic agent

EQUIPMENT
Chemo spill kit
Chemo safety gloves
Protective eyewear and face shield

Disposable gown with long sleeves and elastic cuffs
Mask/respirator with HEPA filter attachment
Shoe covers
Biohazard bags for containing nonsharp waste
Small hand broom and pan for collecting sharps
Biohazard sharps container
Chemotherapy warning labels for placement on outside of biohazard bags
Absorbent towels

OUTCOMES

The client/caregiver will:

▶ Be knowledgeable in emergency procedure
▶ Be able to prevent prolonged exposure to spilled chemo agent

ASSESSMENT DATA

Note exposure of client/caregiver to chemotherapy spill
Assess environment for potential contamination of furniture, clothing, linens
Estimate amount of drug spilled

RELATED NURSING DIAGNOSES

At risk for altered skin integrity
At risk for injury
Knowledge deficit
Anxiety

SPECIAL CONSIDERATIONS

The implementation of this procedure occurs as a result of an unusual occurrence. An incident report will need to be filed. Follow agency policy and procedure for correct reporting.

TRANSCULTURAL CONSIDERATION

An interpreter will be needed for the client unable to speak or understand the English language. Obtain educational materials in the client's native language, if available. Consider use of AT&T Language Line. See also the Culturological Assessment procedure in Unit 2 for general overview of cultural considerations.

▶ INTERVENTIONS

1. Wash hands.	*Prevents transmission of microbes*
2. Open chemo spill kit and don chemo gloves, eyeware, and disposable gown.	*Decreases risk of exposure to cytotoxic agent*
3. Tuck gloves under sleeved elastic cuff of disposable gown.	*Decreases risk of exposure to cytotoxic agent*
4. Use absorbent towels one at a time to absorb spill.	*Ensures thorough removal of spilled chemo agent*
5. Place all contaminated supplies/equipment into leak proof chemo container.	*Decreases risk of exposure to cytotoxic agent*
6. After completely removing chemo spill residue, clean spilled area thoroughly with soap and water.	*Removes any remaining drug*

7. Wash hands thoroughly.

8. Instruct client/caregiver to wash all contaminated clothing/linens separately in hot water.
9. Instruct client/caregiver to don chem gloves to scrub contaminated furniture with soap and water.
10. Dispose of waste in chemical waste container and return container to the agency for disposal do not discard in regular home trash.
12. Have client/caregiver demonstrate procedure.

Ensures removal of drug which may have come in contact with skin surfaces
Prevents transference and drug exposure to family
Prevents transference and drug exposure to family
Keeps the general community safe from contamination

Documents client/caregiver's ability to safely implement the procedure

DOCUMENTATION
The following should be included in the nursing note:

Estimated amount of chemo spill
Document procedure used to clean spill
If exposed, document steps taken to protect client/caregiver
All client/caregiver teaching:
   Topics to include in teaching plan:
      safe and correct equipment handling
      emergency procedures
      underlying disease pathology
      appropriate community resources and contact persons

INTERDISCIPLINARY COLLABORATION
Notify physician of chemo spill and estimated amount of drug not infused
Notify nursing administrator and follow policy and procedure for reporting the incident [6, 7, 17, 40]

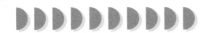

Adult Gastrointestinal System Procedures

4

PROCEDURE
Nasogastric Tube Insertion/Removal

DESCRIPTION

Nasogastric intubation is performed by advancing a tube through the nose into the alimentary canal and through to the stomach. The tube is used for both diagnostic and therapeutic purposes. Small-bore single-lumen, flexible catheters are suitable for long-term management and are preferred for enteral feedings.

PURPOSE

To enable gastric aspiration, decompression, feeding, and administration of medications

EQUIPMENT

Nonsterile gloves
Towel
30–60 cc syringe
Stethoscope
Hypoallergenic tape: 3-inch strip split in half to the center, two 1-inch strips
Litmus paper
Benzoin
Appropriate length/size feeding tube
KY jelly for lubrication
Glass of water
Emesis basin
Alcohol
Safety pin

OUTCOMES

The client/caregiver will:

▶ Maintain a patent airway
▶ Maintain gastric decompression and/or hydration and nutritional balance
▶ Maintain normal bowel function
▶ Maintain regular oral and nasal hygiene
▶ Demonstrate ability to determine tube placement per protocol
▶ Verbalize understanding of complications related to tube placement
▶ Perform tape change every two days

The nurse will:

▶ Change enteral feeding tubes per physician order

ASSESSMENT DATA

Verify NG tube placement before instilling fluids, after coughing, vomiting, or reinsertion
Assess gastrointestinal function
Record type and amount of NG infusion/drainage
Note and report any pulmonary complications and/or skin irritations

RELATED NURSING DIAGNOSES

At risk for ineffective airway clearance
Fluid volume deficit
At risk for ineffective coping
Knowledge deficit

SPECIAL CONSIDERATIONS

In pediatric, geriatric and malnourished clients be aware of sensitivity to tape and skin irritation from the NG tube. Stylets are used with caution in clients predisposed to esophageal puncture. There is an increased risk of aspiration when inserting an NG tube in clients with decreased level of consciousness due to impaired gag reflex.

TRANSCULTURAL CONSIDERATION

An interpreter will be needed for the client unable to speak or understand the English language. Obtain educational materials in the client's native language, if available. Consider use of AT&T Language Line. Consider incorporating religious or cultural practices into the plan of care. See also the Culturological Assessment procedure in Unit 2 for general overview of cultural considerations.

▶ INTERVENTIONS

Intervention	Rationale
1. Verify physician order.	*Reduces risk of error*
2. Wash hands.	*Prevents transmission of microbes*
3. Organize equipment.	*Promotes efficiency*
4. Perform physical assessment.	*Establishes baseline information of physiological data findings*
5. Explain procedure.	*Allays anxiety*
6. Establish a signal for the client to use to denote distress.	*Promotes early recognition of client distress*
7. Position client in upright position or right lateral if sitting is not advised.	*Decrease risk of aspiration*
8. Inspect nare for evidence of obstruction.	*Allows for selection of nostril*
9. Measure the insertion length. Measure the distance from tip of the nose to the tragus (tip of ear) to the xiphoid process	*Ensures proper tube placement*
10. Mark insertion distance with tape or pen and measure.	*Establishes reference line for noncalibrated tubes*
11. Place a towel bib over the client.	*Protects client's clothing/linens*
12. Don gloves.	*Serves as a protective barrier*
13. Prepare tube. a. tube may be warmed in water or chilled in ice per manufacturer's recommendation	*Allows for ease of insertion*
14. Lubricate the tip of the NG tube with KY jelly.	*Allows for ease of insertion*

15. Insert the tube in a downward direction advancing gently.	*Follows the anatomy of the nasal passages*
16. When advancing into the nasopharynx instruct the client to lower head slightly and/or swallow a sip of water.	*Facilitates advancement of the tube*

⚡ **DO NOT FORCE INSERTION. IF RESISTANCE IS MET PULL TUBE BACK SLIGHTLY, TRY REINSERTING. IF UNSUCCESSFUL, REMOVE TUBE AND ATTEMPT TO INSERT IN OTHER NARE. IF CLIENT DISPLAYS DISTRESS, REMOVE TUBE IMMEDIATELY.**

17. When NG tube is fully advanced (remove stylet if applicable), tape to cheek or forehead and cap end.	*Secures the tube until placement is confirmed*

Verification of Tube Placement

1. Visually inspect length of tube inserted.	*Ensures that predetermined length has been inserted*
2. Using a 30- or 60-cc syringe, instill 20 cc of air into the tube while auscultating with stethoscope placed on abdomen over gastric area.	*Provides initial confirmation of tube placement*
3. Aspirate gastric contents for pH testing. a. for pH of 4 or less, tube is in position b. for pH of 6 or more, pull tube back and recheck pH	*Verifies tube placement*
4. Obtain x-ray if ordered.	*Most reliable method of verifying tube placement, must be obtained for pH > 6*

Secure Tube in Place

1. Cleanse skin with alcohol.	*Removes oils*
2. Apply benzoin to nose if not contraindicated.	*Enhances adhesiveness*
3. Apply 3-inch tape with wide end secured to bridge of nose and spiral ends wrapped around tube.	*Secures tube without obstructing airway*
4. Secure tape on bridge of nose by covering with an additional 1-inch piece of tape.	*Provides additional security*
5. Cap distal end of tube if tube is not connected to suction or feeding.	*Prevents siphoning of gastric contents*
6. Secure distal end of tube to client's gown/shirt with safety pin.	*Reduces tension on tube*

Removal of NG Tube

1. Wash hands.	*Prevents transmission of microbes*
2. Organize equipment.	*Promotes efficiency*
3. Perform physical assessment.	*Establishes baseline information of physiological data findings*
4. Explain procedure.	*Allays anxiety*
5. Establish a signal for the client to use to denote distress.	*Promotes early recognition of client distress*

6. Position client in upright position or right lateral if sitting is not advised.	*Decrease risk of aspiration*
7. Don gloves.	*Serves as protective barrier*
8. Check placement as above.	*Verifies position of tube*
9. Irrigate tube with 10-cc NSS.	*Ensures that tube is free of debris*
10. Remove tape gently.	*Reduces risk of injury to skin*
11. Remove slowly and gently while client exhales, when end of tube reaches esophagus remove quickly.	*Decreases risk of aspiration and vomiting*
12. Dispose of tube in appropriate container, follow agency protocol for mercury-tipped catheters.	*Maintains universal precautions*
13. Provide nose and skin care and instruct client in continued skin care as needed.	*Maintains skin integrity*

DOCUMENTATION
The following should be included in the nursing note:

Date, time, type, name and size of tube
Identify nostril used
Record internal length of tube and method used to verify placement
Client's tolerance
Any untoward response and interventions employed to correct
All client/caregiver teaching:
    Topics to include in teaching plan:
        safe and correct equipment handling
        emergency procedures
        underlying disease pathology
        appropriate community resources and contact persons

INTERDISCIPLINARY COLLABORATION
Notify physician of any complications related to tube placement and determine if x-ray is required to verify placement
Anticipate need to reorder supplies from DME vendor [2, 6, 7, 9, 15, 17, 21, 22, 39, 41 50]

PROCEDURE
Nasogastric Tube Feeding

DESCRIPTION
Nasogastric tube feedings are administered to the client unable to eat adequate amounts of foods to maintain nutritional balance. Feeding formulas may be prepared by the nutritionist to meet individual client needs or purchased from commercial vendors to meet the needs of a wide variety of clients. Feedings are classified as blenderized, lactose-free, fiber containing, milk-based, modular, elemental, and disease-specific. See Table 6-3, Adult Enteral Feeding Classification.

PURPOSE
To provide enteral feedings and maintain balanced nutritional status

TABLE 6-3 Adult Enteral Feeding Classification

Category	Indications
Intact Protein Products	Normal digestive and absorptive capacity of the Gastrointestinal Tract (GI)
Intact Protein Products—Fiber Containing	▶ Regulation of bowel function ▶ Long-term feeding ▶ Normal digestive and absorptive capacity of GI tract
Elemental Diets	▶ Minimal digestive capacity ▶ Limited absorptive surface of GI tract (such as short bowel syndrome, celiac sprue, malnutrition) ▶ Protein-losing enteropathy (such as inflammatory bowel disease or radiation enteritis)
Critical Care	▶ Metabolically stressed ▶ Designed to improve maintenance of immunologic functions and/or decrease risk of bacterial translocation
Healing Support Diets	▶ Metabolically stressed ▶ Designed to improve maintenance of immunologic functions and/or decrease risk of bacterial translocation
Condition Specific Diets: Glucose Intolerance	▶ Abnormal glucose tolerance ▶ Selection based on metabolic needs
Hepatic	▶ Hepatic failure patients ▶ Selection based on metabolic needs
Pulmonary	▶ Pulmonary patients ▶ Selection based on metabolic needs
Renal	▶ Renal failure patients ▶ Selection based on metabolic needs
Modulars: Protein	▶ Protein supplementation to limited volume ▶ Normal digestive and absorptive capacity of the GI tract
Carbohydrate	▶ Caloric supplementation ▶ Normal digestive and absorptive capacity of GI tract
Fat	▶ Caloric supplementation ▶ MCT fat modules indicated for fat maldigestion or malabsorption

Free AA = Free Amino Acids

EQUIPMENT
Nonsterile gloves
Feeding formula
Feeding bag
Infusion pump
30–60 cc syringe
Stethoscope
Litmus paper

OUTCOMES

The client/caregiver will:

▶ Maintain patent airway
▶ Maintain normal bowel pattern
▶ Maintain oral and nasal hygiene
▶ Demonstrate ability to verify tube placement
▶ Perform NG feedings independently
▶ Irrigate NG tube as ordered

ASSESSMENT DATA

Note and report any pulmonary complications
Verify NG tube placement
Document amount and type of NG tube intake/output
Assess gastrointestinal system functioning and report evidence of obstruction
Observe for symptoms of fluid/electrolyte imbalance
Obtain diet history: food likes/dislikes, feeding history, food allergies
Review results of relevant blood chemistries and hematology reports

RELATED NURSING DIAGNOSES

Altered nutrition less than body requirements
At risk for ineffective airway clearance
Fluid volume deficit
At risk for ineffective coping
Knowledge deficit

SPECIAL CONSIDERATIONS

In pediatric, geriatric, and malnourished clients, be aware of sensitivity to tape and skin irritation from the NG tube. Observe for any evidence of fluid and electrolyte imbalance. The physician orders will determine the type and amount of feeding formula to use. Tube feedings should be administered at room temperature to avoid abdominal discomfort. Observe for any evidence of lactose intolerance.

TRANSCULTURAL CONSIDERATION

An interpreter will be needed for the client unable to speak or understand the English language.

Obtain educational materials in the client's native language, if available. Consider use of AT&T Language line. Consider incorporating religious or cultural practices into the plan of care. See also the Culturological Assessment procedure in Unit 2 for general overview of cultural considerations.

▶ INTERVENTIONS

1. Wash hands.	*Prevents transmission of microbes*
2. Organize equipment.	*Promotes efficiency*
3. Perform physical assessment.	*Establishes baseline information of physiological data findings*
4. Explain procedure.	*Allays anxiety*

5. Establish a signal for the client to use to denote distress.

Promotes early recognition of client distress

6. Position client in upright position or right lateral if sitting is not advised.

Decrease risk of aspiration

7. Don gloves.

Serves as protective barrier

8. Check tube placement.

Verifies tube position

9. Check for gastric residual: if > 100ml or 10–20% of continuous hourly rate, hold feeding for 1 hour.

Prevents over distension and potential for aspiration

10. If gastric residual persists after 1 hour, notify physician.

To obtain orders for change in therapy

11. If gastric residual does not exceed parameter, pour feeding into feeding bag as prescribed, depending on rate of infusion, feeding solution should hang for no longer than 4 hours.

Retards growth of bacteria

12. Prime the tubing label bag with date and time.

Feeding bag should be changed daily

13. Connect tubing to pump if ordered, or allow to hang by gravity.

Feeding should instill slowly to prevent possible onset of dumping syndrome

14. Uncap NG tube and connect feeding tube.

Initiates infusion

15. Upon completion of feeding, fill feeding bag with ordered amount of water.

Reduces risk of hypertonic dehydration

16. Stop infusion, clamp feeding tube disconnect from NG tube, and cap NG tube.

Prevents siphoning of gastric contents

17. Instruct client to keep head elevated for 30 minutes following feeding.

Reduces risk of aspiration

18. Instruct to check for gastric residual prior to administering bolus feeding and q 4 hours for continuous feeds.

Prevents overdistension and potential for aspiration

19. Clean and flush feeding apparatus per agency protocol.

Prevents contamination

20. Obtain serum specimens for blood chemistries (BUN, glucose, electrolytes, creatinine) as ordered.

Monitors trends in laboratory results

21. Instruct client/caregiver in the procedure and permit return demonstration.

Documents client/caregiver's ability to implement procedure

DOCUMENTATION
The following should be included in the nursing note:

Verification of tube placement
Characteristics of gastric secretions
Client's tolerance of feedings
Client/caregiver's ability to implement procedure
Any untoward response and interventions employed to correct
All client/caregiver teaching:
    Topics to include in teaching plan:
        safe and correct equipment handling
        emergency procedures
        underlying disease pathology
        appropriate community resources and contact persons

INTERDISCIPLINARY COLLABORATION

Notify physician of any complications related to tube placement, abdominal discomfort, hydrational status, vomiting, diarrhea, or large gastric residuals

Consult with nutritionist regarding adequacy of enteral feedings, type of feedings, nutritional assessment [2, 6, 9, 15, 17, 18, 21, 22, 24, 26, 39, 41, 61]

PROCEDURE
Management of Long Term Enteral Feeding Devices

DESCRIPTION

When nasogastric feeding is contraindicated, as in clients with head and neck trauma, with an obstruction of the esophagus, or in need of long-term feeding, placement of a more permanent feeding tube may be an option. Placement of gastrostomy, jejunostomy, or percutaneous endoscopic gastrostomy (PEG) tubes is a medical act. The gastrostomy tube is surgically inserted into the stomach via the abdominal wall. Typically a foley or mushroom catheter with a balloon tip is used. The balloon is inflated with 5–30 cc of sterile saline, depending on type used, to secure the tube in position. Once the stoma site has healed, the changing of the gastrostomy tube is a routine nursing procedure. The PEG tube is placed under endoscopic examination with use of a guidewire treaded through the alimentary canal and brought out onto the abdominal wall. The PEG tube is threaded over the guidewire, brought through the abdominal wall, and positioned securely in place. An adapter is used on the end of the tube to attach to the feeding apparatus. Jejunostomy tubes are placed surgically into the jejunum and sutured into place. While the physician places the first long-term enteral tube, the nurse or family member, who has been properly trained and with orders from the physician, may change the gastrostomy tube according to agency policy. See also Unit 5, Enteral Feeding Tube Care and Management [9, 17, 41].

PURPOSE
To maintain long-term nutritional support

EQUIPMENT
30-cc half-strength peroxide, if ordered
60-cc tap water
Small basin
Cotton-tipped applicators
Gauze
Tape
60-cc catheter-tipped syringe
If changing, new gastrostomy tube or gastrostomy button with obturator
Lubricant
Gloves

OUTCOMES
The client/caregiver will:

▶ Maintain fluid balance
▶ Maintain nutritional status to meet metabolic needs
▶ Maintain a patent airway
▶ Maintain serum proteins
▶ Maintain normal bowel function
▶ Be free of complications associated with long-term feeding tube placement
▶ Demonstrate ability to care for feeding tube

ASSESSMENT DATA

Note and report any pulmonary complications
Document amount and type of feeding tube intake/output
Assess gastrointestinal system functioning and report evidence of obstruction
Observe for symptoms of fluid/electrolyte imbalance
Observe skin surrounding feeding tube for evidence of irritation, inflammation or infection
Determine patency of tube or presence of clogging from formula or medication administration
Assess tolerance of feeding formula
Evaluate results of relevant blood chemistries and hematology reports

RELATED NURSING DIAGNOSES

Altered nutrition less than body requirements
Fluid volume deficit
At risk for alteration in bowel elimination
At risk for ineffective airway clearance
Knowledge deficit
Anxiety

SPECIAL CONSIDERATIONS

High-osmolarity feeding formulas should not be administered via jejunostomy tubes because of potential for poor tolerance. The type of formula used will depend on client's diagnosis and clinical status. Feeding type may also depend on the economic resources of the client.

TRANSCULTURAL CONSIDERATION

An interpreter will be needed for the client unable to speak or understand the English language. Obtain educational materials in the client's native language, if available. Consider incorporating religious or cultural practices into the plan of care. Consider use of AT&T language line. See also the Culturological Assessment procedure in Unit 2 for general overview of cultural considerations.

▶ INTERVENTIONS

1. Wash hands.	*Prevents transmission of microbes*
2. Organize equipment.	*Promotes efficiency*
3. Perform physical assessment.	*Establishes baseline information of physiological data findings*
4. Explain procedure.	*Allays anxiety*
5. Implement the following procedures as appropriate.	*Maintains/manages long-term gastric feeding tubes*

For Routine Feeding-Tube Site Care

a. perform site care	*Reduces skin contaminants*
► pour small amount of half-strength peroxide solution into basin	
► saturate end of cotton-tipped applicators in solution	
► use circular motion to cleanse site with peroxide-soaked applicators	
► continue until site is clean of debris	

   ▸ rinse insertion site by irrigating with tap water using catheter-tipped syringe

   ▸ dry with gauze

b. cover site with a dry dressing or leave open to air depending on agency protocol

   A dressing may not be needed for the well healed stoma site

c. secure tube to abdomen with tape

   Reduces tension on tube

For Gastrostomy Tube Removal/Insertion

a. fill the catheter balloon with 10–20 ml of sterile water, then deflate

   Tests the integrity of the balloon

b. lubricate tip of catheter

   Facilitates ease of insertion

c. assist client to position of comfort

   Reduces discomfort during procedure

d. remove the old tube by deflating the balloon and twisting gently to dislodge

   Reduces trauma to site

e. insert the lubricated tip of the new gastrostomy tube via ostomy site using gentle twisting motion

   Facilitates insertion

f. inflate balloon with 10–20 ml of sterile water

   Secures tube in place

g. aspirate stomach contents, then return

   Checks tube placement

h. tape tube in place

   Prevents accidental dislodgment

For Gastrostomy Feeding Button Removal/Insertion

a. remove button and wash with soap and water per agency policy

   Removes debris

b. check depth of stoma site

   Provides a guide for determining depth of insertion

c. cleanse surrounding area

   Removes debris

d. lubricate obturator, mushroom dome, and stoma site

   Facilitates ease of insertion

e. gently push button through stoma into the stomach (see Figure 6-15)

   Prevents trauma to tissue

f. remove obturator by gently rotating, being sure to note that antireflex valve is in closed position

   Prevents leakage of gastric contents

g. close the safety plug or open and attach adapter to feeding tube to begin infusion

   Plug should remain closed between feedings to prevent loss of gastric contents

6. Wash hands.

   Prevents transmission of microbes

7. Instruct client/caregiver in procedure and permit return demonstration.

   Documents client/caregiver's ability to perform procedure

DOCUMENTATION

The following should be included in the nursing note:

Evidence of site irritation, inflammation, or infection
Characteristics of gastric secretions

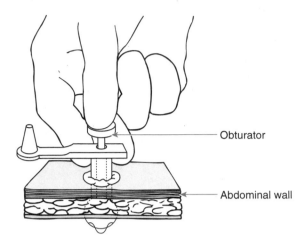

— Obturator

— Abdominal wall

FIGURE 6-15 ▶ Insertion of gastrostomy button.

Client's tolerance of feedings
Any untoward response and interventions employed to correct
All client/caregiver teaching:
    Topics to include in teaching plan:
        safe and correct equipment handling
        emergency procedures
        underlying disease pathology
        appropriate community resources and contact persons

INTERDISCIPLINARY COLLABORATION

Notify physician of any complications related to tube placement, abdominal discomfort, hydrational status, vomiting, diarrhea, or large gastric residuals. Consult wih WOC nurse for management of ostomy.
Anticipate need to reorder supplies and consult DME vendor
Consult with nutritionist regarding client's tolerance/intolerance of feeding regimen [2, 6, 9, 15, 17, 18, 21, 22, 24, 26, 47, 60, 61]

Adult Renal System Procedures

5

PROCEDURE
Peritoneal Dialysis

DESCRIPTION

Currently three methods of peritoneal dialysis are used in the home setting: intermittent peritoneal dialysis (IPD), continuous cyclic peritoneal dialysis (CCPD), and continuous ambulatory peritoneal dialysis (CAPD). All three methods are performed by the trained client or caregiver. IPD is performed using an automatic cycling unit three times per week with treatment durations of 8 to 10 hours. CAPD is performed daily (Figure 6-16). The client performs three to four exchanges during the course of the day and leaves the final exchange in the dwell stage over night. CCPD combines both the IPD and CAPD methods of dialyzing. The client programs the automatic cycling unit to perform three exchanges during the night, and leaves the final exchange in the dwell stage throughout the day. The process of exchanging is resumed in the evening. [2, 17, 25, 39]

PURPOSE

To remove metabolic waste, maintain fluid/electrolyte balance, and control azotemia

EQUIPMENT

Face masks, gloves, and other protective gear as needed
Bottle of povidone-iodine if ordered
Sterile barrier
Tape
Ordered dianeal solution
Clamps
Belted pouch
Sterile barrier
Towel
Tubing set
Syringes
Medication additives if ordered
IV pole
Alcohol wipes
Gauze

OUTCOMES

The client/caregiver will

▶ Maintain fluid/electrolyte balance
▶ Perform fingerstick blood sugar daily

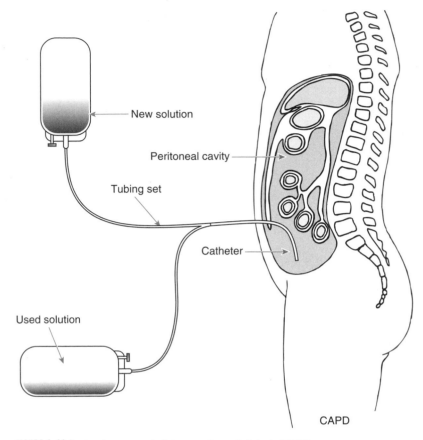

New solution

Peritoneal cavity

Tubing set

Catheter

Used solution

CAPD

FIGURE 6-16 ▶ Continuous ambulatory peritoneal dialysis (CAPD).

▶ Observe for complications of therapy
▶ Perform dialysis exchanges as ordered
▶ Maintain diet as ordered
▶ Verbalize understanding of purpose of therapy
▶ Monitor for symptoms of infection

ASSESSMENT DATA
Assess fluid volume and electrolyte balance
Obtain vital signs and observe for evidence of abnormal findings
Monitor laboratory results and daily weights as ordered
Assess client/caregiver's ability to implement aseptic technique
Evaluate system of dialysis used for malfunction
Evaluate peritoneal catheter site for evidence of irritation, inflammation, infection

RELATED NURSING DIAGNOSES
Fluid volume excess
At risk for decreased cardiac output
At risk for infection
Knowledge deficit

Anxiety
Altered urinary elimination

SPECIAL CONSIDERATIONS

To avoiding chilling of the client, the dialysate should be warmed to room temperature. While dietary and fluid restrictions will be less strict for the client on CAPD than for the client on hemodialysis, the diet should be high in protein, potassium, and fiber. Because of sodium retention, the dietary intake of sodium should be limited. Fluid restriction depends upon residual urinary function.

The dialysate solution is available in several concentrations of dextrose: 1.5, 2.5, and 4.25%. The physician order will determine the schedule of dialysate solution to be used. The client must measure and record fluid loss/gain daily and obtain fingerstick blood glucose readings. [2, 17, 23, 39]

Extensive client teaching is usually provided by a community-based dialysis center.

TRANSCULTURAL CONSIDERATION

An interpreter will be needed for the client unable to speak or understand the English language. Obtain educational materials in the client's native language, if available. Consider incorporating religious or cultural practices into the plan of care. Consider use of AT&T language line. See also the Culturological Assessment procedure in Unit 2 for general overview of cultural considerations.

▶ INTERVENTIONS

Intervention	Rationale
1. Verify physician order.	*Reduces risk of error*
2. Wash hands.	*Prevents transmission of microbes*
3. Organize equipment.	*Promotes efficiency*
4. Perform physical assessment.	*Establishes baseline information of physiological data findings*
5. Explain procedure.	*Allays anxiety*
6. Warm bag of dialysate and inspect the character of the dialysate and integrity of the bag.	*Prevents chilling and detects any flaws in the system*
7. Spike bag, prime tubing, and clamp.	*Prevents loss of dialysate*
8. Put on mask and don gloves.	*Serves as protective barrier*
9. Open transfer set and connect one end to dianeal solution (fill) tubing and other end to drainage bag (drain) tubing keeping all clamps closed.	*Maintains closed system*
10. Open clamp on solution bag, clamp on fill tubing, and clamp on drain tubing and initiate flow of dialysate for 5 seconds.	*Primes tubing and flushes air from system*
11. Close fill tubing clamp.	*Prevents loss of dialysate solution*
12. Remove cap from trocar site and connect primed transfer set.	*Establishes connection of flow system*
13. Open drain tubing clamp.	*Begins drain phase*
14. Remove mask.	*Mask may be safely removed when trocar is either capped or connected to transfer set*
15. Drain abdominal contents for approximately 20 minutes, then clamp drain tubing.	*Empties abdominal cavity of dialysate*
16. Add medications, if ordered, to new dianeal solution.	*Corrects electrolyte imbalance*

17. Open clamp to fill tubing and permit solution to infuse into abdomen.	*Begins* fill phase
18. When fill is complete, close clamp.	*Prevents backflow*
19. Allow solution to remain in abdomen as ordered.	*Begins* dwell phase
20. Repeat procedure to drain, fill, and dwell per physician order.	*Reduces risk of error*
21. Close clamp to transfer set.	*Prevents backflow*
22. Put on mask.	*Serves as protective barrier*
23. Open disconnect cap package, cap trocar/catheter, discard fill, and drain tubing.	*Permits client to ambulate freely without being hampered by connection tubing*
24. Remove mask.	*Mask may be safely removed when trocar is either clamped or connected to transfer set*
25. Check drainage bag for clarity of solution and evidence of sediment, blood, fibrin, etc. If drainage output is poor, reposition client	*Detects presence of exudate*
26. Measure amount of drainage and discard in toilet.	*Monitors fluid losses/gains and maintains universal precautions*
27. Discard all used supplies appropriately.	*Maintains universal precautions*
28. Wash hands.	*Prevents transmission of microbes*
29. Instruct client/caregiver in procedure and permit return demonstration.	*Documents client/caregiver's ability to perform procedure*

If using automated cycling unit connect per manufacturer's recommendations and follow instructions for regulating fill, dwell and drain times. If dialysate returns are cloudy obtain culture per agency protocol.

DOCUMENTATION
The following should be included in the nursing note:

Evidence of trocar/catheter site irritation, inflammation or infection
Characteristics of dialysate returns
Client's tolerance of procedure
Any untoward response and interventions employed to correct
All client/caregiver teaching:
    Topics to include in teaching plan:
        safe and correct equipment handling
        emergency procedures
        underlying disease pathology
        appropriate community resources and contact persons

INTERDISCIPLINARY COLLABORATION
Notify physician of any complications related to dialysis procedure
Consult with social worker to determine client eligibility for financial assistance/reimbursement

Confer with DME vendor for reordering of equipment/supplies. Consult with community-based dialysis center to evaluate client progress [2, 6, 15, 17, 21, 25, 39, 58]

PROCEDURE
Care of Urinary Diversion Devices

DESCRIPTION
Urinary diversions are surgical procedures performed to provide alternate pathways for the flow of urine to correct obstructions of the renal system caused by tumors, trauma, congenital malformations, or other disease states. There are several types of urinary diversion procedures: bladder cystostomy (suprapubic), cutaneous ureterostomy, ileal conduit, colon conduit, ureterosigmoidostomy, and continent ileal bladder conduit.

PURPOSE
To maintain adequate flow of urine

EQUIPMENT
Appropriate pouch
Paste
Skin sealant
Scissors
Wash cloths
Towel
Gloves
Clamp
Drainage container
Tape
Gauze

For continent diversion

Sterile gloves
Antiseptic ointment if ordered
Catheter
Drainage container

OUTCOMES
The client/caregiver will:

▶ Maintain adequate urine flow
▶ Identify presence of skin irritation, inflammation, or infection at stoma site
▶ Measure and record urinary output
▶ Perform procedure as ordered
▶ Verbalize understanding of complications
▶ Maintain adequate fluid/electrolyte balance

ASSESSMENT DATA
Observe condition of skin surrounding stoma site
Observe and document characteristics of urinary output
Note integrity of pouching system used
Monitor urinary laboratory results

Observe for urinary retention

Note client/caregiver ability to implement procedure

RELATED NURSING DIAGNOSES

Altered urinary elimination

Altered body image

At risk for altered skin integrity

At risk for infection

Ineffective coping

Anxiety

Knowledge deficit

SPECIAL CONSIDERATIONS

Cutaneous ureterostomy is surgically created by excising the ureters from the bladder and forming a stoma by bringing one or both ureters to the abdominal surface (See Figure 6-17a). Because of continuous urinary drainage, an appliance must be worn.

Ileal conduit is surgically created by taking a small section of the small intestine and forming a pouch with a stomal opening on the abdominal surface. The ureters are disconnected from the bladder and redirected to drain into the stoma (See Figure 6-17b). This technique carries a high potential for reflux. Again because of continuous urinary drainage, an appliance must be worn.

Colon conduit is surgically created by taking a small section of the sigmoid colon to form a pouch as above. With this procedure, reflux is less of a problem, however an appliance must be worn

Ureterosigmoidostomy is surgically created by disconnecting the ureters from the bladder and implanted them into the rectum where urine is expelled with defecation and the passage of flatus (See Fig. 6-17c). Because of a high risk of infection and electrolyte imbalance, this procedure is seldom performed. When performed, attention must be paid to the increased incidence of anal irritations caused by the constant flow of urine.

Continent ileal conduit is surgically created by forming a pouch with intussuscepting tissue that forms nipple valves to prevent reflux and leakage. While an appliance will not need to be worn, the client must be able to perform intermittent self-catheterization every 2 to 4 hours.

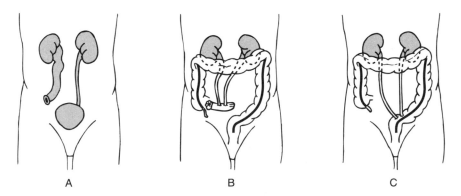

A   B   C

FIGURE 6-17 ▶ Urinary diversion devices. **A.** Cutaneous ureterostomy. **B.** Ileal conduit. **C.** Ureterosigmoidostomy.

TRANSCULTURAL CONSIDERATION

An interpreter will be needed for the client unable to speak or understand the English language. Obtain educational materials in the client's native language, if available.

Consider incorporating religious or cultural practices into the plan of care. See also the Culturological Assessment procedure in Unit 2 for general overview of cultural considerations.

INTERVENTIONS

1. Verify physician order.	*Reduces risk of error*
2. Wash hands.	*Prevents transmission of microbes*
3. Organize equipment.	*Promotes efficiency*
4. Perform physical assessment.	*Establishes baseline information of physiological data findings*
5. Explain procedure.	*Allays anxiety*
6. Position the client for easy access to stoma.	*Provides unobstructed view of site*
7. Perform procedure as indicated below.	

For Continent Urinary Diversion

Secures pouch to prevent leakage
   a. don gloves
   b. remove old dressing
   c. cleanse stoma site using gauze soaked in NSS or antiseptic solution if ordered
   d. insert catheter into soma 2–2.5 inches and allow urine to drain into container
   e. cleanse around stoma with soap and water, pat dry
   f. apply gauze dressing

For Incontinent Urinary Diversion

Secures pouch to prevent leakage
   a. cut pouch opening to size
   b. remove adhesive backing
   c. don gloves
   d. remove old pouch
   e. cleanse stoma site with soap and water, pat dry
   f. apply skin barriers or adhesives, then pouch over stoma and apply pressure for 5 minutes
   g. empty contents of old pouch and measure drainage, discard in toilet
   h. rinse pouch with tap water

8. Wash hands.	*Prevents transmission of microbes*
9. Instruct client/caregiver in procedure and permit return demonstration.	*Documents client/caregiver's ability to perform the procedure*

DOCUMENTATION
The following should be included in the nursing note:

Evidence of stoma site irritation, inflammation, or infection
Characteristics of urinary drainage
Client's tolerance of procedure
Any untoward response and interventions employed to correct
All client/caregiver teaching:
    Topics to include in teaching plan:
        safe and correct equipment handling
        emergency procedures
        underlying disease pathology
        appropriate community resources and contact persons

INTERDISCIPLINARY COLLABORATION
Notify physician of any complications related to urinary drainage procedure
Consult with social worker to determine client eligibility for financial assistance/reimbursement
Confer with DME vendor for reordering of equipment/supplies
Collaborate with the enterostomal therapist or WOCN in the management of all ostomies [2, 6, 15, 21, 25, 39]

PROCEDURE
Suprapubic Catheter Care and Insertion

DESCRIPTION
A suprapubic cystostomy is created by surgically inserting a catheter through the abdominal wall into the abdomen above the symphusis pubis. The catheter is connected to a straight drainage system for collection of urine (Figure 6-18). Once the stoma site has healed, changing of the suprapubic catheter may be a nursing procedure depending on agency policy, state board of nursing practice acts, or complexity of surgical technique.

PURPOSE
To maintain patency of catheter and adequate urine flow

EQUIPMENT
Gloves
Gauze
Antiseptic solution if ordered
Tape
Drainage system
10-m syringe

For Catheter Changing

Sterile catheter kit
Fenestrated drape
Sterile indwelling catheter
Tubing
Sterile 10-ml syringe prefilled with NSS
Lubricant

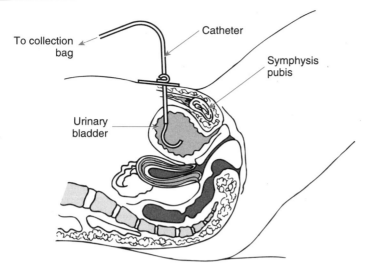

FIGURE 6-18 ▶ Suprapubic catheter

Sterile gloves
Tape
Biohazardous waste bag

OUTCOMES
The client/caregiver will:

▶ Maintain adequate urine flow
▶ Identify presence of skin irritation, inflammation, or infection at stoma site
▶ Be free of urinary tract infection
▶ Measure and record urinary output
▶ Perform procedure as ordered
▶ Verbalize understanding of complications

ASSESSMENT DATA
Observe condition of skin surrounding stoma site
Observe and document characteristics of urinary output
Monitor urinary laboratory results
Observe for urinary retention and symptoms of infection
Note client/caregiver ability to implement procedure

RELATED NURSING DIAGNOSES
Altered urinary elimination
Altered body image
At risk for altered skin integrity
At risk for infection
Ineffective coping
Anxiety
Knowledge deficit

SPECIAL CONSIDERATIONS

The sensitive skin of the elderly or cachetic client may not be able to tolerate harsh antiseptic solutions or adhesive tape. Supra pubic catheters will need to be changed frequently, per agency policy, to reduce risk of obstruction. Clients should be instructed to maintain adequate hydration as ordered and to keep the site clean and dry. Any symptoms of infection, leakage, or catheter obstruction should be reported immediately.

TRANSCULTURAL CONSIDERATION

An interpreter will be needed for the client unable to speak or understand the English language. Obtain educational materials in the client's native language, if available. Consider use of AT&T language line. See also the Culturological Assessment procedure in Unit 2 for general overview of cultural considerations.

▶ **INTERVENTIONS**

1. Verify physician order.	*Reduces risk of error*
2. Wash hands.	*Prevents transmission of microbes*
3. Organize equipment.	*Promotes efficiency*
4. Perform physical assessment.	*Establishes baseline information of physiological data findings*
5. Explain procedure.	*Allays anxiety*
6. Position the client for easy access to stoma.	*Provides unobstructed view of site*
7. Don gloves.	*Serves as protective barrier*
8. Remove old dressing and discard appropriately.	*Maintains universal precautions*
9. Remove gloves and don sterile gloves.	*Serves as protective barrier*
10. Assess insertion site and patency of catheter.	*Ensures absence of obstruction*
11. Cleanse stoma site using circular motion with gauze saturated with antiseptic solution or NSS as ordered (Figure 6-19).	*Removes debris from stoma site*
12. Use gauze pad to cleanse catheter from distal to proximal end.	*Removes debris from catheter*

For Catheter Reinsertion

First follow steps 1 to 12 above, then continue with the following steps:

a. Attach empty 10-ml syringe to balloon port of catheter and remove fluid.	*Deflates balloon for removal of catheter*
b. Gently remove old catheter from supra pubic opening and discard in biohazardous waste.	*Prevents contamination*
c. Remove gloves, wash hands, and open catheter kit using sterile technique.	*Prevents transmission of microbes*
d. Don sterile gloves.	*Prevents transmission of microbes*
e. Organize supplies on sterile field.	*Facilitates efficiency*
f. Lubricate catheter tip.	*Promote ease of insertion*

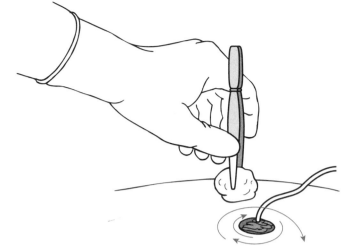

FIGURE 6-19 ▶ Cleanse stoma site using circular motion.

g. Hold catheter 4 inches from tip and gently insert into stoma site, if resistance is met, stop and retry.	*Reduces risk of trauma to stoma site*
h. Attach 10-ml syringe prefilled with NSS to balloon port of catheter and inject solution.	*Secures balloon in place*
i. Connect catheter end to closed drainage system and secure catheter.	*Reestablishes drainage system*
13. Apply dry sterile dressing at stoma site and secure with tape.	*Collects any drainage*
14. Maintain closed drainage system and change drainage bag per agency policy.	*Retards growth of bacteria*
15. Remove gloves and wash hands.	*Prevents transmission of microbes*
16. Instruct client/caregiver in the procedure and permit return demonstration.	*Documents client/caregiver's ability to implement procedure*

DOCUMENTATION

The following should be included in the nursing note:

Evidence of stoma site irritation, inflammation or infection
Characteristics of urinary drainage
Client's tolerance of procedure
Any untoward response and interventions employed to correct
Date and time of catheter reinsertion
Size of catheter used for reinsertion
All client/caregiver teaching:
    Topics to include in teaching plan:
        safe and correct equipment handling
        emergency procedures
        underlying disease pathology
        appropriate community resources and contact persons

INTERDISCIPLINARY COLLABORATION
Notify physician of any complications related to urinary drainage procedure
Consult with social worker to determine client eligibility for financial assistance/reimbursement
Confer with DME vendor for re-ordering of equipment/supplies [6, 15, 21, 25, 39, 41]

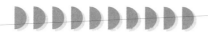

6

Adult Endocrine System Procedures

Diabetes Management: Insulin Administration

DESCRIPTION

The client with insulin dependent diabetes mellitus (IDDM) must be maintained on an exogenous source of insulin for the remainder of his or her life. Clients who are unable to be controlled with diet and/or oral antidiabetic agents, experiencing gestational diabetes, taking steroid medications, experiencing stress, undergoing surgery, or being maintained on high-calorie enteral/parenteral feedings are representative of the clients typically in need of insulin administration. Insulin is manufactured as short-acting preparations, intermediate-acting preparations, and long-acting preparations. Insulin is administered subcutaneously as intermittent doses or continuously with an insulin pump. See also Unit 3, Perinatal Section, on Blood Glucose Monitoring.

PURPOSE

To maintain blood glucose levels within normal limits

EQUIPMENT

Insulin vial
Insulin syringes
Gloves
Alcohol preps
Glucose monitoring device
Lancets
Sharps disposal container
Insulin pump if ordered
Log

OUTCOMES

The client/caregiver will:

▶ Demonstrate correct technique for injection, site rotation, mixing of insulin, and blood glucose monitoring
▶ Maintain blood glucose levels within normal limits, as ordered
▶ Verbalize understanding of complications of therapy
▶ Identify signs and symptoms of hypo/hyperglycemia and interventions to correct

ASSESSMENT DATA

Document site used and amount/type of insulin given
Note signs of lipohypotrophy or lipoatrophy

467

Observe for signs of hypo/hyperglycemia
Obtain diet history
Obtain history of current illness
Evaluate fingerstick blood glucose results
Monitor glycosylated hemoglobin levels as ordered
Observe for evidence of peripheral neuropathy and retinopathy

RELATED NURSING DIAGNOSES
Anxiety
Powerlessness
Altered body image
At risk for ineffective coping
Altered nutrition, less than body requirements
Knowledge deficit
At risk for infection

SPECIAL CONSIDERATIONS
Following specific agency policy, the nurse may prefill the client's insulin syringes with the ordered amount of medication. Prefilled syringes may be stored for up to 3 weeks in the refrigerator and should be stored in the vertical position with the needle up. Prior to administration, the prefilled syringe should be gently rolled between the palms to resuspend the insulin.

Commercially prepared prefilled disposable and reusable insulin pens are also available. These devices obviate the need for multiple-dose vials or separate syringes. The pen is designed to allow the client to dial in the ordered dose of insulin. The client is to change the needle prior to each injection to maintain aseptic technique. These devices can hold up to 300 units of insulin for multiple daily dosing as ordered.

To safely and accurately administer medication for the child or elderly client with limited vision or dexterity, subcutaneous injectors are ideal. These devices use a pressure jet to deliver prescribed doses of regular insulin. The system may come with a replaceable cartridge or may require the client or caregiver to withdraw the appropriate amount of drug. Jet-injected insulin has been shown to be more rapidly absorbed because the medication is more evenly dispersed throughout the subcutaneous tissue, avoiding the puddling effect that often occurs with conventional needle and syringe systems (Figure 6-20).

As part of the teaching plan, the client should be aware that activity levels, and the presence of infection, or other trauma can affect insulin absorption rates.

TRANSCULTURAL CONSIDERATIONS
An interpreter will be needed for the client unable to speak or understand the English language.

Obtain educational materials in the client's native language, if available. Consider use of AT&T language line. Consider incorporating religious or cultural practices into the plan of care. See also the Culturological Assessment procedure in Unit 2 for general overview of cultural considerations.

▶ INTERVENTIONS

1. Verify physician order.	*Reduces risk of error*
2. Wash hands.	*Prevents transmission of microbes*
3. Organize equipment.	*Promotes efficiency*

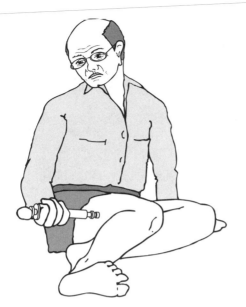

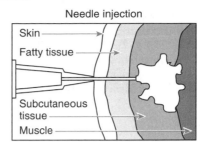

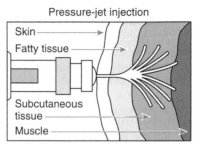

FIGURE 6-20 ▶ **A.** Self-administering insulin using pressure jet. **B.** Needle injection. **C.** Pressure-jet injection.

4. Perform physical assessment.	*Establishes baseline information of physiological data findings*
5. Explain procedure.	*Allays anxiety*
6. Inspect insulin vial noting appearance of solution and expiration date (follow package insert directions for refrigeration guidelines).	*Regular insulin preparations are clear in appearance*
7. Roll insulin vial gently between palms.	*Mixes the contents of the vial*
8. Wipe top of vial with alcohol prep.	*Prevents transmission of microbes.*
9. Remove needle cover and draw back on plunger until amount of air in syringe equals the amount of insulin to be withdrawn.	*Will counteract negative pressure*
10. Inject air into vial, invert the vial, and withdraw plunger to appropriate amount. If mixing two types of insulin into one syringe, inject air into long-acting insulin first, then inject air into short-acting insulin, and withdraw short-acting insulin first.	*Allows for ease of withdrawal*
11. Check for air bubbles in the syringe and expel as necessary.	*Excess air will decrease the amount of insulin to be injected*
12. Don gloves.	*Serves as protective barrier*
13. Cleanse skin at injection site.	*Prevents transmission of microbes*
14. Gently pinch skin and insert needle at 90-degree angle.	*Enables the subcutaneous administration of insulin*

15. Push down on the plunger until all medication has been injected.

Injects the medication

16. Pull needle straight out and press alcohol swab lightly over injection site.

Heavy pressure or excessive rubbing can alter insulin absorption

17. Discard syringe in sharps container.

Maintains universal precautions

18. Wash hands.

Prevents transmission of microbes

19. Instruct client/caregiver to rotate sites.

Alternating sites facilitates drug absorption

20. Instruct in safe management of continuous subcutaneous insulin infusion (CSII), if ordered.

Reduces risk of error

 a. prepare subcutaneous site for insertion.
 b. connect prefilled syringe with ordered amount of regular insulin to pump per manufacturer's instructions
 c. prime line
 d. attach subcutaneous needle to tubing
 e. insert needle into subcutaneous tissue of abdomen
 f. turn on pump and program the device to infuse medication at ordered rate

21. Instruct in protocol for sick-day management.

Reduces potential development of diabetic complications

 a. monitor blood glucose every 2 hours
 b. drink plenty of fluids
 c. get plenty of rest
 d. notify physician for elevated blood glucose, fever, vomiting, diarrhea, dehydration, loss of vision, or abdominal pain

22. Instruct client/caregiver in all related procedures and permit return demonstration.

Documents client/caregiver's ability to perform related procedures

DOCUMENTATION
The following should be included in the nursing note:

Type and amount of insulin
Site used for insulin injection
Blood glucose results
Client's response to procedure
Untoward reactions and interventions employed to correct
All client/caregiver teaching:
    Topics to include in teaching plan:
        safe and correct equipment handling
        emergency procedures
        underlying disease pathology
        appropriate community resources and contact persons

INTERDISCIPLINARY COLLABORATION
Inform physician of all untoward reactions
Consult with nutritionist for diabetic meal planning

Obtain permission from physician for initiation of exercise regimen

Encourage routine foot care by podiatrist, and yearly eye examinations

Consult with social worker to locate community diabetic classes and to determine client eligibility for financial assistance/reimbursement for supplies

Collaborate with the certified diabetic educator in the care and management of the diabetic client

Consult with DME vendor to reorder supplies as needed [6, 15, 20, 21, 25, 39, 41]

PROCEDURE
Diabetes Management: Dietary Regimen

DESCRIPTION
The dietary management of diabetes requires carefully balancing nutrient intake, energy expenditure, and the timing of insulin or oral antidiabetic medications. The client with diabetes must consume a structured diet to prevent the development of hyperglycemia. Clients in need of dietary management of diabetes include those diagnosed with as insulin dependent diabetes mellitus (IDDM) Type I, noninsulin dependent diabetes mellitus (NIDDM) Type II, and impaired glucose tolerance (IGT).

PURPOSE
To guide the person with diabetes in making appropriate food choices and behavioral changes that will aid in improvement of blood glucose levels and overall nutritional status, and thereby enhance diabetes self-management.

EQUIPMENT
Meal planning book/education materials

Weight scale

OUTCOMES
The client/caregiver will:

▶ Maintain near-normal blood glucose levels

▶ Achieve/maintain optimal serum lipid levels

▶ Consume adequate calories to attain/maintain reasonable weight for adults

▶ Identify and treat hypoglycemia and hyperglycemia symptoms

▶ Follow sick-day management guidelines

▶ Identify long-term complications of diabetes such as retinopathy, nephropathy, neuropathy, and cardiovascular disease

ASSESSMENT DATA
General nutrition assessment data obtained from preliminary nursing assessment

Growth pattern

Blood glucose levels

Timing of meals

Nutrition history including current diet pattern

Exercise patterns

RELATED NURSING DIAGNOSES
Anxiety

Powerlessness

Altered body image

At risk for ineffective coping
Altered nutrition, less than body requirements
Knowledge deficit
At risk for infection

SPECIAL CONSIDERATIONS

In collaboration with the physician, the nutritionist will determine the type of meal planning approach that is most appropriate for each individual based on: abilities of client/caregiver, economic resources, nutrition needs and goals, age, activity, medication regime, food preferences, and eating and lifestyle habits.

The client teaching plan should include signs and symptoms of hypoglycemia, hyperglycemia, and complications of the disease. (See Appendix 6-6.)

TRANSCULTURAL CONSIDERATIONS

For clients with predominant ethnic food choices, appropriate list of foods with guidelines on how to incorporate these foods into the meal plan should be provided.

An interpreter will be needed for the client unable to speak or understand the English language. Obtain educational materials in the client's native language, if available. Consider use of AT&T language lien. Consider incorporating religious or cultural practices into the plan of care. See also the Culturological Assessment procedure in Unit 2 for general overview of cultural considerations.

▶ INTERVENTIONS

1. Obtain diet history: Include height, weight, weight history, intake, and calorie/carbohydrate control.	*Basis for individualized meal plan*
2. Determine need for nutrition counseling and client/caregiver understanding of goals.	*Identifies learning deficits and supports consult for registered dietician*
3. Identify initial foods client may need to avoid prior to counseling, i.e., total carbohydrates, treatment of hypoglycemia, and sick-day management.	*Basic nutrition intervention and survival skill information*
4. Initiate request for initial or further nutrition counseling by nutritionist.	*Provides in-depth nutrition intervention and meal planning with determination of type of appropriate meal planning tools*
5. Assess relevant laboratory data.	*Determine past and current diabetes control*

DOCUMENTATION

The following should be included in the nursing note:

Type of diet client currently follows and major concerns to be addressed.
Previous diet instruction, if any
Interim diet/diabetes control advice given
Need for future nutrition counseling
Client/caregiver verbalized understanding of principles of diabetes management
Client's response to procedure
Untoward reactions and interventions employed to correct

All client/caregiver teaching:
  Topics to include in teaching plan:
    safe and correct equipment handling
    emergency procedures
    underlying disease pathology
    appropriate community resources and contact persons

INTERDISCIPLINARY COLLABORATION

The nutritionist will consult with the physician to determine the Kcal needs for prevention of long-term complications

The nutritionist will collaborate with the nurse in addressing special dietary concerns and management of the client's diabetic condition based on lab results, dietary adherence, etc.

Collaborate with a certified diabetic instructor in the planning of care for the diabetic client [6, 18, 47, 60, 61]

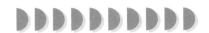

7 Adult Neurological System Procedures

Intraspinal Infusion Pain Management

DESCRIPTION

Intraspinal analgesia is used to control the intractable pain of cancer and other chronic conditions. The intraspinal route may be either intrathecal (into the subarachniod space) or epidural (into the epidural space). The catheter is placed by an anesthesiologist or nurse anesthetist under local anesthesia and connected to an infusion pump for continuous administration of a narcotic analgesic agent. For long-term therapy the catheter is tunneled under the subcutaneous tissue and exits the body on the side of the abdomen (Figure 6-21). For long-term pain management implantable drug delivery pump systems will be used (Arrow, Medtronic, and Synchromed).

See also procedure for Managing Infusion Therapy.

PURPOSE
To manage pain

EQUIPMENT
Gloves
Intravenous equipment
Narcotic infusion/prefilled syringe
Infusion pump
Povidone-iodine swabs
10-cc syringes
Tubing
Tape
Gauze
Arrow, Medtronic, or Synchromed refill kit
External programming unit if needed
Non-coring needle

OUTCOMES
The client/caregiver will:

▶ Verbalize relief of pain
▶ Demonstrate ability to troubleshoot equipment
▶ Maintain vital signs within normal limits
▶ Maintain level of consciousness
▶ Maintain normal bowel/bladder function
▶ Be free of infection

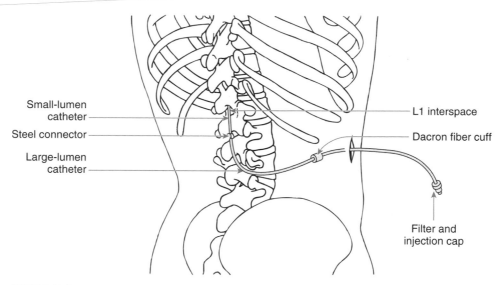

Small-lumen catheter

Steel connector

Large-lumen catheter

L1 interspace

Dacron fiber cuff

Filter and injection cap

FIGURE 6-21 ▶ Intraspinal catheter.

ASSESSMENT DATA
Assess the client's pain intensity
Monitor changes in level of consciousness, vital signs, motor and sensory function
Observe for evidence of infection at catheter insertion/exit site
Obtain history of current illness, noting any history of medication allergy
Assess the length of catheter at each visit and notify physician of any changes in length

RELATED NURSING DIAGNOSES
Pain
At risk for altered thought process
At risk for decreased cardiac output
At risk for ineffective breathing patterns
At risk for altered bowel/bladder elimination
Anticipatory grief
Caregiver role strain
At risk for infection

SPECIAL CONSIDERATIONS
The intraspinal route of administration of medication poses a threat to client safety because of the catheter's proximity to nerves, vessels and potential to migrate through the dura. Only specially trained nurses should be employed to manage the infusion and instruct clients and caregivers in the safe maintenance of therapy.

Synchromed Pump—Programming of this pump is achieved by telemetry and requires the presence of an external programmer, who provides a printout of the programming sequence and final pump operating parameters. A lithium battery is the power source and usually lasts 3–5 years. Upon death, the pump must be removed if the body is to be cremated, and should then be returned to the manufacturer. Before performing an MRI, the pump should be stopped and the reservoir filled with saline to prevent overdosing, underdosing or alteration of the pump memory mechanism. All nurses should be inserviced by the manufacturer and supervised by an experienced nurse prior to implementing this procedure.

Arrow Pump—With this device the nurse should be aware that the flow of drug from the pump can be altered by several factors: an increase in the client's temperature, atmospheric pressure changes, a change in blood pressure, and the degree of concentration and viscosity of the medication. Clients should be instructed to avoid long hot baths, saunas, placing a heating pad over the pump, scuba diving, or traumatic physical activity. Clients should notify their physician when planning air travel or trips to another location with differing altitude, or upon developing a febrile state.

For both types of pumps clients should be instructed to wear a medic alert bracelet and to carry an ID card indicating pump placement.

TRANSCULTURAL CONSIDERATIONS

An interpreter will be needed for the client unable to speak or understand the English language. Obtain educational materials in the client's native language, if available. Consider incorporating ethnic or religious practices into the plan of care. See also the Culturological Assessment procedure in Unit 2 for general overview of cultural considerations.

▶ INTERVENTIONS

1. Verify physician order.	*Reduces risk of error*
2. Wash hands.	*Prevent transmission of microbes*
3. Perform a physical assessment.	*Establishes baseline information of physiological data findings*
4. Obtain history of current illness.	*Assists in the development of an individualized plan of care*
5. Implement appropriate pump procedure as ordered.	*Initiates equipment-specific guidelines*
6. Don mask and gloves.	*Serves as a protective barrier*

For Continuous Infusion

Maintains constant drug levels usually via patient controlled analgesic setups
  a. clean injection cap of epidural catheter with povidone-iodine (do not use alcohol)
  b. dry cap with sterile gauze
  c. attach prefilled syringe to proximal end of infusion pump tubing and prime line
  d. attach distal end of infusion tubing to epidural catheter, tape all connections, initiate pump
  e. verify pump settings

For Arrow Pump System

Used in long-term intraspinal infusion therapy
  a. obtain pump kit and palpate system
  b. confirm physician order
  c. prep pump site with betadine using sterile technique
  d. secure connections on the needle/tubing set and to stopcock (turned to off position)

e. access pump system using a noncoring needle, hold at a perpendicular angle, and advance needle until it is in contact with the needle stop

f. attach empty syringe barrel and open stopcock, pump reservoir will empty automatically

g. when pump is completely empty, close stopcock and remove syringe and stopcock

h. attach a syringe filled with nonperservative NSS and inject 5 cc into the pump, release pressure and allow the 5 cc of NSS to return into the syringe. clamp and remove the syringe

i. attach a prefilled syringe containing prescribed medication, open clamp and begin to fill pump. Inject 5 cc increments and allow 1 cc to return, continue this procedure until pump is filled

j. when pump is filled, clamp tubing and remove needle

For Medtronic or Synchromed Pump System

Used in long-term intraspinal infusion therapy

a. perform telemetry

b. confirm medication dosage with physician order

c. program the appropriate new parameters with the computer

d. prep site with betadine

e. place template over pump, access with a non-coring needle and withdraw remaining drug from pump, clamp tubing and remove syringe

f. attach 0.22 micron filter and pressure monitor to a prefilled syringe and prime line, attach to pump tubing and open clamp, 2–3 cc should automatically be drawn into the pump, then slowly inject remainder of medication into the pump

g. close the stopcock to syringe and check position of fluid meniscus in pressure monitor. If level is acceptable, clamp tubing and deaccess. If level is unacceptable, remove the stopcock and filter, empty pump completely. Obtain new 0.22 micron filter and attach as above

7. Remove mask and gloves

Risk of introducing microbes into the system ends when the port is de-accessed

8. Manage side effects of narcotic administration.

Improves client's ability to tolerate drug therapy

a. Constipation
   (1) implement planned exercise program
   (2) increase intake of fruits and fruit juices
   (3) drink warm beverages at night
   (4) increase water intake
   (5) administer stool softeners and laxatives as ordered

b. Sedation
   (1) slowly increase activity levels
   (2) increase intake of caffeine if not contraindicated
   (3) consult with physician to consider need to reduce dose of narcotic and add nonopoid pain medications

c. Nausea
   (1) administer medications to control motion sickness as ordered
   (2) administer antiemetics as ordered

  d. Pruritus
     (1) avoid harsh soaps
     (2) use cool compresses on affected areas
     (3) wear soft clothing
     (4) protect face and neck from extremes in temperature
  e. Urinary retention
     (1) monitor urinary output
     (2) encourage voiding 3–4 times per day
     (3) report evidence of oliguria
  f. Respiratory depression
     (1) attempt to stimulate client
     (2) perform coughing and deep-breathing exercises
     (3) maintain narcotic antagonist at bedside and instruct
         caregivers in method of administration
9. Instruct client/caregiver in self-management of care and   *Documents client/caregiver's*
   permit return demonstration   *ability to implement inter-*
                                                                      ventions

DOCUMENTATION

The following should be included in the nursing note:

Date, time of procedure
Medication dose and amount
Client tolerance to the procedure
Any untoward reactions
For synchromed pump system, obtain printout from computer documenting telemetry parameters
    and indicate needle size used
All client/caregiver teaching:
    Topics to include in teaching plan:
        safe and correct equipment handling
        emergency procedures
        underlying disease pathology
        appropriate community resources and contact persons

INTERDISCIPLINARY COLLABORATION

Report any untoward reactions to the physician
Consult with the pharmacist to verify pump settings, amount to be withdrawn and computer
    printout documentation of parameters set [1, 2, 6, 7, 13, 15, 17, 21, 25, 39, 41, 62]

REFERENCES

1. Bean, CA. High-tech homecare infusion therapies. *Critical Care Nursing Clinics of North America* 10:287–303, 1998.
2. Boggs, RL, & Wooldridge-King, M. *AACN procedure manual for critical care,* 3rd Ed. Philadelphia, PA: W. B Saunders Company, 1993.
3. Bruderman I, & Abboud S. *Telespirometry: novel system for home monitoring of asthmatic patients.* Telemedicine Journal 3:127, Summer 1997.
4. Carrol, P. Using pulse oximetry in the home. *Home Healthcare Nurse,* 15:88, 1997.
5. Carrol, T. Home care of severe heart failure with intravenous diuretics and inotropes. *Infusion* 13–16, May, 1996.

6. Carpenito, L. *Nursing diagnosis: Application to clinical practice,* 7th edition. Philadelphia, PA: Lippincott, 1997.

7. *Coram healthcare corporation nursing orientation manual.* Denver, CO: The Corporation, 1995.

8. *Coram healthcare corporation clinical panual policy 2.7.1.* Introduction to Inotropic Therapies. Denver, CO: The Corporation, 1998.

9. *Coram healthcare corporation clinical manual.* Enteral Nutrition Policy and Procedure. The Corporation, 1997.

10. Corbett, NA. Homecare, technology and the management of respiratory disease. *Critical Care Nursing Clinics of North America,* 10:305–313, 1998.

11. Feldman, AM. Can we alter survival in patients with congestive heart failure? *Journal of the American Medical Association,* 267:1956–1961, 1992.

12. Fischbach, Frances. *A manual of laboratory & diagnostic tests,* 5th ed. Philadelphia: Lippincott, 1996.

13. Fonteyn, M. The Agency for Health Care Policy and Research Guidelines: Implications for home health care providers. *AACN Clinical Issues* 9:338–354, 1998.

14. Frantz, A. Summary of the nursing practice guidelines for the Cardiac Home Care Patient. *Home Healthcare Nurse,* 16:743–752, 1998.

15. Fuller, J, & Schaller-Ayers, J. *Health assessment: a nursing approach,* 2nd Edition. Philadelphia, PA: Lippincott, 1994.

16. Glass, C, Boling, PA, & Gammon, S. Collaborative support for caregivers of individuals beginning mechanical ventilation at home. *Critical Care Nurse* 16:6:67–72, 1996.

17. Gorski, LA. *High-tech home care manual.* Gaithersburg, MD: Aspen Publishers, Inc. 1997.

18. Gottschlich, MM, Matarese, LE, & Shronts, EP, eds. *Nutrition support dietetics core curriculum,* 2nd edition. Silver Springs, Maryland: A.S.P.E.N. 1993.

19. Green, K. *Home care survival guide.* Philadelphia, PA: Lippincott, 1998.

20. Hodgson, BB & Kizior, RJ. *Saunders nursing drug handbook 1999.* Philadelphia, PA: WB Saunders Company, 1999.

21. Jarvis C. *Pocket companion for physical examination and health assessment.* Philadelphia, PA: W.B. Saunders Company, 1996.

22. Johnson JY, Smith-Temple J, & Carr P. *Nurses' guide to home procedures.* Philadelphia, PA: Lippincott, 1998.

23. Kelley, C, McBride, L, Randolph, S, & Lonergan, J. *Home care management of the blood cell transplant patient.* Sudbury, MA: Jones and Bartlett Publishers, Inc. 1996.

24. Klein, GL, Roger, JZ, Friedman, J, et al. A multidisciplinary approach to home enteral nutrition. *Nutrition in Clinical Practice* 13(4):157–162, 1998.

25. LeMone, P, & Burke KM. *Medical surgical nursing: critical thinking in client care.* Menlo Park, CA: Addison Wesley Publishers, 1996.

26. Loan, T, Kearney, P, Magnuson, B. et al. Enteral feeding in the home environment. *Home Healthcare Nurse.* 15:531–536, 1997.

27. Lowdermilk D. Homecare of the patient with gynecologic cancer. *Journal of Obstetric, Gynecologic, and Neonatal Nursing* 24:157, 1995.

28. Marrelli TM. *Handbook of home health standards and documentation guidelines for reimbursement,* 3rd edition. St Louis, Missouri: Mosby, 1998.

29. McConnell EA. The future of technology in critical care. *Critical Care Nurse Supplement* 3–16, June 1996.

30. McManamen L, & Hendrickx L. Telemedicine: tuning in critical care's future? *Critical Care Nurse* 16:103, 1996.

31. McNeal, GJ. Twenty-four hour ambulatory monitoring: A new electrocardiographic tool. *Nursing Clinics of North America.* 13:3, 437–448, 1978.

32. McNeal, GJ. Tracing arrhythmias. *American Journal of Nursing* 79:1, 98–100, 1979.

33. McNeal GJ. High-tech home care: an expanding critical care frontier. *Critical Care Nurse* 16:51 1996.

34. McNeal GJ. Diversity issues in the homecare setting. *Critical Care Nursing Clinics of North America* 10(3):357, 1998.

35. McNeal GJ. Care of the critically-ill client at home. *Critical Care Nursing Clinics of North America* 10(3):267, 1998.

36. McNeal GJ. Telecommunication technologies in high-tech homecare. *Critical Care Nursing Clinics of North America* 10(3):279, 1998.

37. Mersch J, & Cook K. *Technology whose time has come: The Stanford Transtelephonic arrhythmia network.* Stanford Nurse 18:4, 1996.

38. Miller, LW. Outpatient dobutamine for refractory congestive heart failure: Advantages, techniques and results. *Journal of Heart and Lung Transplantation.* 10:482-487, 1991.

39. Nettina, SM (Ed.). *The Lippincott manual of nursing practice,* 6th edition. Philadelphia PA: Lippincott Publishers, 1996.

40. *Nurse's Handbook of Home Infusion Therapy.* Springhouse, PA: Springhouse Home Care, 1997.
41. *Nurse's Illustrated Handbook of Home Health Procedures.* Springhouse PA: Springhouse Home Care, 1999.
42. O'Neal P, & McFarlin P. Home care goes high tech. *Stanford Nurse* 18:8, 1996.
43. Pait EP, & Pallesen, BJ. Fundamental Considerations in home chemotherapy administration. *Infusion* 2:24, 1996.
44. Petrosky-Pacini, AJ. The automatic implantable cardioverter defibrillator in home care. *Home Healthcare Nurse* 14:238–243, 1996.
45. Pickworth, KK. Long-term dobutamine therapy for refractory congestive heart failure. *Clinical Pharmacology* 11:618–624, 1992.
46. Portillo, C, & Schumacher, K. Graduate Program: Advanced Practice nurses in the home. *AACN Clinical Issues* 9:355–361, 1998.
47. Powers, M.A., ed. *Nutrition guide for professionals: Diabetes education and meal planning.* Chicago: American Dietetic Association and Alexandria, Va: American Diabetes Association, 1988.
48. *Revised Intravenous Nursing Standards of Practice.* Supplement to Journal of Intravenous Nursing, 21(1S): S1–S91.
49. Rice R. Home mechanical ventilator management. *Home Healthcare Nurse* 13:73, 1995.
50. Romano CA. Imaging: an innovative technology. *Computers in Nursing* 11:222, 1993.
51. Rombeau, JL, & Caldwell, DC. *Parenteral Nutrition.* In L. Hall, TL Pipp, PJ Kearns (Eds.). Parenteral Nutrition Devices and Equipment, 16. 334–348, 1993.
52. Schlachta, LM, & Pursley-Crotteau, S. Leaveraging technology:telemedicine in disease management and implications for infusion services. *Infusion* 4:36, 1997.
53. Singh, P. Managing Chronic Congestive Heart Failure in the Home. *Home Healthcare Nurse* 13:11–13, 1995.
54. Smith, C, Mayre, L, Parkhurst, C, Perkings, S, et al. Adaptation in families with a member requiring mechanical ventilation at home. *Heart and Lung* 20:349, 1991.
55. Snyder, M., Chlan, L., Finkelstein, S., et al. Home monitoring of pulmonary function. *Home Healthcare Nurse* 16:388–393,1998.
56. Stackhouse, JC. *Into the community: Nursing in ambulatory and home care.* Philadelphia, PA: Lippincott, 1998.
57. Stanhope, M, & Knollmueller, RN. *Handbook of community and home health nursing.* St. Louis, MO: Mosby, 1996.
58. Susman E. Telemedicine permits overnight dialysis at home. Health care workers watch for problems from office. *Telemedicine Virtual Reality* 2:13, February 1997.
59. Thomas, V, Ellison, K, Howell, E, & Winters, K. Caring for the person receiving ventilatory support at home: Caregivers' needs and involvement. *Heart and Lung* 21:180, 1992.
60. Trujillo, E, Robinson, M, & Jacobs, D. Nutritional assessment in the critically ill. *Critical Care Nurse* 19:67–74, February 1999.
61. *Pediatric manual of clinical dietetics.* Chicago, IL: The American Dietetics Association, 1998.
62. Zang SM, & Bailey NC. *Home care manual: making the transitition.* Philadelphia, PA: Lippincott, 1997.

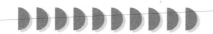

Appendices

Date of visit: _____   Home Care Agent: _____
Follow-up visit: _____

Indicate the correct response by placing a check in the appropriate box.

1. Do you (parent, caregiver) smoke?   ☐ Yes   ☐ No

2. Do other members of the household smoke?   ☐ Yes   ☐ No

3. Are you exposed to smoke at work or other places?   ☐ Yes   ☐ No

4. Does anyone smoke at your child's daycare?   ☐ Yes   ☐ No

5. Do you/your child have asthma symptoms year round?   ☐ Yes   ☐ No

6. Is there mold/mildew or dampness in any room of the house?   ☐ Yes   ☐ No

7. Is there evidence of cockroaches in the home?   ☐ Yes   ☐ No

8. Do you/your child have seasonal asthma symptoms?   ☐ Yes   ☐ No
   If yes, when?
      ☐ Early spring (trees)
      ☐ Late spring (grasses)
      ☐ Late summer to autumn (weeds)
      ☐ Summer and fall (alternaria, cladosporum)

9. Do you use cleaning agents or sprays around the home?   ☐ Yes   ☐ No

10. Do you/your child have constant nasal congestion or runny nose?   ☐ Yes   ☐ No

Home care agent observation:

1. Do you see evidence of cockroaches?   ☐ Yes   ☐ No

2. Do you see evidence of pets?   ☐ Yes   ☐ No

3. Does the home have carpets?   ☐ Yes   ☐ No

4. Do you see evidence of heating problems in the house?   ☐ Yes   ☐ No
   (electric/kerosine heaters)

5. Is the house draft free?   ☐ Yes   ☐ No

APPENDIX 6-1 ▶ Asthma Environmental Assessment

Date of Home Care visit: _____   Home Care Agent: _____
Reschedule date (if applicable): _____

Personal Information:

1. What medical or social concerns do you have?

    _____

    _____

    _____

2. How long has it been since you've experienced chest tightness, cough, shortness of breath, or wheezing?
    ☐ Less than a week
    ☐ Within 30 days
    ☐ In the last 6 months
    ☐ In the last year

3. Do you awaken at night due to chest tightness, cough, shortness of breath, or wheezing?
    ☐ Yes   ☐ No
    If yes, how frequently?
    ☐ Every night
    ☐ Two times a week
    ☐ Weekly
    ☐ Rarely

4. Has your asthma ever restricted your physical activity?
    ☐ Yes   ☐ No
    If yes, when has this occurred? _____
                         (date)

5. How many days have you missed from school/work due to asthma symptoms?
    ☐ Never
    ☐ Once a month
    ☐ 1–4 times per month
    ☐ 5 times or more per month

6. Have you had an emergency room visit for asthma?
    ☐ Never
    ☐ In the last month
    ☐ In the last year
    Date of last visit: ___ _____

7. Have you been hospitalized for "asthma related" problems?
    ☐ Never
    ☐ In the last month
    ☐ In the last year
    Date of hospitalization _____

APPENDIX 6-2 ▶ Asthma Management Program–Homecare Assessment

Medication:

8. Do you take any medications on a constant basis?

☐ Yes ☐ No

If yes, list the medication(s):

_____

_____

_____

9. How many puffs of your "rescue medicine" do you take daily?

_____

APPENDIX 6-2 [CONTINUED] ▶ Asthma Management Program—Homecare Assessment

Implementation of Plan of Action

Have client pick a stop date within the next 7–10 day of initial visit.

Have client sign a commitment letter stating "I will quit smoking on _____ record date.

Discuss with client why they smoke.

Ask client to write down all the reasons he or she want to quit smoking

Encourage the client to maintain a journal listing triggers to smoking, i.e., telephone, stress

Have client to maintain a record of every cigarette smoked

Encourage the client to use the delay technique. Each time a cigarette is desired, wait an extra 10–15 minutes prior to smoking. This will begin elimination of an unnecessary cigarette

Encourage the client to avoid coffee and caffeine-related products. It becomes very difficult for a coffee drinker to have coffee without having the desire for a cigarette.

Avoid alcohol. Alcohol has the ability to lower the defenses and inhibitions. Smokers who use alcohol double or triple their tobacco use when drinking alcohol. Avoid alcohol during the quitting process.

Encourage client to change routine that leads to smoking, i.e., Drink coffee with your left hand if you are right-handed, place coffee in a glass instead of a mug or coffee cup. The most important thing at this time is to break the association

When a cigarette is needed a substitute should be on hand (sugarless gum, sugarless candy, carrot sticks, fresh fruit, chopped ice or fruit juices without sugar)

Shop for healthy food and plan all meals in advance

Deep Breathing

Most smokers are shallow breathers. The only time they take a deep breath is when they are inhaling the smoke of a cigarette.

Encourage practicing deep-breathing exercise:

-it emulates the smoking behavior

-it helps the client relax

Deep breathing increase oxygen causing a decrease in pressure in the chest activities. It also decreases the pressure in the veins. With the increase blood flow, there is an increase in oxygen flowing to the heart and lungs. This increase in oxygen causes the heart to slow down and they feel more relaxed.

Deep breathing is the most important tool you could use when you are teaching someone to stop smoking.

APPENDIX 6-3 ▶ Client Education: Smoking Cessation

Deep-Breathing Technique

Take a deep breath through your nose. Hold it for 3−5 seconds then slowly exhale through you pursed lips. Repeat ten times or more if desired.

Smoking does not relax you. Nicotine is a stimulant.

Remember, deep breathing along with inhaling smoke helps to give the smoker a relaxed sensation.

This relaxed sensation can be achieved by deep breathing and at the same time eliminate the tars and poisons that are in tobacco.

Deep Breathing Helps You:

▶ Cleanse your lungs and helps to get rid of the residual smoke remaining in your lungs.

▶ Overcome your desire to smoke as it emulates what you do when you inhale a cigarette.

▶ Oxygenate your body and provide more energy

▶ Relax

▶ Focus your mind; it helps you feel more in control

▶ Get in touch with your body and your mind and promotes a greater awareness of yourself.

Surveying the Home

Remove all smoking paraphnelia

Remove all visual cues reminding the smoker to smoke

Ashtrays, matches, lighters, and cigarettes

Remove any cigarettes you have lying around. Look through all your hidden places.

Remove the ashtray in the car and lighter. Replace with mints or sugarless candy.

If another smoker is in the home elicit his or her support.

APPENDIX 6-3 [CONTINUED] ▶ Client Education: Smoking Cessation

Catheter: Non-Tunneled Central Catheter

General Information

The catheter:
1. is inserted at the hospital bedside or in an outpatient setting
2. is percutaneously inserted into the vein via the skin and terminates in the superior vena cava.
3. access sites used are typically the jugular or subclavian veins, however, because the jugular site tends to impair client mobility and is difficult to maintain an intact dressing, the subclavian site is preferred
4. is usually made of polyurethane
5. is intended for short term use and may be left in place for a few days to a few weeks
6. the upper chest or neck insertion sites are difficult for the client to self manage
7. has a multiple lumen feature
8. may be secured with sutures
9. may be used for all types of infusion therapies

Routine and Maintainence Flush * [the type of flush solution, amount and frequency will vary, refer to agency standardized flushing protocols]

1. Heparin strength 10 to 1000 unit/ml
2. Heparin volume should be equal to twice the internal volume capacity of the catheter
3. The catheter should be flushed after medication administration and every 12–24 hours to maintain patency

Dressing Type and Change Frequency

1. Dressing change is a sterile technique
2. More frequent dressing changes may be required to keep the dressing intact and occlusive to air
3. Dressing may be gauze or transparent semipermiable membrane
4. Transparent dressings promote stabilization of the catheter
5. Change the dressing immediately if it becomes loose, soiled or damp
6. Evaluate the site with each dressing change for presence of erythema, pain, edema, and drainage

Internal Volume

0.3–0.5 ml plus extension set

Injection Cap Change

The cap:
1. should have a luer lock design to decrease chance of cap becoming dislodged
2. should be made of latex or other material designed to create a closed system
3. should be changed minimally every 7 days, or after blood sampling/withdrawal, or If the integrity becomes compromised

Special Considerations

1. If the nurse is to remove the catheter, ensure that the procedure is covered under the state nurse practice act and that the agency has a written policy
2. Follow the agency policy, if applicable, for removal
3. To reduce risk of air embollsm, have the client lie in a dorsal recumbent position with the head of the bed flat and have the client performed Valsalva's maneuver while the catheter is being removed
4. Apply occlusive dressing after catheter removal to prevent formation of air embolism

Catheter: Tunneled Central Catheter

General Information

The catheter:
1. must be surgically placed
2. tip is positioned in the superior vena cava
3. is tunneled within the subcutaneous tissue and exits the body at the exit site
4. is usually made of silastic
5. is intended for long-term use and may be left in indefinitely
6. has a multilumen feature
7. is designed to promote client self care
8. may be used for all types of therapies

Routine and Maintainence Flush * [the type of flush solution, amount and frequency will vary, refer to agency standardized flushing protocols]

1. Heparin strength 10 to 1000 unit/ml
2. Heparin volume should be equal to twice the internal volume capacity of the catheter
3. The catheter should be flushed after medication administration and every 12–24 hours to maintain patency

Dressing Type and Change Frequency

1. The dressing change is performed using a sterile or aseptic technique
2. The dressing may be made of gauze or may be a transparent semi-permiable membrane with/without gauze
3. Transparent dressings promote stabilization of the catheter and permit direct visualization of the insertion site
4. Depending on the client's immune status, the frequency of dressing change may vary from every 2–7 days
5. The dressing should be changed immediately if it becomes loose, soiled, or damp

Internal Volume

0.15 to 1.8ml plus extension set

Injection Cap Change

The cap:
1. should have a luer lock design to decrease chance of cap becoming dislodged
2. should be made of latex or other material designed to create a closed system
3. should be changed minimally every 7 days, or after blood sampling/withdrawal, or if the integrity becomes compromised

Special Considerations

1. The catheter has an in-line clamp which must be released prior to flushing to avoid risk of catheter rupture
2. Repair a damaged catheter using the manufacturer's repair kit specific for the catheter in use
3. Evaluate the exit site, neck, shoulder, and catheter tunnel, minimally with each dressing change, for presence of pain, erythema, edema, or drainage
4. When used for blood sampling, the catheter should be flushed with 0.9% sodium chloride to remove red blood cells prior to being flushed with heparin solution

APPENDIX 6-4 [CONTINUED] ▶ Infusion Access Devices

Catheter: Groshong Tunneled Central Catheter, Groshong Port or Groshong PICC

General Information

1. The Groshong catheter is a valve-tipped catheter and should never be trimmed at the terminal end
2. The three-way Groshong valve opens inward for aspiration, opens outward for infusion, and remains closed when not in use to prevent blood backup into the catheter
3. The valve, when closed, prevents air flow into the system so the hub can be opened to air without having an adverse effect
4. The catheter may be used for all types of therapies
5. No clamping of the catheter is necessary

Routine and Maintenance Flush

1. Flush with 5 ml of 0.9% sodium chloride before and after each intermittent infusion
2. Flush each lumen weekly for tunneled and PICC lines, and flush each implanted port monthly
3. Post blood draw, flush with 20ml 0.9% sodium chloride

Dressing Type and Change Frequency

1. The dressing change is performed using a sterile or aseptic technique
2. The dressing may be made of gauze or may be a transparent semi-permiable membrane with/without gauze
3. Transparent dressings promote stabilization of the catheter and permit direct visualization of the insertion site
4. Depending on the client's immune status, the frequency of dressing change may vary from every 2–7 days
5. The dressing should be changed immediately if it becomes loose, soiled, or damp

Internal Volume

0.9ml plus extension set for tunneled or port
0.33ml plus extension set for Groshong PICC

Injection Cap Change

The cap:
1. should have a luer lock design to decrease chance of cap becoming dislodged
2. should be made of latex or other material designed to create a closed system
3. should be changed minimally every 7 days, or after blood sampling/withdrawal, or if the integrity becomes compromised

Special Considerations

1. A clamp should not be used, will damage the three-way valve
2. DO NOT USE VACUTAINER SYSTEM FOR BLOOD DRAW, may damage the three-way valve over a period of time

APPENDIX 6-4 [CONTINUED] ▶ Infusion Access Devices

Catheter Implanted Reservoirs (Ports)

General Information

1. The implantation procedure is surgically performed
2. The device is placed under the surface of the skin
3. Ports can be made of plastic, titanium, steel, or silicone rubber
4. The device consists of a reservoir with latex rubber septum with an attached silicone catheter
5. The septum is the point of injection and helps in stabilizing the needle when the port is in use

Routine and Maintainance Flush

1. Heparin strength 100units/ml
2. Heparin volume is 3–5 ml
3. After blood draw, catheter should be flushed with 10-20ml of NSS followed by the ordered amount of heparin flush solution
4. Frequency of changing the Huber needle is based on the manufacturer's guidelines
5. When port is not being used, it is accessed and flushed every 4 weeks with 10ml NSSS followed by ordered amount of heparin flush solution

Dressing Type and Change Frequency

1. The dressing change is performed using a sterile technique
2. The dressing may be made of gauze or may be a transparent semi-permiable membrane with/without gauze
3. Transparent dressings promote stabilization of the catheter and permit direct visualization of the insertion site
4. Depending on the client's immune status, the frequency of dressing change may vary from every 2–7 days
5. The dressing should be changed immediately if it becomes loose, soiled, or damp

Internal Volume

0.5ml to 1.5ml plus extension set

Injection Cap Change

Performed with every Huber needle change

The cap:
1. should have a luer lock design to decrease chance of cap becoming dislodged
2. should be made of latex or other material designed to create a closed system
3. should be changed minimally every 7 days, or after blood sampling/withdrawal, or if the integrity becomes compromised

Special Considerations

1. DO NOT use a traditional needle to access port. May damage the septum by coring the latex, causing damage
2. USE ONLY NON-CORING NEEDLE also called Huber needle
3. The Huber needle is angled at 90 degrees and has a bevel which opens on the side of the needle rather than on the end, and permits self-sealing of the latex when de-accessed
4. The Huber needle comes in a variety of lengths and gauge sizes. Make sure to use the appropriate size for the port to prevent dislodging of the needle, which could cause an infiltration
5. The port catheter may be placed intraarterially for chemotherapy, such types of ports are flushed weekly, or more frequently, with a Heparin 1000units/ml to maintain patency

APPENDIX 6-4 [CONTINUED] ▶ Infusion Access Devices

Catheter PICC, Midclavicular, Midline

General Information

1. The PICC is a long (20–25 inches), flexible, radiopaque catheter that is inserted in an antecubital fossa vein with the tip extending into the superior vena cava. Sizes range from 16 to 28 gauge
2. Tip placement is verified by x-ray
3. The basilic and cephalic antecubital fossa veins are sites for PICC line insertion. The basilic is the largest and is the preferred vein for PICC insertion. The cephalic vein is smaller and has a greater curvature
4. PICC line insertion requires a physician order. Check with the state nurse practice act to verify authorization for placement by a professional nurse
5. Informed consent is required for PICC line insertion
6. PICC lines may only be inserted by nurses with advanced therapy skills and specific training
7. The insertion procedure is dependent on the manufacturer's guidelines
8. If the catheter is placed in the superior vena cava it can be used for all therapies. If placed as a midclavicular line use only therapies appropriate for peripheral access
9. Midline catheters are peripherally inserted catheters in which the tip does not extend beyond the axilla, in adults the average length is 6–8 inches. They are not to be used for concentrated solutions of TPN, hyperosmolar solutions or chemotherapy
10. Obtain a physician order to apply intermittent warm compresses to upper forearm to prevent the occurrence of phlebitis and provide client comfort
11. A PICC line insertion is contraindicated when:
    ► inadequate vein in the antecubital area
    ► source of potential infection at the selected site of placement
    ► trauma or injury to the upper extremity
    ► client noncompliance
    ► coagulopathies (unless specified by the physician)

Routine and Maintainance Flush

1. Most commonly used concentration is Heparin 100units/ml flush solution
2. Flushing frequency varies with agency policy
3. The amount of heparin will vary depending on length and gauge. Remember to consider the extension set and injection cap when determining heparin volume

Dressing Type and Change Frequency

1. The dressing change is a sterile procedure
2. For the first 24 hours after the initial insertion, place a sterile 2×2 gauze dressing to soak up any oozing of blood, and cover with transparent dressing
3. When removing the transparent dressing, stabilize the end of the catheter and peel the transparent dressing toward the insertion site parallel to the skin to prevent catheter dislodgement
4. Part of the site assessment should include a measurement of the external catheter, due to the possibility of catheter migration, and a midupper arm circumference measurement to assess for complications
5. Transparent dressings promote stabilization of the catheter and visualization of the insertion site
6. Depending on dressing type frequency of dressing change varies from every 2–7 days
7. Change the dressing immediately if it becomes loose, soiled, or damp
8. Application of an antimicrobial ointment to exit site may compromise adherence of the transparent dressing

Internal Volume

PICC 0.04–0.4ml plus extension set
Midline 0.12–0.25ml plus extension set

Injection Cap Change

It is recommended that an extension set be added to the catheter to prevent tugging on the PICC line when starting and stopping the IV medication
    If the extension set is attached to the catheter as part of the sterile insertion, a scheduled change may not be necessary, follow agency protocol

The cap:
1. should have a luer lock design to decrease chance of cap becoming dislodged
2. should be made of latex or other material designed to create a closed system
3. should be changed minimally every 7 days, or after blood sampling/withdrawal, or if the integrity becomes compromised

Special Considerations

1. Blood sampling from catheters smaller than 3.8 Fr is not recommended
2. Know the length of the PICC line prior to removal. If the catheter is shorter at removal than at insertion and no documentation of catheter repair or having been trimmed, notify the physician immediately
3. If repairing a damage, catheter use only the manufacturer's repair kit
4. Evaluate exit site, neck and shoulder, minimally with each dressing change, for presence of erythema, pain, edema, or drainage
5. Know the catheter tip placement prior to initiating any therapies

Catheter Intraspinal (epidural, intrathecal)

General information

1. Intraspinal catheters are inserted into the epidural or intrathecal spaces by the physician
2. These catheters are 10–30 inches long with 22–36 gauge
3. They are made of polyurethane or silicone-like polymers
4. If intended for long term use, they can extend several inches into the epidural space
5. They can exit directly from the spinal puncture, or they can be threaded subcutaneously to exit on the anterior surface of the abdomen
6. The tunneled catheter may terminate in a subcutaneously implanted pump as the Infusaid®, Arrow®, or Medronic®
7. Insertion of these catheters is a medical act
8. Nursing responsibilities include medication administration, site care, and client education
9. Continuous infusions should be administered using an electronic infusion pump
10. Medications infused must be preservative free
11. A 0.22 micron filter should be used for intraspinal infusions and changed according to the manufacturer's recommendations
12. The intraspinal access is primarily used for pain management and occasionally for chemotherapy

APPENDIX 6-4 [CONTINUED] ▶ Infusion Access Devices

Routine and Maintainence Flush

1. The epidural catheter should be aspirated prior to administration of medication to ascertain the absence of spinal fluid and blood
2. The intrathecal catheter should be aspirated prior to medication administration to ascertain the presence of spinal fluid and the absence of blood
3. When an intrathecal catheter is attached to an implanted pump follow the manufacturer's guidelines for aspiration
4. Intraspinal catheters do not clot so no routine flush is required

Dressing Type and Change Frequency

1. Dressing change is a sterile procedure
2. Alcohol is contraindicated for the site preparation because of the potential for alcohol migration into the epidural or intrathecal space. Hydrogen peroxide may be used but must have a physician order
3. Frequency of site care and dressing change will be established according to agency policy and state nurse practice act guidelines
4. Assess site for erythema, swelling, drainage, or change in catheter position

Internal Volume

not applicable

Injection Cap Change

If an injection cap is used, strict aseptic techniques will be used to change the cap

Special Considerations

1. The delivery of medications, maintenance, and care of intraspinal catheters is performed in accordance with agency policy and nurse practice acts
2. Monitoring for adverse effects of intraspinal catheters and infusions include the following:
    - catheter related systemic sepsis
    - drug related problems
    - local infections
    - mechanical complications
    - meningitis
    - occlusion
    - pump malfunction

APPENDIX 6-4 [CONTINUED] ▶ Infusion Access Devices

Class I	No limitation on physical activity; ordinary activity does not produce symptoms
Class II	Slight limitation on physical activity; no symptoms at rest, but symptoms occur with ordinary physical activity
Class III	More severe limitations; the client is usually comfortable at rest; clinical manifestations occur with less than ordinary physical activities
Class IV	Unable to carry on normal physical activity without producing symptoms; discomfort is increased when any physical activity is undertaken

APPENDIX 6-5 ▶ New York Heart Association Functional Classification of Persons with Congestive Heart Failure

Hypoglycemia

Hypoglycemia occurs when blood sugar levels drop below normal

Causes
Taking too much diabetic medication
Skipping meals or snacks
Eating meals or snacks at the wrong time
Exercising more than usual

Symptoms
Feeling shaky
Feeling tired
Feeling hunger
Fast heartbeat
Irritability or moodiness
Feeling of numbness or tingling in the mouth or lips
Experiencing blurred vision or headaches
Skin feeling moist and sweaty

Treatment of Hypoglycemia
Low blood sugar must be treated immediately. Test your blood, if the value is less than 70mg/dl or below the
   level set by your physician, eat something that contains real sugar immediately to increase your level.
Remember when in doubt, eat carbohydrates (CHO):
   $\frac{1}{2}$ cup of fruit juice
   $\frac{1}{2}$ cup of regular soda
   three glucose tablets
   1 cup of skim milk

Hyperglycemia

Hyperglycemia occurs when blood sugar levels rise above normal. High blood sugar may have a gradual onset,
but may continue to increase over a period of time.

Causes
Insufficient amount of insulin or oral diabetic medication
Illness or stress
Limit or lack of exercise
Overeating

Symptoms
Increased thirst or hungry
Frequent urination
Vision problems
Dry or itchy skin
Infection, yeast or viral
Increased tiredness or sleepiness

APPENDIX 6-6 ▶ Client Education: Diabetes Management

Treatment of Hyperglycemia

If your blood sugar level remains over 240mg/dl or the level set by your physician and when you feel sick, notify your healthcare provider

Take the correct amount of diabetes medication as scheduled

Check and record your blood sugar everyday or as often as your healthcare provider requests

Exercise regularly

Eat meals according to a scheduled meal time

Remember, you can prevent high blood sugar levels from becoming dangerous for your health

Test your blood sugar regularly, and let your healthcare provider know when your blood sugar gets out of control

Complications of Diabetes Mellitus

Long term complication will occur if diabetes remains out of control. It is important to develop healthy lifestyle changes to prevent these complications from becoming life threatening

Eye problems: about 12,000 new cases of blindness caused by diabetes occur in the U.S. each year. Prevention or treatment can help with yearly complete eye exams.

By maintaining blood pressure and blood sugar levels near to normal, you will help prevent eye damage

See an ophthalmologist or eye care specialist if these symptoms occur:

Blurred or double vision

Feeling of pressure or pain in the eyes

Seeing dark spots

Kidney problems: about 4,000 cases of kidney failure occur each year in the U.S. among people with diabetes.

Controlling blood sugar and blood pressure levels and treating infections immediately can help prevent kidney damage.

Early kidney damage can be treated with diet and medicines.

Kidney failure can only be treated with dialysis or kidney transplant.

Foot or leg problems: about 20,00 people in the U.S. with diabetes have a foot or leg amputated each year.

Early treatment of foot and leg problems can many times prevent the need for removal of these limbs.

Diabetes damages blood vessels, thereby causing poor blood flow to your lower extremities.

Always wear proper fitting shoes, examine your feet regularly, and contact your healthcare provider if a sore or cut is slow to heal.

Prevention of Diabetes Complications

Some diabetics never develop any of these long-term complications. Others may have only one. Still others have all and very severe complications. The risk of developing any of these complications can be reduced by:

Understanding your disease

Maintaining good blood sugar control

Maintaining blood pressure levels within normal limits

Maintaining good weight control

Controlling blood fat levels, including cholesterol and triglycerides

Avoiding cigarette smoking

APPENDIX 6-6 [CONTINUED] ▶ Client Education: Diabetes Management

UNIT

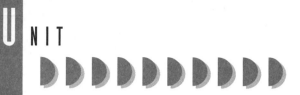

7

Geriatric Homecare

1

Geriatric Musculoskeletal System Procedures

PROCEDURE
Pressure-Relieving Beds and Support Surfaces

DESCRIPTION
Pressure-relieving devices are classified as static or dynamic. Static pressure-relieving devices refer to beds and mattresses that are motionless, and that reduce pressure by redistributing the client's weight with position changes. Dynamic pressure-relieving devices refer to beds and mattresses that have moving parts and that require electrical power to mobilize. While the use of such equipment requires a medical order because of associated costs, decisions to utilize these devices are dictated by the eligibility requirements of the third-party payor.

PURPOSE
To reduce pressure on skin surfaces to prevent tissue ischemia

EQUIPMENT
Bed linen and protective sheets
Specialty bed or mattress as ordered
Lift, slide or other device for transferring
Pressure ulcer risk management assessment form

OUTCOMES
The client/caregiver will:

▶ Be free of pressure ulcers
▶ Maintain skin integrity
▶ Improve peripheral circulation
▶ Demonstrate ability to manage pressure-relieving device
▶ Verbalize knowledge of complications of immobility

ASSESSMENT DATA (see Appendix 7-1)
Perform and document risk assessment for pressure ulcer formation
Measure and stage all wounds
Inspect all skin surfaces for evidence of altered integrity
Assess client's level of discomfort
Assess client/caregiver's understanding of purpose of therapy and ability to manage the device as ordered

Assess for complications of immobility: decubitus ulcers, renal calculi, deep vein thrombosis, pneumonia, paralytic ileus, anorexia, and depression

RELATED NURSING DIAGNOSES

Impaired mobility

Pain

At risk for infection

At risk for altered tissue perfusion

At risk for altered urinary/bowel elimination

At risk for altered breathing patterns

Altered skin integrity

At risk for altered nutrition less than body requirements

At risk for ineffective coping

At risk for diversional activity deficit

SPECIAL CONSIDERATIONS

In the home setting, the use of specialized beds and mattresses constitutes a significant cost to the third-party payor. Such expense must be evaluated against the cost of care associated with the complications of altered skin integrity. Some reimbursers will not authorize payment for such devices unless the client has already experienced pressure ulcer formation staged at level 3 or above.

TRANSCULTURAL CONSIDERATIONS

An interpreter will be needed for the client unable to speak or understand the English language.

Obtain educational materials in the client's native language, if available. Consider use of AT&T Language Line. See also the Culturological Assessment procedure in Unit 2 for general overview of cultural considerations.

▶ INTERVENTIONS

1. Verify physician order.	*Reduces risk of error*
2. Wash hands.	*Prevents transmission of microbes*
3. Perform physical assessment.	*Establishes baseline information of physiological data findings*
4. Explain procedure.	*Allays anxiety*
5. Obtain order for hospital bed.	*Required to initiate therapy*
6. Determine adequacy of the structural integrity and electrical supply of the home environment.	*The size, weight and energy needs of the device must be factored into the home's ability to support use*
7. Obtain ordered mattress and position client as appropriate.	*Assures protection of bony prominences.*

For Foam Mattress Overlay

- ▶ place foam mattress overlay over hospital bed mattress, cover with protective linen
- ▶ apply sheet and tuck under bed mattress, avoiding wrinkles
- ▶ transfer client to bed

For Air Mattress Overlay

- ► apply deflated air mattress over hospital bed mattress
- ► secure air mattress with straps
- ► inflate air mattress per manufacturer's instruction
- ► apply sheet and tuck under hospital bed mattress

For Air Fluidized Bed

- ► transfer client to air fluidized bed using appropriate transfer technique
- ► depress power switch and regulate temperature
- ► position client with foam wedges as needed
- ► use fluidization switch to harden the bed for turning and other procedures

8. Reposition the client every two hours and prn.   *Maintains circulation*
9. Perform ROM to all extremities.   *Maintains flexibility of joints*
10. Observe for hazards of immobility.   *Ensures early detection of complications*

11. Instruct caregiver in implementing the procedure and permit return demonstration.   *Documents caregiver's ability to implement procedure*

DOCUMENTATION
The following should be included in the nursing note:

Nutritional status
Pressure ulcer risk management assessment
Range of motion exercises
Skin integrity
Caregiver's ability to implement procedure
Any untoward reactions and appropriate interventions implemented
All client/caregiver teaching:
   Topics to include in the teaching plan:
      safe and correct equipment handling
      emergency procedures
      underlying disease pathology
      appropriate community resources and contact persons

INTERDISCIPLINARY COLLABORATION
Report all untoward responses to physician
Consult with DME vendor for reordering of supplies as needed
Confer with social worker regarding client's eligibility for financial assistance/reimbursement for equipment
Consider need to assist the caregiver with the services of a home health aide
Confer with the enterostomal therapist or WOCN for assessment and evaluation of altered skin integrity
Consult with physician regarding need to have physical therapist provide range of motion and strengthening exercises

Consider conferring with rehabilitation nurse to assist with client teaching in self-care management, bowel/bladder training, and reinforcement of physical therapy exercises

Consider conferring with occupational therapist to provide adaptive devices to use in maintaining ADLs [1, 2, 5–7, 11, 13]

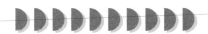

Geriatric Integumentary System Procedures

PROCEDURE
Complex Wound Management

DESCRIPTION
Wound healing is a complex, dynamic process that occurs in three progressive phases: reaction, regeneration, and remodeling. Complex wound healing is a long-term process sometimes taking more than a year to complete. Three basic principles govern the goals of wound care: keep the wound clean, moist, and protected. Debridement and exudate management will keep the wound clean. A moist environment facilitates the proliferation of epithelial cells. Protection from both mechanical and chemical trauma is achieved with the application of specialized dressings. Surgical incisions and some traumatic wounds heal by primary intention. Because the wound edges are well approximated, new capillary circulation bridges the wound and healing occurs in 3–4 days. Burns, infected wounds and deep pressure ulcers heal by secondary intention, where the wound is left open to allow granulation tissue and epithelialization to heal the injury. Wound healing by tertiary intention, or delayed primary intention, occurs when a contaminated wound is left open to drain, and is sutured closed once the infectious process has been controlled; or, when a primary wound becomes infected, is reopened, allowed to granulate and then sutured closed.

PURPOSE
To facilitate wound healing and prevent infection

EQUIPMENT
Gloves and other protective gear as needed
Container for contaminated waste
Protective pad
NSS
Irrigation kit
Gauze
Collecting basin for returns
Suture/staple removal kit
Ointment
Specialized dressings as ordered
   films
   hydrocolloids
   foams
   hydrogels
   exudate absorbers
   composites

skin sealants
leg ulcer wraps
packing gauze

OUTCOMES

The client/caregiver will:

- ▶ Demonstrate evidence of wound healing
- ▶ Be free of infection
- ▶ Maintain adequate nutrition
- ▶ Demonstrate improved peripheral circulation
- ▶ Demonstrate ability to manage pressure-relieving device
- ▶ Verbalize knowledge of complications of wound healing

ASSESSMENT DATA

Perform and document risk assessment for pressure ulcer formation
Measure and stage all wounds
Inspect all skin surfaces for evidence of altered integrity
Assess client's level of discomfort
Assess nutritional status
Assess client/caregiver's understanding of purpose of therapy and ability to maintain dressings as ordered
Assess for complications of wound healing
Monitor laboratory studies: CBC, albumin, transferring, electrolyes, blood glucose, creatinine, culture reports, and other studies as ordered

RELATED NURSING DIAGNOSES

Impaired mobility
Pain
Altered skin integrity
At risk for altered nutrition less than body requirements
At risk for infection
At risk for ineffective coping
At risk for altered tissue perfusion
Knowledge deficit

SPECIAL CONSIDERATIONS

Wound healing is a complex process affected by the client's nutritional status, medication therapy, circulatory status, and presence of co-morbid disease states. Wound healing depends upon adequate oxygenation and perfusion. A tissue PaO_2 of 40 mmHg is required to support fibroblast proliferation and collegen synthesis. Compromised tissue perfusion interferes with the delivery of oxygen and nutrients to the area of altered skin integrity. NSAIDs, antineoplastics, steroids, and anticoagulants, depending on dose, are medications that may adversely affect the healing process. Adequate nutrition is essential for wound healing. The intake of carbohydrates, vitamins, proteins, fats, and minerals is necessary for cell metabolism. The presence of chronic and/or debilitating disease, such as Diabetes Mellitus and cancer, will significantly slow the healing process.

TRANSCULTURAL CONSIDERATIONS

An interpreter will be needed for the client unable to speak or understand the English language.

Obtain educational materials in the client's native language, if available. Consider use of AT&T Language Line. Also see the Culturological Assessment procedure in Unit 2 for general overview of cultural considerations.

) INTERVENTIONS

1. Verify medical order.	*Reduces risk of error*
2. Wash hands.	*Prevents transmission of microbes*
3. Perform physical assessment.	*Establishes baseline information of physiological data findings*
4. Explain procedure.	*Allays anxiety*
5. Don gloves.	*Serves as protective barrier*
6. Remove dressings and discard.	*Maintains universal precautions*
7. Measure and stage the wound.	*Establishes baseline for comparison*
8. Remove gloves and wash hands.	*Prevents transmission of microbes*

For Wound Measurement

Needed to establish wound diagnosis, plan treatment, and document results

1. Measure length of wound along horizontal axis and record in cm.
2. Measure the width of wound along the vertical axis and record in cm.
3. Measure the depth of the wound from skin surface to deepest part of wound bed and record in cm.
4. If undermining or tunneling has occurred, gently probe under the wound edges with a cotton-tipped applicator.
5. Measure depth of each track in clockwise fashion aligning the 12 o'clock position with the client's head.

For Wound Staging of Pressure Ulcers (Display 7-1)

Classifies wound severity
 Use following parameters to determine stage:

Stage I   = nonblanchable erythema with intact skin surfaces
Stage II = partial thickness tissue loss
Stage III = full thickness tissue loss
Stage IV = full thickness tissue loss with involvement of fascia, muscle, and bone

For Wound Cleaning and Flushing

1. Place protective barrier under affected body part.	*Keeps bedlinen clean*
2. Don gloves and other protective gear as needed.	*Serves as protective barrier*
3. Assess wound bed for need to culture.	*Ensures early detection of presence of infection*
4. Open irrigation kit.	*Facilitates access*
5. Fill container with ordered solution.	*Softens debris for ease of removal*
6. Withdraw solution into syringe and gently flush ordered solution onto wound.	*Removes debris*

Stages of Pressure Ulcers

Stage I

- ► Blood stasis in underlying tissues (hyperemia)
- ► Not relieved by massage or pressure relief
- ► Reddened skin color
- ► Warm to touch

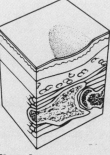

Stage I

Stage II

- ► Epidermal tissue loss
- ► May be damage to the dermis
- ► Moist and depressed skin erosion

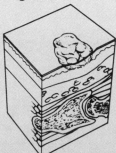

Stage II

Stage III

- ► Full-thickness skin loss
- ► Dermal ulceration may extend to the subcutaneous layer
- ► Serosanguineous or purulent drainage common

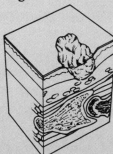

Stage III

Stage IV

- ► Full-thickness skin destruction
- ► Ulceration into deeper tissue structures (fascia, connective tissue, muscle, bone)

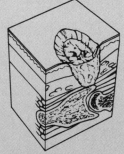

Stage IV

7. Dry surrounding skin with gauze.	*Prevents maceration*
8. Apply dressing as ordered.	*Provides wound protection*
9. Dispose of contaminated supplies.	*Maintains universal precautions*
10. Remove gloves and wash hands.	*Prevents spread of microbes*

Dressing Wounds with Drains

1. Create sterile field.	*Maintains aseptic technique*
2. Open ABDs, and split gauze dressings and place on sterile field.	*Facilitates access*
3. Don gloves and other protective gear as needed.	*Serves as protective barrier*
4. Irrigate wound as above.	*Removes debris*
5. Remove gloves, wash hands, change gloves.	*Prevents spread of microbes*
6. Apply split gauze dressings around drains.	*Absorbs drainage*
7. Apply ABDs.	*Absorbs drainage*
8. Secure with Montgomery straps.	*Secures dressings*
9. Remove gloves and wash hands.	*Prevents spread of microbes*

Dressing Open Wounds

1. Create sterile field.	*Maintains aseptic technique*
2. Open ABDs, and gauze dressings and place on sterile field.	*Facilitates access*
3. Pour NSS onto gauze.	*Provides moisture to dressing*
4. Don gloves and other protective gear as needed.	*Serves as protective barrier*
5. Irrigate wound as above.	*Removes debris*
6. Remove gloves, wash hands, change gloves.	*Prevents spread of microbes*
7. Pack wound with NSS-soaked gauze.	*Provides moisture to wound bed*
8. Cover with dry ABDs.	*Supports and maintains moist dressings*
9. Secure with Montgomery straps.	*Secures dressings*
10. Remove gloves and wash hands.	*Prevents spread of microbes*

For Removal of Staples

1. Create sterile field and open staple removal kit.	*Maintains aseptic technique*
2. Don gloves.	*Serves as protective barrier*
3. Remove dressing, cleanse wound as ordered.	*Removes debris*
4. Inspect and measure wound edges.	*Determines approximation of wound edges*
5. Remove gloves, wash hands, and change gloves.	*Serves as protective barrier*
6. Insert lower tip of staple remover under first staple (Figure 7-1).	*Isolates staple from skin*
7. Press handle close (Figure 7-2).	*Elevates staple*
8. Angle the staple remover side to side, lift staple out, place on sterile field.	*Permit visualization of staple*
9. Repeat steps 6 to 8 until all of the staples have been removed.	*Completes the process*
10. Cover wound edges with steri strips leave open to air.	*Maintains approximation of suture line*

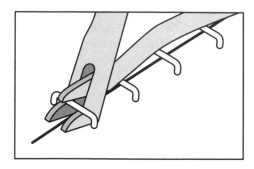

FIGURE 7-1 ▶ Insert staple remover.

11. Instruct client to keep wound dry until steri-strips begin to pull away.

Facilitates wound healing and assures that wound edges remain intact

For Removal of Sutures

1. Create sterile field and open suture removal kit.
2. Don gloves.
3. Remove dressing; cleanse wound as ordered.
4. Inspect and measure wound edges.

5. Remove gloves, wash hands, and change gloves.
6. Take scissors in dominant hand and forceps in nondominant hand.
7. Grasp suture with forceps and slip scissors under suture and snip (Figure 7-3).
8. Pull knotted end of suture out and place on sterile field.

9. Repeat steps 6 to 8 until all of the sutures have been removed.
10. Cover wound edges with steri strips leave open to air and keep wound dry.

Maintains aseptic technique
Serves as protective barrier
Removes debris
Determines approximation of wound edges
Serves as protective barrier
Enhances control of instruments

Cuts suture

Allows for visualization of suture

Completes the process

Maintains approximation

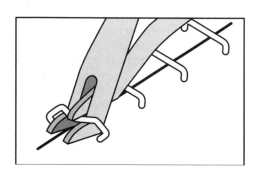

FIGURE 7-2 ▶ Press handle of staple remover to elevate staple.

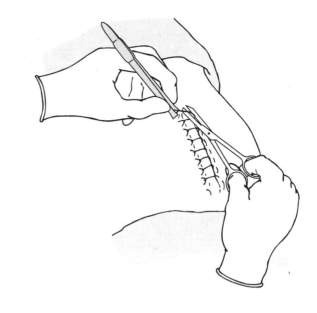

FIGURE 7-3 ▶ Removing sutures.

DOCUMENTATION
The following should be included in the nursing note:

Nutritional and fluid status
Staging and size of wound
Wound appearance
Type of dressing applied
Pressure ulcer risk management assessment
Range of motion exercises
Skin integrity
Caregiver's ability to implement procedure
Any untoward reactions and interventions made to correct
All client/caregiver teaching:
    Topics to include in the teaching plan:
        safe and correct equipment handling
        emergency procedures
        underlying disease pathology
        appropriate community resources and contact persons

INTERDISCIPLINARY COLLABORATION
Report all untoward responses to physician
Consult with DME vendor for reordering of supplies as needed
Confer with social worker regarding client's eligibility for financial assistance/reimbursement for
    equipment

Consult with enterostomal therapist or WOCN for recommended wound care therapy

Consider conferring with physical therapist for range of motion and strengthening exercises

Consider conferring with rehabilitation nurse to assist with client teaching in self-care management, bowel/bladder training, and reinforcement of physical therapy exercises

Consider conferring with occupational therapist to provide adaptive devices to use in maintaining ADLs

PROCEDURE
Dietary Wound Care Management

DESCRIPTION

The dietary management for wound care requires the careful balancing of nutrient intake with energy expenditure. The client with a complex wound must consume a structured diet to promote the development of wound healing. Careful monitoring of laboratory data and body weight will be important assessments of the adequacy of the dietary regimen.

PURPOSE

To provide nutritional intervention to promote wound healing and improved nutrition status.

EQUIPMENT

Health Assessment forms
Weight scale
Meal planning guide
Educational materials

OUTCOMES

The client/caregiver will:

▶ Maintain adequate calorie, protein, vitamin, and mineral intake to assist with wound healing and improve nutritional status

▶ Be able to identify when nutritional intake has declined which may lead to poor nutrition status and wound healing

ASSESSMENT DATA

Note decreased levels of laboratory values that may indicate protein and/or generalized malnutrition

Note current weight and weight history and determine if there has been unintentional weight loss

Document potential nutritional food categories that may be lacking, i.e., total calories, protein, and or whole food groups missing

Monitor: ability to self-feed, food intake, fluid intake, and food preferences and tolerances.

RELATED NURSING DIAGNOSES

Impaired mobility
Pain
Altered skin integrity
At risk for altered nutrition less than body requirements
At risk for infection
At risk for ineffective coping
At risk for altered tissue perfusion
Knowledge deficit

SPECIAL CONSIDERATIONS

If potential triggers for malnutrition occur, the client should be evaluated by the nutritionist for calorie, protein, vitamin, and mineral intake. For the morbidly obese client, recognize that the wound healing process will be slower, mobility will be significantly impaired, and the client will have an increased risk for the development of infection.

TRANSCULTURAL CONSIDERATIONS

An interpreter will be needed for the client unable to speak or understand the English language.

Obtain educational materials in the client's native language, if available. Consider use of AT&T Language Line. See also the Culturological Assessment procedure in Unit 2 for general overview of cultural considerations.

▶ INTERVENTIONS

1. Obtain nutritional assessment including parameters discussed above.

   Correlate the decline in parameters of nutritional status, such as body weight and circulating proteins, with the risk and incidence of pressure ulcers

2. Initiate request for further nutrition evaluation if nutritional parameters are decreased.

   Intervention to include estimation of nutrition needs and possible use of medical nutritional products and/or tube feeding

3. Instruct client/caregiver on meal planning following ordered dietary therapies.

   Establishes dietary regimen

DOCUMENTATION

The following will be noted in nursing note:

Potential nutritional inadequacies
Nutritional parameters not in compliance
Past or interim nutritional intervention
Need for further nutrition evaluation
All client/caregiver teaching:
    Topics to include in the teaching plan:
        safe and correct equipment handling
        emergency procedures
        underlying disease pathology
        appropriate community resources and contact persons

INTERDISCIPLINARY COLLABORATION

Report client's nutritional status to the physician
Consult with the nutritionist regarding nutritional concerns and potential medical nutritional interventions [1, 4, 5, 7, 8, 10–12, 18]

REFERENCES

1. Agency for Health Care Policy and Research (AHCPR), *Treatment of Pressure Ulcers. Clinical Practice Guideline, No. 15.* AHCPR Publications Clearinghouse, 1994.

2. Boggs, RL, & Wooldridge-King, M. *AACN Procedure Manual for Critical Care,* 3rd Ed. Philadelphia, PA: W.B. Saunders Company, 1993.
3. Boswick, JA. *The art and science of wound care.* Rockland, MD: Aspen Publishers, 1987.
4. Campbell, SM. *Pressure ulcer prevention and intervention: A role for nutrition.* Columbus, OH: Products Division, Abbott Laboratories, 1994.
5. Carpenito, LJ. *Nursing diagnosis: Application to clinical practice.* Philadelphia, PA: Lippincott, 1997.
6. Catanzaro, J, & Serembus, JF. High-tech wound and ostomy care in the home setting. *Critical Care Nursing Clinics of North America* 10(3):327, 1998.
7. Fuller, J, & Schaller-Ayers, J. *Health assessment: A nursing approach.* 2nd Edition. Philadelphia, PA: Lippincott, 1994.
8. Gottschlich, MM, Matarese, LE, & Shronts, EP, eds. *Nutrition support dietetics core curriculum,* 2nd ed. Silver Springs, MD: A.S.P.E.N. 1993.
9. Hodgson, BB, & Kizior, RJ. *Saunders Nursing Drug Handbook 1999.* Philadelphia, PA: W.B. Saunders Company, 1999.
10. Jaffe, MS, & Skidmore-Roth, L. *Home health nursing assessment and care planning.* St. Louis, MO: Mosby, 1997.
11. Jarvis C. *Pocket companion for physical examination and health assessment.* Philadelphia, PA: W.B. Saunders Company, 1996.
12. Johnson JY, Smith-Temple J, Carr P. *Nurses' guide to home procedures.* Philadelphia, PA: Lippincott, 1998.
13. LeMone, P, & Burke KM. *Medical surgical nursing: Critical thinking in client care.* Menlo Park, California: Addison Wesley Publishers, 1996.
14. Marrelli, TM. *Handbook of home health standards and documentation guidelines for reimbursement,* 3rd edition. St. Louis, Missouri: Mosby 1998.
15. *Nurses Illustrated Handbook of Home Health Procedures.* Springhouse, PA: Springhouse Corporation, 1999.
16. Stanhope, M, & Knollmueller, RN. *Handbook of community and home health nursing.* St. Louis, MO: Mosby, 1996.
17. Sussman, C, & Bates-Jensen, B. *Wound care: A collaborative practice manual for physical therapists and nurses.* Gaithersburg, MD: Aspen Publications Inc, 1998.
18. *Pediatric manual of clinical dietetics.* Chicago, IL: The American Dietetic Association, 1998.
19. Zang SM, & Bailey NC. *Home care manual: making the transitition.* Philadelphia, PA: Lippincott, 1997.

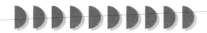

Appendices

Sample pressure ulcer assessment guide

Patient Name: _____ Date: _____ Time: _____

Ulcer 1:
Site _____
Stage[a] _____
Size (cm)
  Length _____
  Width _____
  Depth _____   No   Yes

Ulcer 2:
Site _____
Stage[a] _____
Size (cm)
  Length _____
  Width _____
  Depth _____   No   Yes

Ulcer 1 checklist (No / Yes):
Sinus Tract ☐ ☐
Tunneling ☐ ☐
Undermining ☐ ☐
Necrotic Tissue ☐ ☐
  Slough ☐ ☐
  Eschar ☐ ☐
Exudate ☐ ☐
  Serous ☐ ☐
  Serosanguineous ☐ ☐
  Purulent ☐ ☐
Granulation ☐ ☐
Epithelialization ☐ ☐
Pain ☐ ☐
Surrounding Skin:
Erythema ☐ ☐
Maceration ☐ ☐
Induration ☐ ☐
Descripton of Ulcers(s):

Ulcer 2 checklist (No / Yes):
Sinus Tract ☐ ☐
Tunneling ☐ ☐
Undermining ☐ ☐
Necrotic Tissue ☐ ☐
  Slough ☐ ☐
  Eschar ☐ ☐
Exudate ☐ ☐
  Serous ☐ ☐
  Serosanguineous ☐ ☐
  Purulent ☐ ☐
Granulation ☐ ☐
Epithelialization ☐ ☐
Pain ☐ ☐
Erythema ☐ ☐
Maceration ☐ ☐
Induration ☐ ☐

Indicate Ulcer Sites:

Anterior   Posterior
(Attach a color photo of the pressure ulcer(s) [Optional])

[a]Classification of pressure ulcers:
Stage I: Nonblanchable erythema of intact skin, the heralding lesion of skin ulceration. In individuals with darker skin, discoloration of the skin, warmth, edema, induration, or hardness may also be indicators.
Stage II: Partial thickness skin loss involving epidermis, dermis, or both.
Stage III: Full thickness skin loss involving damage to or necrosis of subcutaneous tissue that may extend down to, but not through, underlying fascia. The ulcer presents clinically as a deep crater with or without undermining adjacent tissue.
Stage IV: Full thickness skin loss with extensive destruction, tissue necrosis, or damage to muscle, bone, or supporting structures (e.g., tendon or joint capsule).

APPENDIX 7-1 ▶ Sample pressure ulcer assessment guide.

Asthma is a life-long lung disease that affects the way you breathe. When you inhale, air is taken in through your nose and mouth. The air goes into your lungs through your windpipe and into your bronchial (bron-kee-al) tubes and air sacs. When you breathe out, stale air leaves your lungs.

Mucus makes a thin, moist lining inside your airways, such as your nose. When you have an asthmatic attack, your bronchial tubes and other airways get small and tight. This blocks the air from moving in and out of your lungs and makes it difficult to breathe normally. The muscles constrict. The lining becomes swollen, puts out extra thick mucus, and becomes inflamed. When this happens, more mucus is made and this makes it harder for the air to pass through.

Symptoms and Signs of Asthma

▶ Wheezing
▶ Trouble breathing or shortness of breath
▶ Chest tightness or suffocating feeling
▶ Retractions
▶ Interrupted sleep
▶ Peak flow meter in yellow (cautious) or danger range (red zone)
▶ Blue or gray coloring around mouth and fingernails - late sign
▶ Worsening of cough and/or mucous production
▶ Increased respiratory rate

When to Treat Your Symptoms

An asthmatic attack can start out with the mildest of symptoms and increase in severity. Treatment should begin with the onset of mild symptoms. **The earlier the better!**

How to Treat Your Symptoms

▶ Develop an asthma treatment plan with your healthcare provider and follow it
▶ Use prescribed medicines as directed by MD or RN
▶ Decrease activity and increase rest
▶ Drink normal amounts of fluids frequently
▶ Eat small, frequent well balanced meals

APPENDIX A5-3 ▶ Client Education: Asthma Facts

What causes an attack?

People with asthma have very sensitive airways. **To control your asthma you must know and control your triggers.** Learn which triggers bother you and learn to avoid them.

Common Triggers

Listed below are some of the common triggers for an asthmatic attack. Make a mental note or place an "X" next to the triggers that bother you and talk to your health care provider about them.

Allergens

☐ Dogs
Cats
Birds
Small rodents
☐ House dust (mites)
(in curtains, beds, carpets, furniture
and stuffed animals)

☐ Bugs that live inside (cockroaches)

☐ Molds that grow in damp places,
like sinks and bath tubs, cellars, kitchens.

Irritants

☐ Cigarette smoke, smog,
hairspray, perfumes, cosmetics,
paint, and air pollution

☐ Colds and flu–infections

☐ Weather and temperature (cold
dry, warm, or wet)

How to Avoid Asthma Triggers

An asthmatic attack may be caused by triggers. Learn what your triggers are and avoid them. Here are some things you can do to avoid asthma triggers.

Animal Dander

▶ Keep cats, dogs, and birds outside. If you can't do that, think about giving them away. If you must have a pet, keep it out of your bedroom at all times.
▶ Give cats and dogs weekly baths.
▶ Avoid a pet with fur or feathers.
▶ Avoid products made with feathers, like pillows or comforters .

Dust Mites

▶ Bare floors are better than carpet.
▶ Use rugs that can be washed.
▶ Remove carpets laid on concrete.
▶ Cover mattresses, box springs, pillows or polyester pillows in airtight plastic covers.
▶ **Avoid sleeping or lying** on upholstered furniture.
▶ Wash sheets, clothes, and stuffed toys once a week in hot water.

Insects

▶ Have someone else use an insect spray when you are outside of the house.
▶ Air your house for a few hours after spraying.
▶ Use roach traps.
▶ Ask exterminator to use low irritant chemical.

APPENDIX A5-4 ▶ Client Education: Asthma Triggers

Pollens and Molds (Outdoors)

▶ Stay indoors during midday and afternoon when pollen counts are high.

▶ Use air conditioning if possible.

▶ Keep windows closed during seasons when pollen and molds are highest.

▶ Avoid sources of molds (wet leaves, garden debris).

▶ Don't hang clothes or sheets outside to dry. Pollen can stick to them.

▶ Shower at bedtime - rinses off pollen and mold stuck to body and hair.

Molds (Indoors)

▶ Use dehumidifer in basement. Empty and clean them regularly.

▶ Keep bathroom, kitchen and basement well aired.

▶ Clean damp areas like the shower, tub and sinks regularly.

▶ Do not use humifiders. They make molds grow faster.

▶ Avoid using recycled mattresses.

▶ Keep temperature in winter at maximum of 66–68 degrees, lowers need of use of humidifer or vaporizer.

Dirty Air

It is hard to stay away from perfume, smoke and polllution. Try some of these tips:

Tobacco Smoke

▶ Do not smoke.

▶ Do not allow smoking in your home.

▶ Have household member or guests smoke outside.

▶ Sit in non-smoking areas when you go out.

Smoke from Indoor Heaters

▶ Avoid wood burning stoves/fireplaces.

▶ Avoid using kerosene heaters.

Strong Odors/Sprays

▶ Do not stay in your home when it is being painted. Allow time for paint to dry.

▶ Avoid perfumes, moth balls, hairspray, spray deodorant, and air freshners.

▶ Avoid baby powder or talcum powder.

▶ Use non-perfumed cleaning products.

▶ Reduce strong cooking odors by opening windows or using a fan.

Colds and Infection

▶ Do not take non-prescription cold medicine without talking to your healthcare provider. These medicines may interact with your asthma medications

▶ Avoid people with colds or flu - and wash hands frequently.

▶ Talk to your healthcare provider about flu shots.

APPENDIX A5-4 [CONTINUED] ▶ Client Education: Asthma Triggers

Things to do at Home to Prevent Asthma Attacks

▶ Develop a plan with your doctor for early treatment of symptoms. Use the medicines and the peak flow meter as directed by your doctor.

▶ Schedule regular check ups, even when symptoms do not exist. Seek early treatment for colds, the flu, sinus infections and other respiratory infections.

▶ Make sure that you get adequate rest, eat a healthy diet, and engage in regular physical activity/exercise.

▶ Know the early symptoms of an asthmatic attack.

▶ Identify your own "asthma triggers" and avoid them.

Really Managing Your Asthma

Although asthma cannot be cured, you can often prevent, control and relieve the symptoms. It is very important that you work with your healthcare provider to develop a treatment plan suited just for you. The type of plan will depend on your asthma history and how you respond to treatment.

Medications

There are two kinds of medicine used to treat asthma.

Bronchodilators (bron-ko-die-lay-tors) are medicines that help you breathe by opening up narrow or clogged bronchial tubes. Bronchodilators relax muscles that have tightened up around your airways. They relieve your asthma symptoms. They may be pills, liquid, inhalers (breathed in) or nebulizer. **Take this medicine at the first sign that your asthma is getting worse.** If you are using the medicine more than prescribed it may mean your asthma is getting worse. **Call your healthcare provider right away.**

Anti-imflammatory medicine is used to prevent airway swelling, and will reduce airway swelling when you are having an attack. Anti-Inflammatory medicine may be pills, liquid, or inhaler (breathed in). **Take your anti-inflammatory medicine exactly as it is orders, even if you have no symptoms.**

Medications can help manage your asthma.

Take the *right medication at the correct time*. Call your healthcare provider if you have any unusual reaction to your medication, such as nausea, vomiting, fast heart beat, anxiety, jitters. **Do not tak any non-prescription drugs before discussing with your healthcare provider.**

Exercise

Exercise can help improve your health in general, increase your lung capacity, and relieve stress. It will be helpful to follow these general guidelines

▶ Work out an exercise plan with your healthcare provider.

▶ Warm up before exercising and cool down afterwards.

▶ Take medicines before exercising.

▶ During cold weather—wear scarf over nose and mouth.

Checking Your Breathing

Depending on your condition, part of your treatment plan may be to check your peak flow. If this is prescribed, your health care provider will show you how to use the peak flow meter and how to interpret the reading.

APPENDIX A5-5 ▶ Client Education: Asthma Management

What You Can Do

1. Know your warning signs.
2. Identify and avoid *your triggers*.
3. Take the right amount of medicine at the right time.
4. **Relax.**
5. Eat a balanced diet.
6. Follow your exercise program developed by your health care provider.
7. **See your health care provider regularly.**
8. *Avoid running out of your medicine.*

GO TO THE EMERGENCY ROOM AND CALL PROVIDER IMMEDIATELY WHEN:

1. *Your chest and neck are pulled or sucked in with each breath.*
2. *You are struggling to breath.*
3. *You cannot walk or talk.*
4. *Your fingernails and lips are gray or blue*
5. *Your symptoms get worse even after you have given your medicine a chance to work.*
6. *Your peak flow numbers go down or do not improve after you take your medicine.*

APPENDIX A5-5 [CONTINUED] ▶ Client Education: Asthma Management

Metered Dose Inhaler

Definition: A hand held inhaler that delivers a pre-measured dose of medicine with each use.

Directions to use Inhaler:

▶ Remove the cap and hold the canister upright.

▶ Shake the canister containing the medication

▶ Tilt you head back slightly and exhale completely.

▶ Hold the inhaler about 1 inch in front of your open mouth. Or you may place the inhaler in the open mouth but your lips should not be sealed around the mouth piece.

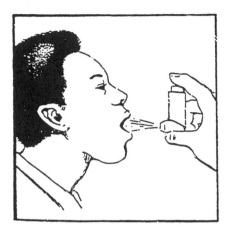 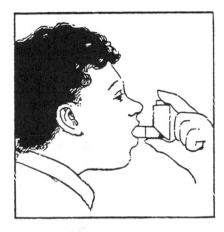

▶ Press down on the inhaler to release the medicine, while starting to breathe in slowly and deeply.

▶ Hold breath for 5-10 seconds to allow the medicine to reach deeply into the lungs.

▶ Repeat puffs as ordered. Waiting 1-2 minutes between puffs may help the second puff to go deeper into the lungs.

Cleaning the Inhaler

▶ Once a day clean the mouth-piece and cap by rinsing it in warm running water Let it air dry before you use it again. Have a second inhaler to use while the first is drying.

▶ Every 3–4 days wash the plastic mouthpiece with mild dishwashing soap and warm water. Rinse and air dry.

APPENDIX A5-6 ▶ Client Education: Use of the Metered Dose Inhaler

Spacers

A Spacer or holding chamber is a device that attaches to a metered dose inhaler (MDI). It holds the medicine in its chambers long enough to inhale it in one or two slow deep breaths. Younger children or infants are unable to take deep breaths and hold 3-4 deep breaths or 6 regular breaths.

Directions to use the Spacer:

1. Attach the inhaler to the spacer or holding chamber.
2. Shake well.
3. Press the button on the inhaler. This will put one puff of medicine in the holding chamber.
4. Place the mouthpiece of the spacer in the mouth and breathe in slowly. A face mask may be helpful for a young child.
5. Hold breath for 5–10 seconds and then exhale slowly through pursed lips.
6. Wait 1–2 minutes, then repeat inhalation steps 2–5 above for a second puff, if prescribed.
7. Rinse out mouth with water.

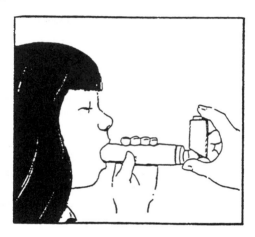

Cleaning the Spacer:

1. Wash mouthpiece with warm water every day and air dry.
2. Wash mouthpiece with mild dishwashing soap and warm water every 3–4 days and air dry.

APPENDIX A5-7 ▶ Client Education: Use of the Spacer

How to Use a Peak Flow Meter

A Peak Flow Meter is a device that measures how well air moves out of your lungs. During an asthmatic attach, the lungs begin to narrow causing decreased movement of air out of lungs. The peak flow meter can be used to detect narrowing of the airways, hours, even days before any signs or symptoms of an asthma attack appear.

Directions to use the Peak Flow meter:

1. Place the indicator at the base of the numbered scale.
2. Take a deep breath.
3. Place the meter in the mouth and close lips around the mouthpiece. Keep tongue out of the hole.
4. Blow out hard and fast (like blowing out candles on a cake).
5. Read the scale by noting the number that the arrow on the indicator is pointing to and record that number on a piece of paper.
6. Repeat steps 1–5 two more times.
7. Write down the highest of the three numbers obtained in your asthma log.

*To find you or your child's personal best peak flow meter number, take peak flow readings before and after taking medication. Take peak flow readings in the morning and evening for at least the first two weeks.

Cleaning the Peak Flow Meter:

1. Rinse the mouthpiece with warm water every day and air dry.
2. Wash the mouthpiece with mild dishwashing soap and water every 3–4 days. Rinse thoroughly. Allow to air dry.

APPENDIX A5-8 ▶ Use of the Peak Flow Meter

PEAK FLOW ZONES

Develop the following plan of action in collaboration with your healthcare provider

Green Zone: (80 to 100 percent of personal best) Signals **all clear**. No asthma symptoms present. Take asthma medicines as usual.

    This is where you or your child should be every day.

    Peak flow _____ (80–100% of personal best)

    No symptoms.

    Normal activities and sleep without symptoms.

    Take these medicines: (dose, time)

    _____

    _____

Yellow Zone: (50 to 80 percent of personal best) signals **caution**. You or your child may be having symptoms of asthma that require a change in medication therapy. Follow your asthma treatment plan. If peak flow meter readings continue in yellow zone, for one day, contact your physician or as ordered.

    This is *not* where you or your child should be every day. Take action to get you or your child's asthma under control (50–80% of personal best).

    Symptoms may be mild or moderate.

    May have decreased activity or sleeping.

    First, take this medicine (dose, time):

    _____

    _____

    If you or your child notice no improvement in symptoms in 20 to 60 minutes and the peak flow is over _____ (70% of personal best) take these medicines (dose, time):

    _____

    _____

    Keep taking your green zone medicine(s).

    If you or your child notice no improvement in symptoms 20 to 60 minutes or the peak flow meter is under _____ (70% of personal best), follow the Red Zone Plan. Notify you or your child's doctor if he/she continues to go to Yellow Zone.

APPENDIX A5-9 ▶ Client Education: Plan for Monitoring Peak Flow Zones

Red Zone: (below 50 percent of personal best) signals an **urgent medical condition**. You or your child need to be seen by the physician immediately.

This is an **EMERGENCY! GET HELP IMMEDIATELY!**

You or your child's asthma symptoms are serious.

Peak flow _____ (below 50% of personal best).

First, take this medicine (dose, time):

_____

_____

Call the doctor to fnd out what to do next.

Tell him/her this is an emergency.

Go to the emergency room.

See the doctor right away, or go to the hospital if you or your child note any of these symptoms:

▶ Blue lips or fingernails.

▶ Struggling to breathe.

▶ No improvement in 20–30 minutes after taking the extra medicine and peak flow is still under _____ (50% of personal best).

▶ Can't talk.

This is a general guideline. Discuss any specific instructions with you or your child's physician.

Remember to keep track of Peak Flow Meter results in your asthma diary.

APPENDIX A5-9 ▶ Client Education: Plan for Monitoring Peak Flow Zones

Glossary

Accreditation—A process of evaluation of a home health agency's standard of care by an external group. In the homecare industry, this function is performed by JCAHO and CHAP

ABD—Abdominal dressing

ADLs—Activities of daily living

Adventitious—Abnormal

Air Fluidized Therapy—A dynamic pressure-relieving bed or support mattress: high air loss, bead, or sand bed

Albumin—An intravascular volume expander obtained from pooled human plasma

Alignment—Positioning in a straight line, as bones following a fracture

Allen Test—Test to assess perfusion through the ulnar and radial arteries

Amino Acids—Basic components of protein molecules

Antihemolytic Factor (AHF)—Used to replace Factor VIII in the treatment of bleeding disorders

Arterial Blood Gas (ABG)—The sampling of arterial blood to determine acid-base balance, oxygenation, and level of carbon dioxide

Artificial Airway—Any mechanical device used to maintain a patent airway

Aseptic Technique (also, sterile technique)—Procedures used to render an environment or objects free of microorganisms

Assist Control (AC)—A ventilator mode that delivers a preset tidal volume in response to the client's inspiratory effort and provides an automatic breath when the client fails to initiate respiration

Automatic Implantable Cardioverter Defibrillator (AICD)—A surgically implanted device that continuously monitors the heart and delivers an electrical shock to terminate lethal dysrhythmias

Autonomic Dysreflexia—An abnormal sympathetic response in clients with spinal cord lesions at C6 and above, often precipitated by bowel/bladder distension leading to a hypertensive crisis, relieved by removal of the causing factor

Barrier Precautions—Infection control procedures used for all clients to reduce the risk of transmission of infectious agents

Baseline—The initial assessment parameter obtained

Bevel—Slanted opening at the tip of a catheter or needle

BiPAP—Bi-positive airway pressure system designed to assist the client's respiratory cycle during rest and sleep

Body Cast—A rigid mold of plaster, plastic, or other substance enclosing the body from the neck to the groin for the purpose of immobilization

Bolus—An amount of fluid or medication administered intermittently or as an addition to the maintainence dose or requirements.

Bolus Feeding—The administration of an ordered amount of feeding formula by gravity via a feeding tube over a 5- to 15-minute duration

Cardiac Dysrhythmia—Irregular heart activity caused by the erratic discharge of cardiac electrical impulses

Cardiac Index (CI)—A measure of cardiac output expressed in liters/minute/square of body surface area

Cardiac Output (CO)—Amount of blood ejected by the ventricles each minute expressed in liters/minute

Cardiac Profile—Measurement and calculation of cardiac output (CO), cardiac index (CI) and systemic vascular resistance (SVR)

Cast—Immobilization of a body part with plastic or plaster to repair a fracture or strain

Catheter Infection—Microbial growth obtained from a catheter tip or from a blood culture drawn from the catheter with no growth of the same organisms in the peripheral blood

Central Venous Catheter (CVC)—A catheter introduced thorough a large peripheral vein, jugular, or subclavian vein and advanced to the superior vena cava for the purpose of administering parenteral solutions

Cerebral Perfusion—The ability of the circulatory system to deliver blood to the cerebral structures

Chest Drainage System—A system which removes air, fluid, or blood from the intrapleural space using water seal, gravity, and suction-collection chambers to restore negative pressure

Chest Tube—A thoracic catheter inserted into the pleural space to collect drainage or permit the escape of air

Chronic Obstructive Pulmonary Disease (COPD)—Any one of three diseases which cause a decrease in pulmonary function: asthma, bronchitis, and emphysema

Compartment Syndrome—A condition in which increased pressure within a compartment interferes with circulation to that compartment, often following trauma or surgery

Community Health Accreditation Program (CHAP)—A subsidiary of the National League for Nursing that accredits homecare agencies

Congestive Heart Failure (CHF)—Inability of the myocardium to pump effectively to meet body demands

Continuous Ambulatory Peritoneal Dialysis (CAPD)—The process of instilling dialysate into the peritoneal cavity four times per day with dwell times of 4 to 10 hours

Continuous Feeding—The slow administration of enteral feeding at a constant rate over 24 hours

Continuous Positive Airway Pressure (CPAP)—The administration of positive pressure during inspiration and expiration via mask or mechanical ventilation

Controlled Mandatory Ventilation (CMV)—The ventilator mode that delivers a preset tidal volume and rate regardless of the client's inspiratory effort

Cycler—An automatic device that controls the infuse and drain phases of the dialysate used in intermittent peritoneal dialysis

Debridement—The removal of necrotic tissue from a wound surgically or with use of an enzymatic topical agent

Dialysate—A solution used in dialysis to move toxic waste products across a semipermiable membrane

Diffusion—The movement of solutes from greater to lesser areas of concentration

Disinfection—The process of eliminating or weakening pathogenic organisms found on inanimate surfaces

Diuretics—Drugs used to reduce body fluid by decreasing renal tubular reabsorption

Dwell Time—The time the dialysate remains in the peritoneal cavity to permit the processes of osmosis and diffusion to occur

Electrocardiogram (ECG)—Recording of the heart's electrical activity and conduction of impulses

Epidural Catheter—An intraspinal catheter surgically placed in the epidural space for the administration of medication

Eschar—The necrotic tissue covering a burn wound

Exchange—The complete cycle of peritoneal dialysis includes the time to infuse, dwell, and drain the dialysate solution

Extraocular Movements (EOM)—Tests the client's ability to move the eye in six cardinal positions to evaluate cranial nerve function

Extravasation—The leakage of intravenous fluid into the subcutaneous tissue

Fraction of Inspired Oxygen (FIO$_2$)—The concentration of oxygen in inspired gas expressed as a percentage

Gastric Residual—The volume of gastric contents which can be aspirated via an enteral feeding tube. Obtained to determine the client's ability to tolerate feedings.

Granulation Tissue—Pink healing tissue formed in response to a deep wound injury to bring about wound closure

Health Care Financing Administration (HCFA)—The federal agency that governs the Medicare Program. It is a branch of the U.S. Department of Health and Human Services

Heimlich Valve—A one-way exit valve which permits air/fluid to exit from the pleural space and prevents atmospheric pressure from entering the pleural space

Hematoma—A collection of blood in a body cavity, tissue, or organ secondary to leakage from a vascular wall

Hemopneumothorax—A collection of blood and air in the pleural space

Huber Needle—A curved beveled needle used to access implanted ports designed to prevent coring of the silicone port septum

Hydrocolloid Dressing—An occlusive dressing which forms a protective cover over a wound site, interacting with the wound exudate to maintain a moist environment for wound healing

Hyperextension—Overextension of a body part

Hyperflexion—Overflexion of a body part

Hyperosmolar—Increased solute concentration of solution in excess of 400 mOsm/L

Hyperventilation—An increased rate/depth of ventilation

Hypoventilation—A decreased rate/depth of ventilation usually associated with hypoxia

Hypovolemia—A decrease in circulation blood volume

Hypoxemia—A decrease in $PaCO_2$ as measured by arterial blood gas analysis

Hypoxia—Decreased tissue oxygenation

Ileal Conduit—The surgical creation of an artificial urinary bladder which drains urine via a stoma opening onto the abdomen

Implanted Access Port—A long-term access device surgically implanted and attached to a silastic catheter leading to any one of the following endpoints: intrathecal, intravenous, intraarterial, intraperitoneal, or intrapleural.

Inotropic Agent—A drug which increases the contractility of the cardiac musculature

Infectious Waste—Biohazardous substances, usually defined by state or federal law, which require special handling

In-line IV filter—A specialized membrane that is placed in an intravenous administration set, used to protect against particulate matter formation, air emboli and contaminants

Inspiratory to Expiratory Ratio (I:E).—The proportion of the length of time of the inspiratory and expiratory phases expressed as a ratio of seconds, normal is 1:2

Intermittent feeding—the administration of a bolus of enteral feeding administered via a tube using gravity drainage over 30–60 minutes

Intermittent Mandatory Ventilation (IMV)—A ventilator mode setting which delivers a preset tidal volume and rate over and above the client's spontaneous respirations, expressed as frequency per minute

Intracranial Pressure (ICP)—A measure of the pressure within the cranium

Intrathecal—Within the subarachnoid space

Intraventicular—Within the lateral ventricles of the brain

Ischemia—Decreased blood flow via a blood vessel to a body part secondary to altered perfusion

JCAHO—Joint Commission on Accreditation of Healthcare Organizations

LEDs—Light-emitting diodes placed in a sensor to give off specific wavelengths of light at the red and infrared ranges of the light spectrum

Leukocyte-Poor Packed Red Blood Cells—A process to remove leukocytes and plasma proteins from packed RBCs for the client with a history of transfusion reactions

Mechanical Debridement—The removal of necrotic tissue by scrubbing, irrigating, or surgically excising

Mechanical Sigh—The delivery of intermittent deep breaths using either a ventilator mode or self-inflating resuscitation bag

Medical Social Worker (MSW)—The health professional who manages the client's psychosocial problems

Mental Status Examination—An assessment of a client's orientation, thinking, judgement, and mood using a series of structured questions

Nasoenteral Feeding—The administration of feeding formula via a tube inserted into the nares and positioned in the small intestine

Nasogastric Feeding—The administration of feeding formula via a tube inserted into the nares and positioned in the stomach

Neurogenic Bladder—Loss of voluntary and reflex innervation to the urinary bladder resulting in overdistension

Neurogenic Bowel—Loss of voluntary and reflex innervation to the bowel resulting in indiscriminate bowel emptying

Neurovascular Check—A series of assessments performed to measure neurological and circulatory status of peripheral tissues

Nitrogen Balance—A measure of the amount of dietary, intravenous, and/or enteral nitrogen intake and the amount of stool, urine, and/or drainage nitrogen output calculated over a 24-hour period to determine protein metabolism

Occupational Therapist (OT)—The health professional who assists the client in performing activities of daily living

Outcome Assessment Information Set (OASIS)—A series of standardized risk-adjusted client outcome measures

Osmosis—The movement of fluid from an area of lesser solute concentration to an area of greater solute concentration across a semipermiable membrane

Packed Red Blood Cells (PRBCs)—The process of centrifuging red cells from whole blood used to restore oxygen-carrying capacity and intravascular volume

PaCO$_2$—The partial pressure of CO$_2$ in arterial blood expressed in mmHg, normal is 35–45

Parenteral Nutrition—The intravenous administration of nutrient products

PaO$_2$—The partial pressure of oxygen in arterial blood expressed in mmHg, normal is 80–100

Patient Controlled Analgesia (PCA)—An infusion system which permits the client to self-administer pain medication

Percutaneous Endoscopic Gastrostomy (PEG)—An implanted feeding tube placed via a small opening into the stomach

Peripheral Enteral Nutrition—The intravenous administration of nutrients via a peripheral vein using solutions with dextrose concentrations below 10–15%

Peritoneal Dialysis—The process of removing metabolic waste products and fluid from the body by instilling into and draining a dialysate solution from the peritoneal cavity

Personal Protective Equipment—Protective gear worn to reduce risk of exposure to health care workers

Petalling—A technique used to cover the rough edges of a plaster cast to prevent skin irritation

Phototherapy—A high-intensity fiberoptic unit used to treat jaundice in the newborn

Physical Therapist (PT)—The health professional who assists the client with mobility, strengthening exercises and pain management

PICC—Peripherally inserted central catheter

Plan of Treatment (POT)—The physician order form authorizing the treatment regimen

Plasmanate—An intravascular volume expander administered adhering to guidelines for blood component infusions

Platelets—Replacement therapy administered to increase platelet count following guidelines for blood component infusions

Positive End Expiratory Pressure (PEEP)—A ventilator mode setting which maintains positive pressure at the end of expiration preventing the intrathoracic pressure from returning to atmospheric pressure, used to maintain alveolar ventilation

Pulse Oximetry—A noninvasive method of measuring arterial oxygen saturation expressed as SaO$_2$, normal is 95–100%

Reimbursement—Payment for healthcare services usually provided by a third-party payor

Silastic Tube—Catheter made of soft, flexible rubber

Speech Language Pathologist and Audiologist—The health professional who assists clients with phonation, swallowing, communication, and hearing loss

Spica Cast—A hardened structure used to immobilize an extremity incorporating the trunk of the body with the injured part

Stoma—A surgically created opening onto the body surface

Subcutaneous Emphysema—The abnormal presence of air/fluid in the subcutaneous tissue

Synchronized Intermittent Mandatory Ventilation (SIMV)—The ventilator mode setting which permits the delivery of a preset volume in synchrony with the client's respiratory effort

Systemic Vascular Resistance (SVR)—Measurement of left ventricular afterload, normal is 900–1,200 dyne sec/cm^5

Telemetry—A monitoring system which uses telecommunication technology to transmit electrical signals from a device to a remote site

Tidal Volume—The amount of inspired/expired air during normal respiration expressed in ml, normal is 350–500

Total Parenteral Nutrition (TPN)—the intravenous administration of nutrients

VAD—Vascular access device

Vital Capacity (VC)—Maximal amount of air that can be expired after a maximal inspiration expressed in ml, normal is 4,500 to 5,000

WOCN—Wound, ostomy continence nurse

Index